AF334628

International Ophthalmology Clinics

International Ophthalmology Clinics (ISSN 0020-8167) (ISBN 0-316-45596-2). Published quarterly by Little, Brown and Company, 34 Beacon Street, Boston, Massachusetts 02108-1493. Send address changes and subscription orders to Little, Brown and Company, Subscription Department, 34 Beacon St, Boston, MA 02108. Subscription rates per year: personal subscription, U.S. and possessions, $90; foreign (includes Mexico), $116; Canada, $103, PLEASE ADD 7% CANADIAN GST FOR ALL CANADIAN SUBSCRIPTIONS (Registration No. R128537917); institutional, U.S., $113; foreign, $147; Canada, $125. Special rates for students, interns and residents per year: U.S., $61; foreign, $84; Canada, $72. Single copies: $31 for subscribers, $39 for nonsubscribers. In Japan please contact our exclusive agent: Medsi, 1-2-13 Yushima, Bunkyo-ku, Tokyo 113, Japan. Subscription rates per year in Japan: individual, ¥24,200; institutional, ¥28,800 (air cargo service only). Second-class postage paid at Boston, Massachusetts, and at additional mailing offices.

Postmaster: Send address changes to International Ophthalmology Clinics, 34 Beacon St, Boston, MA 02108.

International Ophthalmology Clinics is indexed in Index Medicus, Current Contents/Clinical Practice, Excerpta Medica, and Current Awareness in Biological Sciences.

International Ophthalmology Clinics

Volume 33
Number 2
Spring 1993

Advances in Ophthalmic Genetics and Heritable Eye Diseases

EDITED BY

Frederick A. Jakobiec, M.D.

Massachusetts Eye and Ear Infirmary and Harvard Medical School, Boston, Massachusetts

AND

Jeffrey C. Lamkin, M.D.

Former Chief Resident, Massachusetts Eye and Ear Infirmary, Harvard Medical School, and The Retinal Institute, Mt. Sinai Medical Center, Cleveland, Ohio

Little, Brown and Company
BOSTON

Editors

Gilbert Smolin, M.D.
F.I. Proctor Foundation, San Francisco
Department of Ophthalmology,
University of California, San Francisco
Medical Center

Mitchell H. Friedlaender, M.D.
Division of Ophthalmology,
Scripps Clinic and Research Foundation,
La Jolla, California

Editorial Office
1001 Sneath Lane, Room 206
San Bruno, CA 94066

Publisher
Little, Brown and Company, Boston, Massachusetts

Publishing Staff

Publisher
Thomas A. Manning

Executive Editor
David Dionne

Managing Editor
Sherri Frank

Sales and Marketing Manager
Anne Orens

Production Manager
Fredda Purgalin

Contents

Contributing Authors

Frederick A. Jakobiec, M.D., EDITOR
Department of Ophthalmology
Massachusetts Eye and Ear Infirmary
243 Charles Street
Boston, MA 02114

Jeffrey C. Lamkin, M.D., EDITOR
Former Chief Resident
Massachusetts Eye and Ear Infirmary,
    Harvard Medical School, *and*
The Retinal Institute
Mt. Sinai Medical Center
Cleveland, OH
Address correspondence to:
The Retinal Institute
Mt. Sinai Medical Center
1 Mt. Sinai Drive
Cleveland, OH 44106

Daniel M. Albert, M.D.
Department of Ophthalmology
University Hospital and Clinics
600 Highland Avenue, F4/334
Madison, WI 53792

Neal P. Barney, M.D.
Department of Ophthalmology
University Station Clinics
2880 University Avenue
Madison, WI 53705-0902

Eliot L. Berson, M.D.
Berman-Gund Laboratory for the Study of
    Retinal Degenerations *and*
The Electroretinography Service
Massachusetts Eye and Ear Infirmary
243 Charles Street
Boston, MA 02114

Robert J. Brockhurst, M.D.
Massachusetts Eye and Ear Infirmary
Boston, MA
Address correspondence to:
Zero Emerson Place
Suite 3-D
Boston, MA 02114

Sanford Chen, M.D.
Retina Associates *and*
Department of Ophthalmology
Massachusetts Eye and Ear Infirmary
Boston, MA
Address correspondence to:
Department of Ophthalmology
Massachusetts Eye and Ear Infirmary
243 Charles Street
Boston, MA 02114

M. Ronan Conlon, M.B., B.Ch.
University of Iowa
Department of Ophthalmology
University of Iowa Clinics
Iowa City, IA 52242

Donald J. D'Amico, M.D.
Massachusetts Eye and Ear Infirmary
243 Charles Street
Boston, MA 02114-3096

Sashi K. Dharma, M.D.
627 Allen Street
Coppell, TX 75019

Claes H. Dohlman, M.D.
Massachusetts Eye and Ear Infirmary
243 Charles Street
Boston, MA 02114

Evan B. Dreyer, M.D., Ph.D.
Department of Ophthalmology
Massachusetts Eye and Ear Infirmary
243 Charles Street
Boston, MA 02114

Thaddeus P. Dryja, M.D.
Howe Laboratory of Ophthalmology
Massachusetts Eye and Ear Infirmary
243 Charles Street
Boston, MA 02114

Eleanore M. Ebert, M.D., M.P.H.
Department of Ophthalmology
Box 475
University of Virginia Health Sciences Center
Charlottesville, VA 22908

Philip M. Falcone, M.D.
West Reading Ophthalmic Associates
206 South 6th Avenue
West Reading, PA 19611

Judith A. Ferry, M.D.
Department of Pathology
Massachusetts General Hospital
Boston, MA 02114

C. Stephen Foster, M.D.
Massachusetts Eye and Ear Infirmary
243 Charles Street
Boston, MA 02114

Gary D. Haynie, M.D.
Retina Service
Massachusetts Eye and Ear Infirmary
243 Charles Street
Boston, MA 02114

Tatsuo Hirose, M.D.
Retina Associates
100 Charles River Plaza
Boston, MA 02114

Deborah S. Jacobs, M.D.
Massachusetts Eye and Ear Infirmary
243 Charles Street
Boston, MA 02114

Alex E. Jalkh, M.D.
Retina Associates,
    Schepens Eye Research Institute, *and*
Massachusetts Eye and Ear Infirmary
Boston, MA
Address correspondence to:
Retina Associates
100 Charles River Plaza
Boston, MA 02114

Nancy C. Joyce, Ph.D.
Pharmacology Unit
Schepens Eye Research Institute
20 Staniford Street
Boston, MA 02114

Harry R. Koster, M.D.
36 East 36th Street
New York, NY 10016

C. William Lavin, M.D.
54 Harrison Street
Quincy, MA 02169

Simmons Lessell, M.D.
Department of Ophthalmology
Massachusetts Eye and Ear Infirmary
243 Charles Street
Boston, MA 02114

Cynthia Mattox, M.D.
Massachusetts Eye and Ear Infirmary
and
Tufts University
School of Medicine-New England Eye Center
Boston, MA
Address correspondence to:
750 Washington Street
Box 450
Boston, MA 02111

Craig A. McKeown, M.D.
Department of Ophthalmology
Massachusetts Eye and Ear Infirmary
243 Charles Street
Boston, MA 02114

Shizuo Mukai, M.D.
Retina Service
Massachusetts Eye and Ear Infirmary
243 Charles Street
Boston, MA 02114

Peter A. Netland, M.D., Ph.D.
Glaucoma Consultation Service
Massachusetts Eye and Ear Infirmary
243 Charles Street
Boston, MA 02114

John H. Niffenegger, M.D.
Vitreoretinal Consultants, Inc.
1001 Beacon Street, Suite 3E
Brookline, MA 02180

Mark A. Pavilack, M.D.
1532 Lititz Pike
Lancaster, PA 17601

Michael J. Potter, M.D.
McLaren Regional Medical Center
401 South Ballenger Highway
Flint, MI 48532-3685

Mohammad T. Shokravi, M.D.
Howe Laboratory of Ophthalmology
Massachusetts Eye and Ear Infirmary
Boston, MA
Address correspondence to:
P.O. Box 1373
Boston, MA 02117

Eric A. Sieck, M.D.
Ophthalmology Clinic
Fitzsimons Army Medical Center
Aurora, CO 80045

Edward M. Stroh, M.D.
Retina Associates,
   Schepens Eye Research Institute, *and*
Massachusetts Eye and Ear Infirmary
Boston, MA
Address correspondence to:
Retina Associates
100 Charles River Plaza
Boston, MA 02114

Trexler M. Topping, M.D.
Ophthalmic Consultants of Boston
50 Staniford Street
Boston, MA 02114

Robert C. Urban, Jr., M.D.
University of South Florida
12901 Bruce B. Downs Boulevard
MDC, Box 21
Tampa, FL 33612-4799

Nicholas J. Volpe, M.D.
Department of Ophthalmology
Massachusetts Eye and Ear Infirmary
243 Charles Street
Boston, MA 02114

Michael D. Wagoner, M.D.
Department of Ophthalmology
Cornea Service
Massachusetts Eye and Ear Infirmary
243 Charles Street
Boston, MA 02114

Kenneth J. Wald, M.D.
Retina Associates
Schepens Eye Research Institute
Harvard Medical School
100 Charles River Plaza
Boston, MA 02114

David S. Walton, M.D.
Massachusetts Eye and Ear Infirmary
243 Charles Street
Boston, MA 02114

William L. White, M.D.
Ophthalmology Service
Department of Surgery
Beach Pavilion
Brooke Army Medical Center, Fort Sam
Houston, TX 78234-6200

Janey L. Wiggs, M.D., Ph.D.
Department of Ophthalmology
Massachusetts Eye and Ear Infirmary
243 Charles Street
Boston, MA 02114

Jacqueline M. S. Winterkorn, M.D., Ph.D.
Department of Neuro-ophthalmology
North Shore University Hospital-
   Cornell University Medical College
300 Community Drive
Manhasset, NY 11030

Preface

On January 25, 1992, the Clinical Fellows of the Massachusetts Eye and Ear Infirmary, with the assistance of their preceptors, gave a course on "Advances in Ophthalmic Genetics and Heritable Eye Diseases." A capacious and scholarly syllabus was reviewed by the chief editors of *International Ophthalmology Clinics*, who thought the updated coverage of this rapidly developing subject would be of interest to the journal's readers. The Fellows' course is now an annual affair and is coupled with the Dohlman Lectureship at the Massachusetts Eye and Ear Infirmary, which this year was delivered by Richard Allen Lewis of the Baylor College of Medicine.

Medical knowledge proceeds from the intellectual insights and intuitions of great clinicians and scientists, but is also spurred by major technological advances. As we look back over the past 30 years in medicine, and in ophthalmology as well, we see phases of growth that were greatly stimulated by breakthroughs in imaging (transmission and scanning electron microscopy, along with CT and MRI scanning), virology, immunology (particularly with the advent of monoclonal antibodies), and now molecular genetics.

The 22 papers in this issue are preceded by an overview of advanced techniques in ophthalmic molecular genetics that will become staple items throughout the next two decades. The other papers are grouped into sections on genetics of cellular replication in neoplasia; genetics and immunology; genetics of glaucoma; gene localization; x-linked disorders and the carrier state; retinal degenerations; and oculosystemic disorders. Although all of the contributors to this issue were residents at the Massachusetts Eye and Ear Infirmary at the time of this course, several of them, as indicated in the Contributing Authors section, have moved on to other professional or academic appointments.

If the era of molecular genetics is truly upon us, it is also expanding at a vertiginous rate. Its techniques and breakthroughs are very close to ushering in a new period of genetic therapy. No trainee or clinician can afford to be ill-informed about molecular genetics, which will increasingly frame our knowledge and perspectives about ocular diseases. The new vocabulary underwriting genetic concepts is daunting: restriction enzymes leading to restriction fragment length polymorphisms; macro-satellite repeats; polymerase chain reaction; DNA sequencing; intron/exon structure of genes; Southern analysis; and genetic linkage analysis.

Those not fluent with these concepts and conversant with the techniques will be unable to keep up with clinically relevant genetic discoveries. We hope this volume will make readily accessible, and present in a practical manner, the beauty of a burgeoning field which holds great promise for ophthalmology and for unraveling the diseases we want to better treat in our patients.

Frederick A. Jakobiec
Jeffrey C. Lamkin

Molecular Genetics and Ocular Disease

Janey L. Wiggs, M.D., Ph.D.

The recent applications of the novel techniques of molecular genetics to problems in clinical medicine have led to dramatic new insights into the pathophysiology of human disease. Molecular genetic technology has become the dominant approach to the study of many basic biological questions, particularly those questions concerning the nature of genes and how they work in eukaryotic cells. The genes responsible for many of the 3,000 known hereditary disorders that affect humans have been mapped in the human genome, and a number of these genes have been cloned [1]. Many of these disorders involve ocular tissues and can cause blindness. Identification of the genes and of the resultant abnormal protein products responsible for hereditary ocular conditions will provide valuable information about the pathophysiology of these conditions and will have an enormous impact on the clinical diagnosis and treatment of affected individuals. If specific abnormal proteins can be demonstrated to be the cause of a disease, then selective drug therapy targeted for that particular protein activity might be developed. Finding DNA mutation(s) responsible for a disorder can form the basis of new, DNA-based diagnostic tests. Such tests may allow affected individuals to be detected at earlier stages of their disease when medical management may be more effective.

As ophthalmologists, we frequently care for patients affected with hereditary conditions that will benefit from this new technology. It is important that all ophthalmologists recognize the patterns of inherited ocular disorders as well as be aware of advances in the diagnosis and treatment of these conditions. This chapter provides an overview of the basic principles of molecular genetics and some of the techniques commonly used for such studies.

■ Principles of Molecular Genetics

The discipline of molecular genetics is based on the concept that all the information necessary for the function of living cells exists in the mole-

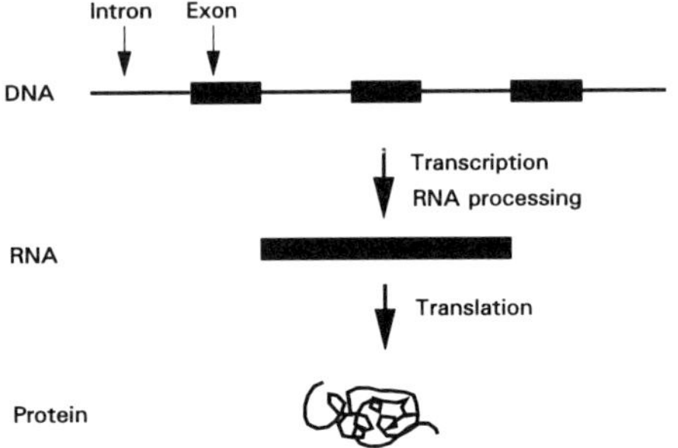

Figure 1 *Structure and expression (the central dogma) of a eukaryotic gene. Eukaryotic genes consist of introns (DNA sequences that are not expressed) and exons (DNA sequences that are expressed). Transcription of a gene produces an initial RNA molecule that contains both intron and exon sequences. This "pre-mRNA" is processed to create the mRNA that serves as a template for protein synthesis (translation).*

cules of DNA that reside in each cell's nucleus. DNA molecules consist of two strands of nucleotide bases joined by hydrogen bonds to form a double helix. Each strand is formed by a sequence of any one of four bases, adenine (A), guanine (G), cytosine (C), and thymine (T), joined to a sugar deoxyribose and a phosphate. The bonding between the two strands is specific, such that A always pairs with T and G always pairs with C. If the sequence of bases along one strand is known, the sequence along the complementary strand can be inferred [2]. The information coded in DNA is arranged as individual genes, which are situated at specific sites, or *loci*, on chromosomes. Each gene is generally responsible for the production of a single protein, and each protein's role in the cell may be structural, regulatory, or enzymatic. The sequence of events that regulates the expression of genes as proteins has been termed the *central dogma of molecular biology* (Fig 1). To enable the information in DNA to be used, the sequence of bases in the DNA is first transferred to an intermediate molecule, called *messenger RNA* (mRNA), by a highly specific and selective biochemical reaction called *transcription*. The sequence of the newly synthesized RNA will be complementary to one of the DNA strands except that the base uracil (U) is substituted for the base thymine (T). Transcription of DNA to RNA is carried out by the enzyme RNA polymerase and is subject to many regulatory processes so that the appropriate genes are transcribed into RNA at the precise moment that this information is required for the direction of critical cellular processes. Once the mRNA is formed, it is used as a template to produce the selected protein product. This process is called *translation* and requires ribosomes, transfer RNA (tRNA), and amino acids, in addition to mRNA. The newly synthesized protein may be modified by additional chemical reactions before it is ready to perform its specific cellular activity.

Human DNA is packaged in the nucleus of most cells of the body as *chromosomes*, which represent DNA that is wound and coiled in an orderly fashion with proteins called *histones*. Most cells in the human body contain nuclei that house two copies of each of the twenty-two autosomes (paired chromosomes alike in women and men) plus two X chromosomes (women) or an X and a Y chromosome (men). (Exceptions to this rule include reproductive cells, which contain only one copy of each chromosome, and red blood cells, which do not have nuclei.) All the information necessary to create a human being is included in this set of chromosomes, which is called the *human genome*. In order that a cell can divide or replicate (mitosis), the entire human genome is copied during a process called *DNA replication*. The new strands of DNA are synthesized according to the specific sequence of the original DNA by the enzyme DNA polymerase. Once the DNA is copied, the old and new copies of the chromosomes pair and the cell divides such that one copy of each chromosome pair belongs to each cell (Fig 2).

Much of the DNA sequence present in human cells is not ultimately transcribed or translated. These sequences are known as *introns* and are spliced out of mRNA during the transcription process. The DNA se-

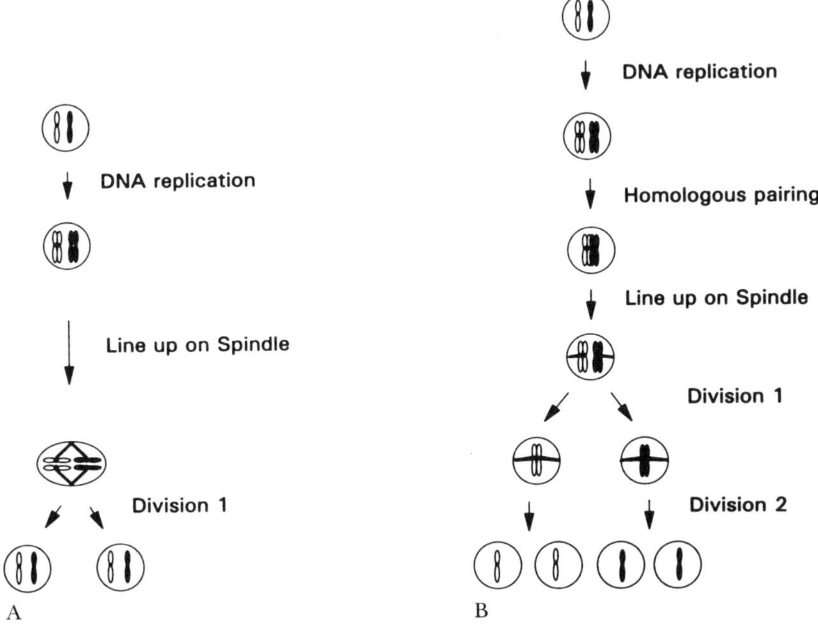

Figure 2 *Mitotic and meiotic cell division. (A) Mitosis. DNA replication results in a doubling of the genetic material. The replicated chromosomes line up on a microtubule spindle, and the cell divides such that a single copy of each chromosome remains in each daughter cell. (B) Meiosis. After DNA replication, the maternal and paternal doubled chromosomes pair (homologous pairing) and exchange genetic material by the recombination process (see Fig 15). The homologous chromosome pairs line up on the microtubule spindle and divide such that the maternal and paternal copies of the doubled chromosomes are distributed to separate daughter cells. A second cell division occurs, and the doubled chromosomes divide so that the daughter cells (gametes) have half the genetic material of somatic (tissue) cells.*

quences that are transcribed and translated are referred to as *exons* (see Figure 1).

■ Basic Inheritance Patterns

Many of the disorders discussed in this issue follow simple modes of inheritance according to basic mendelian genetics. Two general rules—Mendel's two laws of inheritance—govern these hereditary patterns. First, genes are units whose alleles randomly segregate during meiosis, which is the cell division process required for the creation of the reproductive cells (gametes) (see Fig 2). This means that the two copies (alleles) of a gene present in the cells that are precursors of the gametes separate when those cells divide. Second, genes assort independently—that is, alleles from different genes segregate independently of one another. Figure 3 shows the possible offspring from matings at the hypothetical loci A and B.

Genetic traits may be dominant or recessive. A dominant trait manifests the phenotypical trait when the dominant allele is present in either the homozygous or the heterozygous state. A recessive trait will demonstrate the phenotypical trait only when it is present as two copies (homozygous state).

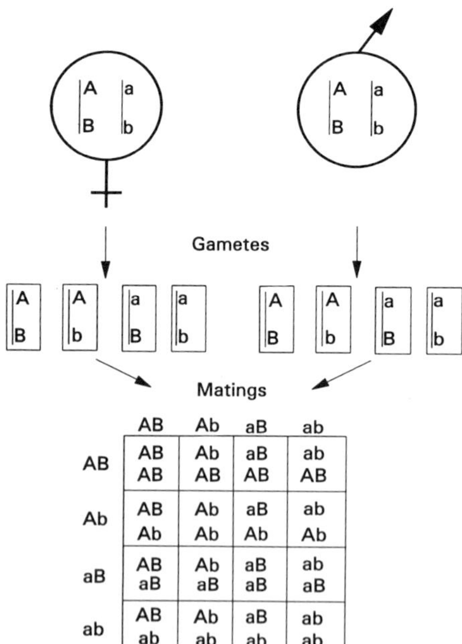

Figure 3 *Independent assortment of genetic traits (Mendel's second law of hereditary).*

Autosomal Dominant Inheritance

Pedigrees exhibiting autosomal dominant inheritance tend to have affected individuals present in every generation. If the penetrance of the condition is near 100%, approximately 50% of the members of each generation will be affected. If the penetrance is less than 100%, fewer than 50% of the family members at risk will be phenotypically affected; however, 50% of the family members at risk will either be affected or unaffected carriers of the disease. Each child born of an affected parent has a 50% chance of inheriting the disease or of becoming an unaffected carrier (Fig 4A).

Autosomal Recessive Inheritance

For an individual to be phenotypically affected by an autosomal recessive disease, both parents must either be affected with the disease or be heterozygous carriers. If both parents are heterozygous carriers, each child has a 25% chance of inheriting the disease and a 50% chance of becoming an unaffected carrier. If one parent is affected and the other parent is a carrier, each child has a 50% chance of inheriting the disease and a 100% chance of becoming a carrier (Fig 4B).

X-Linked Inheritance

A defect on the X chromosome usually is not fully expressed in the female subject because the copy of the X chromosome carrying a mutation is often inactivated (Lyon's hypothesis). Hence, women frequently are

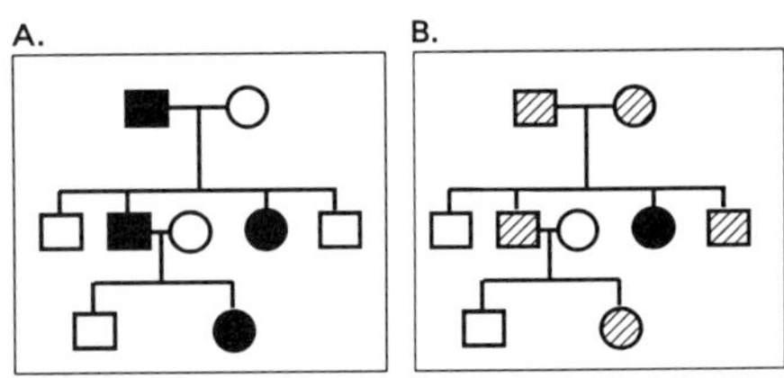

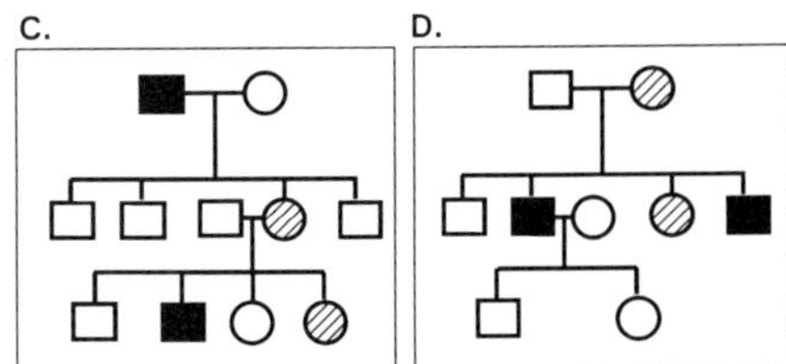

Figure 4 *Basic patterns of inheritance: (A) autosomal dominant, (B) autosomal recessive, (C) X-chromosome linked, and (D) mitochondrial. Affected individuals are shown as solid circles (female individuals) or squares (male individuals). Unaffected carriers are shown as cross-hatched circles or squares.*

asymptomatic carriers of X-chromosome-linked conditions. The defective X chromosome can be passed to both male and female offspring, who will be either carriers of the disease (female offspring) or affected by the disease (male offspring). In pedigrees affected with an X-linked disorder, 50% of the female offspring of a female carrier and a normal man will be phenotypically normal carriers of the defective gene, and 50% of the male offspring will be phenotypically abnormal. All the female offspring of an affected man will be carriers of the disease, and none of the male offspring will be affected. In many X-linked ocular disorders, female carriers can be detected by a specific clinical trait (Fig 4C).

Mitochondrial Inheritance

Mitochondria are organelles found in the cytoplasm of cells. They contain their own DNA, which is related to the ancestral bacteria from which the mitochondria originated [3]. Because mitochondria are located in the cellular cytoplasm, they are always maternally inherited, since the cytoplasm of the human zygote is derived entirely from the female egg and not at all from the male sperm. Consequently, mitochondrial mutations are always passed from either an affected mother or a female carrier to her children, never from an affected father (Fig 4D).

■ Methodology

DNA Preparation

A fundamental requirement for molecular genetic studies is the ability to obtain DNA samples from individuals affected with hereditary conditions and their unaffected relatives. Total human DNA can be prepared from individuals of any age group from a small blood sample [4]. Peripheral whole blood (10 to 30 ml), usually drawn from the arm, is collected in purple-top tubes (the purple top indicates that heparin is present to prevent clotting). The collected blood can be kept for 24 to 48 hours in these tubes. The first step toward the isolation of DNA is separation of the white blood cells from the red blood cells by selective cell lysis and centrifugation. After removal of the red blood cells and blood serum, the white blood cells are collected as a small pellet. These cells can be stored for prolonged periods of time in a freezer at $-70°C$ (or liquid nitrogen tanks) or may be used immediately for the preparation of DNA. To purify DNA, the white cells in the pellet are lysed and the residual cellular components (proteins, RNA) are removed from the DNA by phenol extraction and ethanol precipitation. DNA prepared by this technique may be used for other studies including the polymerase chain reaction (PCR) and Southern blot analysis.

Figure 5 *Schematic representation of gel electrophoresis. A sample of biological material (DNA, RNA, or protein) is applied to the gel and is subjected to an electrical current such that the material is forced through the gel matrix. The sample molecules pass through the matrix at different rates of speed, depending on the size, shape, and intrinsic electrical charge of the individual molecule. In general, smaller molecules (lower molecular weight [MW]) pass through the matrix faster than those of high molecular weight.*

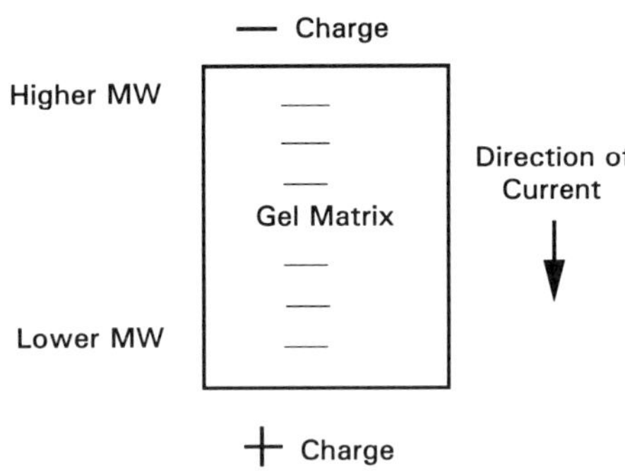

Gel Electrophoresis

Electrophoresis is a technique used to separate molecules of DNA, RNA, or protein. The separation may be based on the total electrical charge of the molecule, the size of the molecule, or the secondary and tertiary structure (shape) of the molecule. In general, electrophoresis is accomplished by subjecting the selected sample to an electrical field such that the molecules are attracted to an electrical charge. The focus of the charge is typically located at the opposite end of a neutral gel matrix (usually agarose or polyacrylamide) so that the electrical attraction forces the molecules to pass through the matrix (Fig 5). Because the matrix offers resistance to the passage of the molecules to be separated, some molecules move faster than others depending on their size, shape, and electrical charge. The type and concentration of gel matrix, the gel shape, the chemical buffers used to create the electrical field, the type and strength of the electrical field, and the preparation of the sample are all factors that can be varied to accomplish maximum separation of the desired biological component. Once a population of molecules is separated in a gel matrix, the molecules can be visualized by a variety of methods.

The Polymerase Chain Reaction

The PCR is a recently developed method for synthesizing many copies of a selected short DNA fragment from a small amount of template (patient) DNA [5]. The technique depends on the activity of a bacterial DNA polymerase that is resistant to elevated temperatures. The first step in the reaction is the synthesis of oligonucleotide primers that flank the DNA fragment to be amplified (Fig 6). Next, all the components of the reaction are heated so that the DNA is denatured and becomes single-stranded. The reaction is allowed to cool and, as it cools, the DNA renatures and again becomes double-stranded. Since an excess of oligonucleotide primers is present, every molecule of template DNA hybridizes with the flanking primer sequences. The primers serve as initiation sites for the thermostable

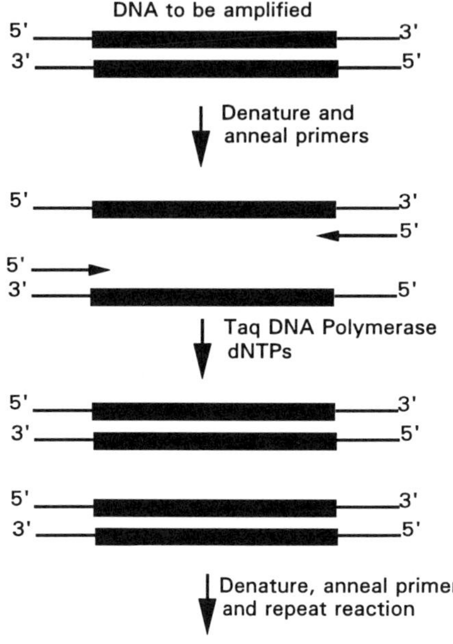

Figure 6 *The polymerase chain reaction (PCR), which provides for rapid amplification of small amounts of a desired segment of DNA. The reaction comprises three steps. In the first phase, the DNA is denatured and then allowed to reanneal with an excess of short oligonucleotide primers. Next, these primers serve as a site of synthesis of DNA by Taq DNA polymerase (a thermostable DNA polymerase). At the completion of these steps, a doubling of DNA has occurred. The cycle is repeated and, after each round of PCR, the number of copies of the sequences between the primer sites is doubled and accumulated exponentially.*

DNA polymerase, which synthesizes a new strand of DNA from the end of each primer and extends the newly synthesized strand across the DNA sequences that are to be amplified. Thus, two new copies of the specified DNA fragment are created. The reaction is repeated and, with each repetition, an exponential increase of newly synthesized DNA fragments is generated. After approximately thirty cycles, the desired DNA sequences have been amplified 10^5 to 10^6 times. The amplified sequences can be visualized directly by electrophoresis in agarose gels stained with ethidium bromide (an intercalating dye that binds DNA). Alternatively, during the amplification process, radioactive deoxynucleotide triphosphates can be incorporated into the synthesized DNA, and the radioactive amplification products can be visualized after polyacrylamide gel electrophoresis and exposure to x-ray film.

The ability to amplify a particular segment of DNA many times is an extremely powerful tool for molecular genetic studies. For example, if one suspected that a specific mutation (change in DNA sequence) was located in a particular region of DNA, and if the DNA sequence around that region was known (in order that the flanking primer oligonucleotide sequences could be synthesized), that region of DNA could be amplified and either directly sequenced or subjected to electrophoretic conditions such that the presumed mutation could be demonstrated. DNA amplified by PCR can also be cloned and used for other important techniques. The only requirement for PCR is that at least a portion of the DNA of interest be sequenced so that the flanking primer sequences can be synthesized. Because PCR makes the identification of specific base pair changes in DNA so rapid, this procedure will play an important role in DNA-based diagnostic procedures.

Southern Blot Analysis

In 1975, Edwin Southern [6] devised a method to allow visualization of a selected fragment of DNA belonging to the whole human genome. This technique had a dramatic impact on the ability to analyze total human DNA. Two additional concepts, restriction endonucleases and DNA probes, are fundamentally important to this technology.

Restriction endonucleases are a type of DNA nuclease with the unique ability to cleave DNA at a specific site after the recognition of a specific DNA sequence, which serves as a signal to cut the DNA [7]. These enzymes are typically found in bacteria and are named according to the organism from which they are purified. For example, restriction enzyme EcoR1 is purified from *Escherichia coli*. EcoR1 recognizes the DNA sequence GAATTC as a site to cleave DNA (Fig 7), and every time this enzyme encounters this sequence it will cut the DNA into two fragments. Hundreds of restriction endonucleases have been characterized and these enzymes have become very important tools for dissecting DNA.

A *DNA probe* is a unique DNA sequence whose location in the human genome is known. Frequently, DNA probes are fragments of human genomic DNA that have been cloned into bacterial vectors, which allows many copies of the selected DNA fragment to be generated (see the next section). Probes are used to identify the presence of the DNA sequence that is

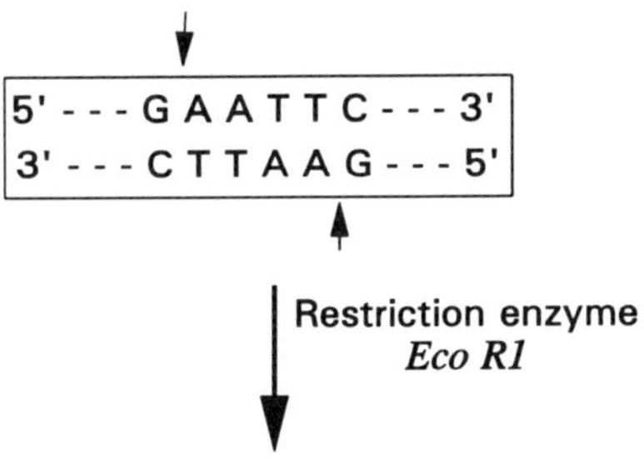

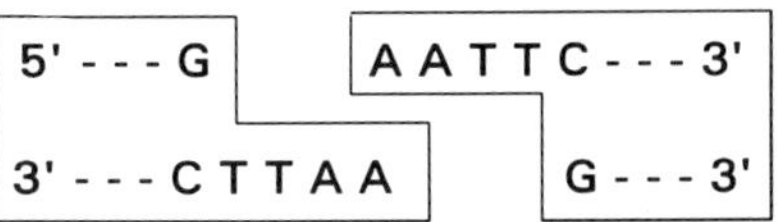

Figure 7   *Specific cleavage of DNA by the restriction enzyme EcoR1. This restriction endonuclease recognizes the DNA sequence 5' GAATCC 3' and cleaves the DNA between the 5' G and A as indicated.*

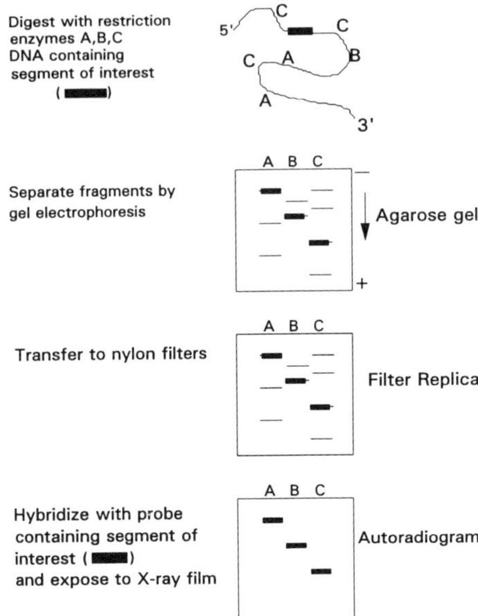

Figure 8 *Southern blot analysis, a method to transfer DNA fragments from an agarose gel to nylon or nitrocellulose filters. The first step in this procedure is to digest total genomic DNA with a specific restriction endonuclease. Next, the DNA fragments are separated by agarose gel electrophoresis. Using the Southern procedure, the DNA fragments are then transferred from the agarose gel to the nylon or nitrocellulose filters. The DNA on the filter is hybridized with a purified radioactive DNA probe designed to indicate which DNA fragment(s) contain the DNA sequences of interest. The radioactive bands are visualized after exposure of the filter to x-ray film.*

complementary to the probe DNA by DNA hybridization, usually using the Southern technique.

For Southern blot analysis, total human genomic DNA is digested with a particular restriction endonuclease so that a specific spectrum of DNA fragments is generated. These fragments are separated by agarose gel electrophoresis and then transferred from the agarose gel to nitrocellulose or nylon paper (Fig 8). The DNA is denatured, or made single-stranded, in the agarose gel before it is transferred. Next, a DNA probe is radioactively labeled, denatured, and allowed to hybridize with the digested total genomic DNA fixed to the nylon or nitrocellulose. The nitrocellulose (now also containing the radioactive sequences) is used to expose x-ray film, which allows visualization of the DNA fragments on the gel that hybridized with the specific radioactive DNA probe. This technique has many applications, including identifying and using restriction fragment length polymorphisms and searching for gene deletions or rearrangements.

DNA Cloning

Cloning a fragment of human DNA is another way of isolating a selected piece of DNA and amplifying it many times so that it may be used in other experiments [8, 9]. The cloning process is dependent on recombinant DNA technology. A typical procedure joins together two pieces of DNA, usually a cloning vector and the selected piece of human DNA (Fig 9). A *cloning vector* is a DNA molecule that can replicate autono-

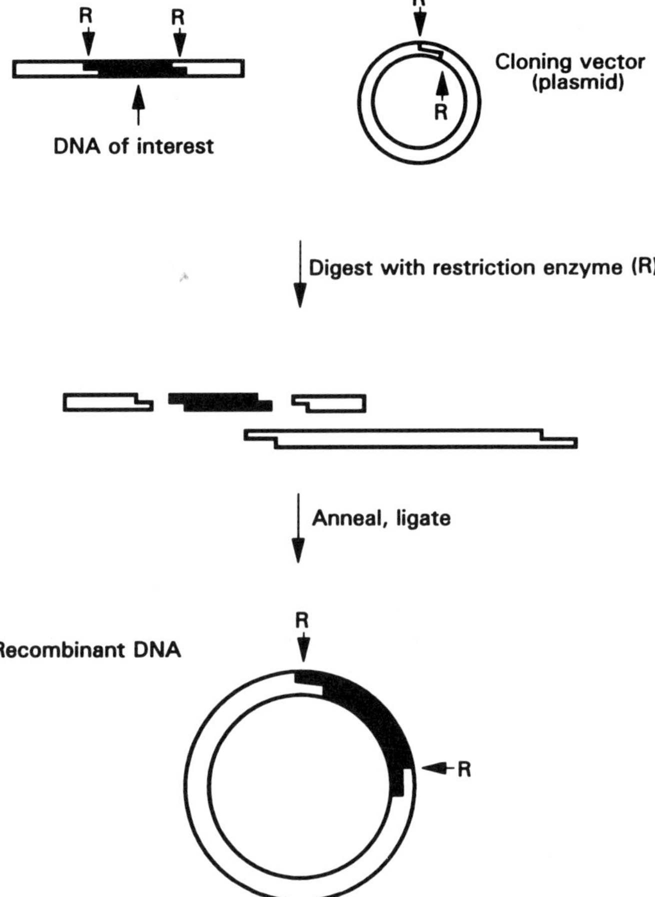

Figure 9 *DNA cloning. To clone a specific fragment of DNA, total human genomic DNA containing that fragment and a selected cloning vector are cleaved with a particular restriction endonuclease (R). Because restriction enzymes cleave DNA at specific sequences, leaving overhanging ("sticky") ends (see Fig 7), the vector DNA and cleaved human genomic DNA can be reannealed and ligated with the enzyme DNA ligase to create recombinant molecules. The recombinant molecules are allowed to replicate many times in a host organism, after which the population of recombinant molecules is isolated and the desired DNA fragment purified.*

mously in a host cell such as a bacteria or yeast. Before two fragments of DNA can be joined, they are first digested with a specific restriction endonuclease, which leaves characteristic "sticky ends" at the termination of each DNA fragment. This population of treated DNA is allowed to anneal (renature) and is treated with another DNA enzyme, DNA ligase, whose function is to make a covalent bond between the sticky ends. The recombinant DNA molecule is then introduced into the host cell where it will be replicated many times. After adequate amplification, the recombinant DNA can be purified from the host cell and used for the desired experiments.

Sequence Analysis

Direct DNA Sequencing   Frequently, studies of molecular biology ultimately require the ability to determine exact nucleotide sequences in DNA or RNA. A specific mutation responsible for a disease often cannot be demonstrated unless the DNA is sequenced. The discovery of restriction enzymes, which cleave DNA into small, consistently reproducible sets of fragments, was an important step in the development of DNA sequencing techniques. A second advance was the refinement of gel electrophoretic techniques, which can separate DNA fragments that contain from 1 to 500 bases and that differ in length by only one residue. One method for rapid sequencing of DNA is called the *dideoxy method* (Fig 10) [10]. In this procedure, a selected fragment of DNA is purified, denatured (to produce single-stranded DNA), and radiochemically labeled on one of its ends. (The radiochemical labeling can be accomplished using a variety of procedures; one method uses an enzyme called *polynucleotide kinase*.) This radiolabeled "primer" DNA is allowed to anneal with a selected purified fragment of denatured "template" DNA. Four samples of the terminally labeled fragment hybridized with the template DNA are used for four different enzymatic reactions that include DNA polymerase and the four deoxynucleoside triphosphates (which are required for DNA synthesis). In addition, each reaction will contain a different dideoxynucleoside triphosphate, which will terminate the newly synthesized DNA chain as soon as it is incorporated by the DNA polymerase. Because the dideoxynucleoside triphosphates are incorporated randomly, each reaction mixture contains fragments of DNA that are labeled at one end and stretch to their terminated ends at each occurrence of one of the four bases. Together, the four reaction mixes contain fragments that stretch from the labeled end to each base in the original segment. Parallel gel electrophoresis of the newly created labeled fragments from the four different samples produces four different lanes of bands. The bands in each lane correspond to all of the fragments that end in a particular nucleotide, arranged in order of length. Because the fragments in different samples end in different nucleotides, the fragments in different columns are never the same length, and the bands formed are never in the same position in any two lanes. Thus, the layout of the bands reveals the order of the nucleotides in the original DNA samples. Modifications of this procedure have been developed so that specific regions of human genomic DNA can be amplified by PCR and then directly sequenced [11].

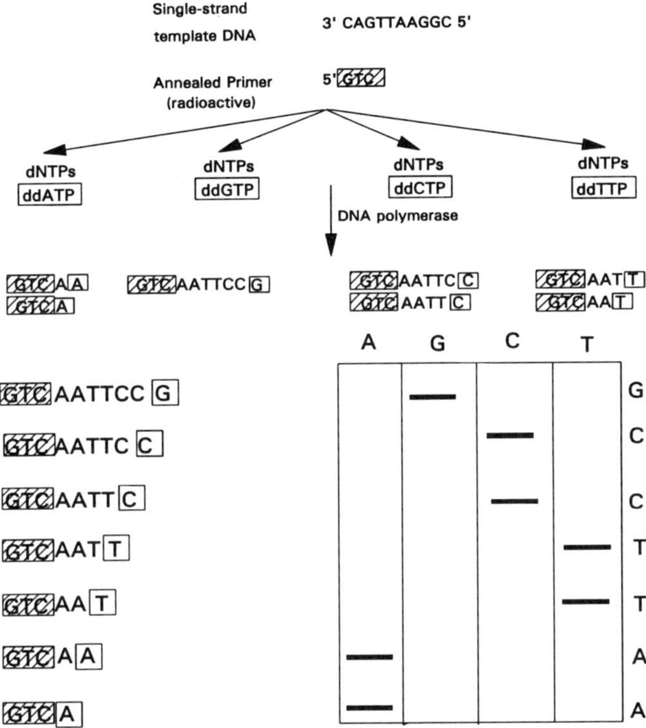

Figure 10 *DNA sequencing by the Sanger (dideoxy) method. A selected, purified fragment of "template" DNA is denatured and allowed to anneal to a radiolabeled primer. This mixture is divided into four separate reactions, each containing the four deoxyribonucleoside triphosphates (dNTP) as well as one of the four dideoxyribonucleoside triphosphates (ddNTP). DNA synthesis by DNA polymerase is allowed to proceed in each of the four reaction mixtures. The dideoxynucleoside triphosphates create a chain termination event and, because the dideoxynucleoside triphosphates are incorporated randomly, each reaction mixture contains fragments of DNA that are labeled at one end and stretch to their terminated ends at each occurrence of one of the four bases. The spectrum of synthesized DNA fragments is separated by gel electrophoresis and, after exposure of the gel to x-ray film, the DNA sequence is read from the gel.*

Single-Strand DNA Gel Electrophoresis   Although direct DNA sequence analysis eventually will demonstrate any mutation that results in a base pair change in the DNA sequence, it is not always convenient to sequence a particular DNA segment. In situations where large numbers of patient DNA are screened for biologically significant mutations, it is easier to use methods that can quickly indicate a base pair change (mutation) in a selected segment of DNA. One such technique is single-strand DNA gel electrophoresis [12]. For analysis using this technique, a homogeneous sample of a selected DNA fragment is prepared either by PCR amplification or by cloning. Next, the native double-strand DNA is denatured to produce two single strands. The single-strand DNA population is subjected to gel electrophoresis under nondenaturing conditions so that the inherent secondary structure of the single-strand DNA fragments will be preserved (Fig 11). The secondary structure of single-strand DNA is very dependent on the base sequence of the DNA. If a mutation creates a base pair change

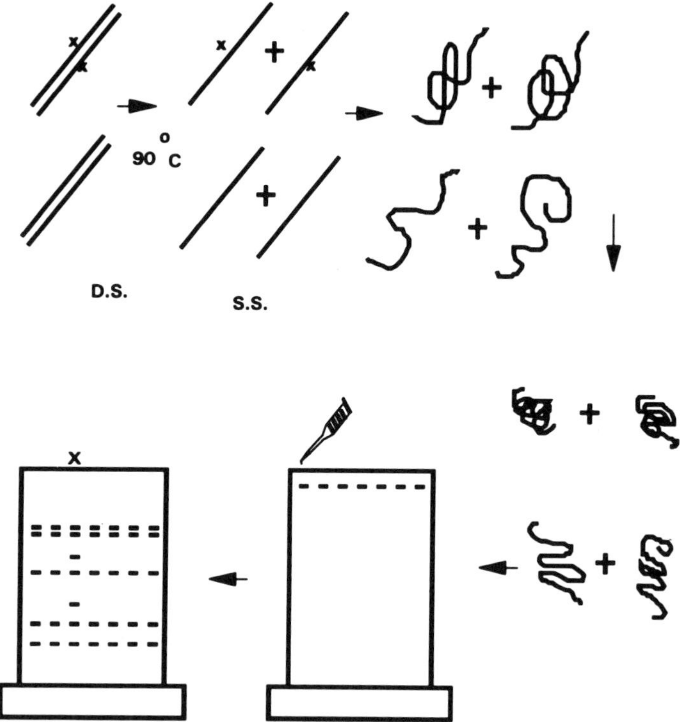

Figure 11 *Single-strand DNA gel electrophoresis demonstrating single-strand DNA conformation polymorphisms (SSCP) resulting from a single base pair change. To perform this technique, selected DNA fragments are amplified by the polymerase chain reaction (PCR). The amplified DNA is denatured to produce single strands and then is subjected to gel electrophoresis under conditions that preserve the inherent secondary structure of the single-strand DNA. Since the secondary structure of single-strand DNA is dependent of the sequence of the DNA, those fragments of DNA that contain a sequence change will travel through the gel at a different rate from those DNA fragments that do not contain the sequence change. If the DNA fragments are radiolabeled during PCR, the gel can be directly exposed to x-ray film and the pattern of DNA fragments after electrophoresis can be visualized. (S.S. = single-strand DNA; D.S. = double-strand DNA.)*

within the DNA fragment under investigation, the fragments containing the base pair change will have a different single-strand secondary structure and a different mobility when subjected to nondenaturing gel electrophoresis. The change in mobility of a DNA fragment can be visualized after the electrophoresis is completed. A change in mobility of a DNA fragment under these conditions suggests that the fragment contains a base pair change in the DNA sequence. These results can be confirmed by directly sequencing the DNA as outlined previously.

Denaturing Gradient Gel Electrophoresis Denaturing gradient gel electrophoresis is yet another technique for screening large populations of DNA for single base pair changes that may represent biologically significant mutations [13]. In this technique, double-strand DNA samples are subjected to electrophoresis through a gradient of a denaturing agent such as urea. Depending on the sequence of a particular DNA fragment, each fragment will reach a point in the gel where that fragment will denature. This point will vary if a change in DNA sequence has occurred. DNA fragments that contain a base pair change will demonstrate a different electrophoretic mobility under these conditions compared with DNA fragments that do not contain a DNA sequence change.

Genetic Markers

Genetic markers are regions of naturally occurring DNA sequence variability found scattered throughout the human genome. These regions typically occur in introns of genes; thus they are not transcribed into RNA or translated into protein. They are probably the result of random DNA mutations, but once created they are inherited as stable genetic elements. If the locations of these regions of variable DNA sequence in the human genome are known, they can function as markers for gene mapping and genetic linkage experiments. Several categories of genetic markers are currently in use.

Restriction Fragment Length Polymorphisms Restriction fragment length polymorphisms (RFLPs) depend on the specificity of DNA restriction endonucleases. These enzymes have the ability to recognize a specific DNA sequence as a site to cleave DNA. A mutation causing a single base pair change within this recognition sequence can alter the DNA cleavage site so that a larger or smaller DNA fragment is produced when the DNA is digested with a particular restriction enzyme (Fig 12). Random mutations involving a restriction enzyme site will occur in some individuals and not others. Once such a polymorphic restriction enzyme site is established, it is inherited by subsequent generations in a mendelian fashion. The DNA fragments generated from digestion at these sites represent the alleles of these polymorphic loci. RFLPs can be used as genetic markers to test for

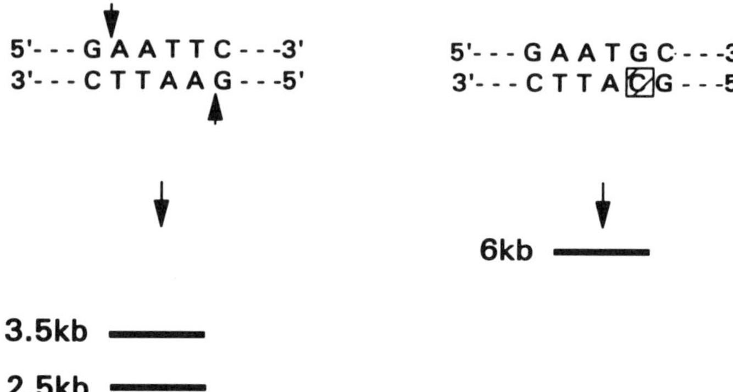

Figure 12 *Restriction fragment length polymorphism (RFLP). A random mutation within the recognition sequence of a DNA restriction endonuclease can result in an alteration of the cleavage of DNA by that enzyme. In this example showing the recognition sequence for the restriction enzyme EcoR1, a G has been changed to a C, thus eliminating the cleavage site. DNA samples purified from a population of individuals and analyzed for this polymorphism would demonstrate two patterns of DNA fragments: Those individuals with the enzyme site would have two smaller DNA fragments, and those without the enzyme site would have one larger fragment.*

linkage relationships in human pedigrees. DNA from members of kindreds in which certain inherited traits are known to segregate can be analyzed, making possible the mapping of the gene responsible for the trait with respect to the DNA marker.

Variable Number of Tandem Repeat Polymorphisms Polymorphic loci are useful for genetic linkage studies only when the parents of the pedigree to be studied are heterozygous for alleles at the marker loci. Standard RFLPs usually have only two different-sized fragments (alleles) at each polymorphic loci. In addition, even when two different-sized fragments are generated, they are not always present in the population in equal amounts. For example, at a given RFLP, two fragments may be found in the general population, but one fragment might be present in 70% of individuals and the other in only 30% of individuals. Given the resultant allele frequencies, only 42% of individuals will be heterozygous. Consequently, the usefulness of such a polymorphic marker in genetic linkage analysis is very limited.

In an attempt to avoid this problem, polymorphic loci with many alleles, and therefore a higher frequency of heterozygosity in the general population, were sought. Variable number of tandem repeats (VNTR) polymorphisms represent regions of DNA where a particular short se-

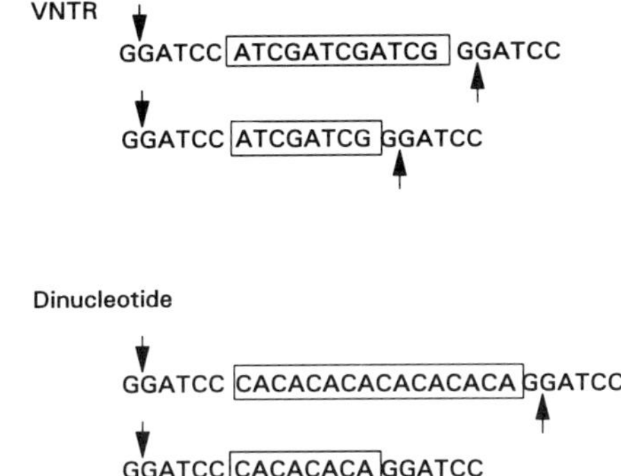

Figure 13 *Variable number of tandem repeats (VNTR) polymorphisms and dinucleotide repeats. A short DNA sequence is repeated many times; however, the exact number of repeats is variable among a population of individuals, thus creating a polymorphic region of DNA. The repeated sequences in this example are ATCG (VNTR) and CA (dinucleotide repeat).*

quence of DNA is repeated many times (Fig 13). These DNA segments are polymorphic because the precise number of repeats from person to person is highly variable. DNA analysis at these loci in a population of individuals may reveal as many as ten different alleles, and the fraction of heterozygous individuals could be as high as 70 to 80%, making these loci extremely useful for genetic linkage analysis [14].

Dinucleotide Repeats Dinucleotide repeats are similar to VNTR polymorphisms in that they represent regions of genomic DNA where a particular short DNA sequence is repeated many times. The repeated sequence is frequently CA, and these regions have been referred to as *CA repeats* or *dinucleotide repeats* [15]. The number of times the dinucleotide sequence is repeated among a population of individuals is extremely variable and, as a result, these regions produce polymorphisms with many different alleles. Patient DNA is analyzed at these polymorphic sites by direct amplification of the region containing the dinucleotide repeat, using PCR. With this procedure, dinucleotide repeats can be used as genetic markers for linkage analysis. This category of genetic markers has the advantage of being extremely polymorphic (typically 80% of the population is heterozygous), and analysis of DNA using PCR requires less time than does the Southern procedure, which must be used with RFLP or VNTR polymorphisms.

Linkage Analysis

Linkage analysis is a method that is used to determine the location of a gene responsible for a particular disease trait in the human genome. This technique is dependent on the genetic concept that two genes located in near proximity on the same chromosome will be inherited together. For example, if a marker locus is located near a disease locus in a family af-

A

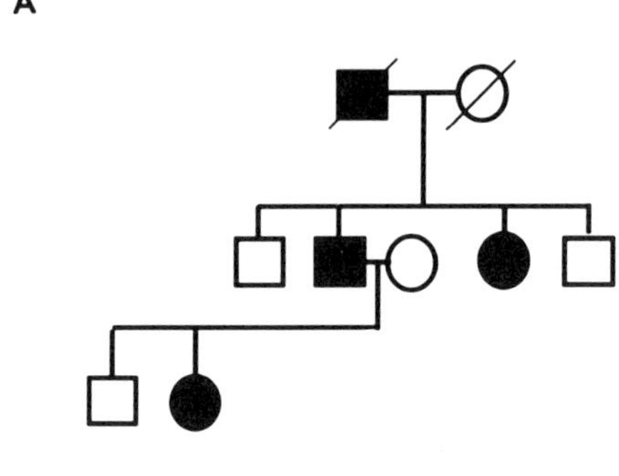

B

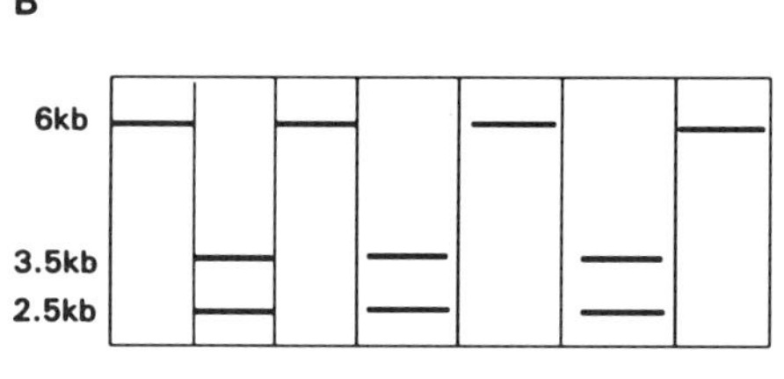

Figure 14 *Genetic linkage analysis using a restriction fragment length polymorphism. (A) Pedigree of a family affected with a genetic disorder inherited in an autosomal dominant fashion. Affected individuals are indicated by the solid squares (male) or circles (female). Circles or squares with a line represent deceased individuals. (B) Results of DNA analysis from living family members at a selected restriction fragment length polymorphism. This restriction enzyme site is polymorphic, so that two fragments of DNA are found in some individuals (those who have the site), whereas some individuals have only one larger DNA fragment (those who no longer have the site because of a DNA sequence change). In this family, the affected individuals all have two DNA fragments of 3.5 kb and 2.5 kb, whereas the unaffected individuals all have only the larger 6-kb DNA fragment. Therefore, the genetic trait in this family shows substantial genetic linkage to this DNA polymorphism.*

fected with a particular disease, the inheritance of the disease trait can be followed in that family by following the inheritance of certain alleles at the marker locus (Fig 14). If the chromosomal location of the marker locus is known, one can infer the location of the disease gene if genetic linkage between the two loci can be demonstrated. Once a genetic marker is shown to be genetically linked to a particular disease gene, that marker can also be used to develop DNA-based diagnostic tests for the condition since it is possible to predict which individuals at risk will develop the disease by determining whether the marker alleles linked to the disease gene have been inherited.

The distance of the marker locus from a disease gene is determined by measuring the degree of genetic recombination that occurs between these two loci during meiosis. At the completion of meiosis, the pairs of chromosomes present in somatic cells are halved to form the gametes (see Fig 2). During the early stages of meiosis, homologous chromosomes exchange segments in a process called *recombination,* which results in crossing over between the pairs of chromosomes so that hybrid chromosomes are generated that contain a portion of the maternal and paternal genetic material (Fig 15). The order of genes is altered and, because crossing over is more likely to occur between genes that are far apart, genes close together will tend to remain undisturbed on the same chromosome but genes farther apart may become separated. If a marker and disease gene are close to each other, recombination will occur rarely between them; if they are far apart, a recombination event will be a common occurrence. The

Homologous Chromosome Pairs

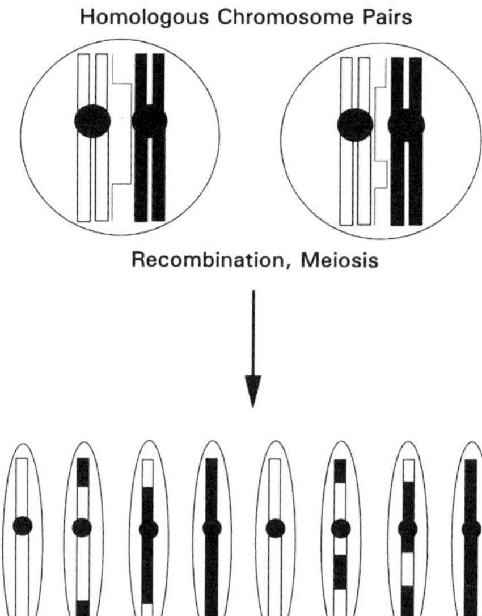

Figure 15 *Meiotic recombination. During the cell division process of meiosis, the homologous chromosomes pair and exchange segments so that hybrid chromosomes are generated that contain a portion of the maternal and paternal genetic material.*

frequency of recombination between two genes, or between one gene and a genetic marker, is a measure of the distance between them. By convention, 1% of recombination is equal to a unit called the *centimorgan* (cM), and the centimorgan is equivalent approximately to the megabase (Mb) [1 Mb is equal to 1,000 kilobases or 1,000,000 base pairs (bp)].

Genetic linkage is calculated as the ratio of the likelihood of linkage versus the likelihood of no linkage based on a range of recombination values. The log 10 of this likelihood ratio is called the *LOD score,* and this method of linkage analysis is called the *LOD method* [16]. Genetic linkage of a particular phenotypical trait to a polymorphic genetic marker is accepted if the likelihood ratio is 1,000:1 or the LOD score is 3.00 [17]. The LOD score for two linked markers is dependent on the number of individuals in a given kindred, the recombination fraction (i.e., the DNA distance) between two markers, and the structure of the family pedigree [18]. Large pedigrees and parents heterozygous for alleles at the marker loci provide the greatest amount of linkage data and, consequently, the highest LOD scores. Polymorphic loci need be no greater than 0.2 Morgans apart to allow demonstrable linkage to a new gene, given a reasonable family size. Thus, given that the approximate size of the human genome is 33 Morgans, roughly 150 polymorphic genetic markers are necessary to establish the chromosomal location of a new gene. Hundreds of genetic markers are currently available for studies of this type [19].

If a polymorphic marker can be demonstrated to be linked to the gene responsible for a hereditary condition, a DNA-based diagnostic test can be developed using the linked genetic marker. The accuracy of these tests depends heavily on the proximity of the marker to the disease gene. Markers that are closest to the disease gene will be most accurate because the likelihood of a recombination event separating the marker and disease gene is small. Figure 16 shows a schematic representation of the markers surrounding a particular disease gene. In this example the diagnostic information arising from markers M2 and M3 would be more accurate than that information from M1.

Linkage Disequilibrium

Linkage disequilibrium is the tendency of specific alleles of one locus (gene) to occur with specific alleles of another locus more frequently than would be expected by chance alone [20]. This is another method that can be used to identify the location of the genes responsible for a particular disease. Genes linked to alleles of the major histocompatibility complex (human leukocyte antigens [HLA]) are examples of linkage disequilibrium. If an allele such as a particular HLA antigen can be shown to be linked to a disease trait, such as the observed linkage between HLA-B27 and Reiter's syndrome [21], the linked allele can serve as a marker that may be diagnostically useful.

■ Chromosomal Assignments of Some Ocular Disorders

Using many of the techniques described, the genes or the location of the genes responsible for a number of ocular disorders have been determined in the human genome [22–93]. The table summarizes these recent findings.

■ Advances in Diagnosis

Molecular genetic technology has led to tremendous advances in the molecular diagnosis of many ophthalmic conditions based on the identification of DNA mutation(s) that are responsible for a disease or the identification of a DNA marker that is genetically linked to the disease gene. If the location in the human genome of a gene responsible for a particular condition is known, it may be possible to identify many affected patients by genetic linkage analysis using DNA markers known to be "genetically close" to the disease gene. This analysis requires a small, simple, blood sample from the affected patient and related family members. Some ophthalmic disorders that can currently be diagnosed in this way include X-linked juvenile retinoschisis, X-linked retinitis pigmentosa, Lowe's syn-

Selected Hereditary Human Disorders with Ocular Manifestations

Disease	Inheritance	Chromosomal Location	Reference
Adenomatous polyposis of the colon	AD	5q22-q23	Nakamura, 1988 [22]
Aicardi's syndrome	XL	Xp22	Ropers, 1982 [23]
Aland island eye disease	XL	Xp21.3-p21.1	Pillers, 1990 [24]
Albinism, tyrosinase-negative	AR	11q14-q21	Barton, 1988 [25]
Alport's syndrome	XL	Xq22-q24	Flinter, 1989 [26]
Aniridia 2	AD	11p13	Glaser, 1986 [27]
Aniridia 1	AD	2p25	Ferrell, 1980 [28]
Anophthalmos, X-linked	XL	Xq27-q28	Graham, 1989 [29]
Anterior segment mesenchymal dysgenesis	AD	4q28-q31	Ferrell, 1982 [30]
Ataxia-telangiectasia	AR	11q22-q23	Gatti, 1988 [31]
Batten's disease (neuronal ceroid-lipofuscinosis)	AR	16q22	Eiberg, 1989 [32]
Cataract, anterior polar	AD	2p25	Moross, 1984 [33]
Cataract, zonular pulverulent (Coppock)	AD	1q21-q25	Conneally, 1978 [34]
Choroideremia	XL	Xq21.2	Cremers, 1990 [35]
Color blindness, blue-cone monochromacy	XL	Xq28	Lewis, 1987 [36]
Color blindness, deutan (green cone pigment)	XL	Xq28	Nathans, 1989 [37]
Color blindness, protan (red cone pigment)	XL	Xq28	Nathans, 1986 [38]
Cone-rod dystrophy	AD	18q21.1-q22.2	Waarburg, 1991 [39]
Corneal dermoids	XL	Xp22.2-p22.1	Igbal, 1987 [40]
Craniosynostosis	AD	7p21.3-p21.2	Garcia-Esquivel, 1986 [41]

Selected Hereditary Human Disorders with Ocular Manifestations (continued)

Disease	Inheritance	Chromosomal Location	Reference
Dyslexia 1	AD	15q11	Fain, 1985 [42]
Fabry's disease	XL	Xq22	Astrin, 1989 [43]
Focal dermal hypoplasia (Goltz's syndrome)	XL	Xp22.31	Friedman, 1988 [44]
Galactosemia 1	AR	9p13	Shih, 1982 [45]
GM_1 gangliosidosis	AR	3p21-cen	McKusick, 1988 [46]
GM_2 gangliosidosis, AB variant	AD	5	Burg, 1985 [47]
Goldenhar's syndrome	AD	7p	Hodes, 1981 [48]
Green/blue eye color	AR	19	Eiberg, 1987 [49]
Gyrate atrophy	AR	10q26	Mitchell, 1988 [50]
Homocystinuria	AR	21q22.3	Skovby, 1984 [51]
Hurler-Scheie syndrome	AR	22q11	Schuchman, 1984 [52]
Incontinentia pigmenti	XL	Xq27-q28	Sefiani, 1989 [53]
Iris coloboma	AD	2pter-p25.1	Arias, 1984 [54]
Kearns-Sayre syndrome	mtDNA		Zeviani, 1988 [55]
Krabbe's disease (galactocerebrosidase)	AR	17	Lyerla, 1989 [56]
Leber's hereditary optic neuropathy	mtDNA		Wallace, 1988 [57]
Lowe's oculocerebrorenal syndrome	XL	Xq25	Reilly, 1990 [58]
Macular dystrophy, atypical vitelliform	AD	8q24	Ferrell, 1983 [59]
Marfan's syndrome (collagen type 1)	AD	17q21.3-q22.05	Sykes, 1990 [60]
Marfan's syndrome 1	AD	15q15-q21.3	Dietz, 1991 [61]

Disease	Inheritance	Location	Reference
Maroteaux-Lamy syndrome (mucopolysaccharidosis VI)	AR	5q11-q13	Litjens, 1989 [62]
Megalocornea	XL	Xq12-q26	Chen, 1989 [63]
Morquio's syndrome B (mucopolysaccharidosis IVB)	AR	3p21-cen	Spranger, 1977 [64]
Multiple endocrine neoplasia I	AD	11q23	Nakamura, 1989 [65]
Multiple endocrine neoplasia II or IIA	AD	10q21.1	Simpson, 1987 [66]
Multiple endocrine neoplasia III or IIB	AD	10q21.1	Jackson, 1988 [67]
Myopia, X-linked	XL	Xq28	Schwartz, 1990 [68]
Myotonic dystrophy	AD	19q13.1	Brunner, 1989 [69]
Nance-Horan cataract dental syndrome	XL	Xp22.3-p21.1	Lewis, 1990 [70]
Neurofibromatosis 1	AD	17q11.2	Cawthon, 1990 [71]
Neurofibromatosis 2 (bilateral acoustic neuroma)	AD	22q11-q13.1	Rouleau, 1990 [72]
Nevoid basal cell carcinoma syndrome	AD	1p	Fryburg, 1989 [73]
Niemann-Pick disease (sphingomyelinase)	AD	17	Konrad, 1987 [74]
Ocular albinism, Nettleship-Falls type	XL	Xp22	Schnur, 1991 [75]
Optic atrophy, Kjer type	AD	2p	Kivlin, 1983 [76]
Phenylketonuria	AR	12q22-q24.1	Woo, 1984 [77]
Retinitis pigmentosa 1	AD	3q21-q23	Farrar, 1990 [78]
Retinoblastoma	AD	13q14.1-14.2	Sparkes, 1980 [79]
Retinoschisis	XL	Xp22	Alitalo, 1991 [80]
Rieger's syndrome	AD	4q23-q27	Ligutic, 1981 [81]

Selected Hereditary Human Disorders with Ocular Manifestations (continued)

Disease	Inheritance	Chromosomal Location	Reference
Sandhoff's disease	AR	5q13	Fox, 1984 [82]
Sanfilippo's syndrome	AR	12q14	Robertson, 1988 [83]
Stickler's syndrome	AD	12q13.1-13.3	Knowlton, 1989 [84]
Tay-Sachs disease	AR	15q22-q25.1	Nakai, 1987 [85]
Tritan color blindness	AD	7q22-qter	Nathans, 1986 [86]
Tuberous sclerosis 2	AD	11q23	Haines, 1989 [87]
Tuberous sclerosis 1	AD	9q33-q34	Fryer, 1987 [88]
Usher's syndrome, type II	AR	1q	Kimberling, 1990 [89]
von Hippel-Lindau syndrome	AD	3p25-p24	Vance, 1989 [90]
Waardenburg's syndrome	AD	2q35	Asher, 1991 [91]
Wilson's disease	AR	13q14-q21	Bonne-Tamir, 1986 [92]
Zellweger's syndrome	AR	7q11.12-q11.23	Naritomi, 1988 [93]

AD = autosomal dominant; AR = autosomal recessive; mtDNA = mitochondrial DNA, XL = X-linked.

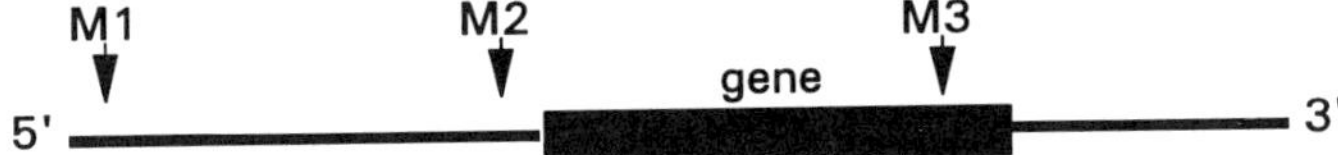

Figure 16 *Hypothetical disease gene with three polymorphic genetic markers (M1, M2, M3), which could be used diagnostically to identify individuals at risk for the disorder.*

drome, Stickler's syndrome, Norrie's disease, ocular albinism, choroideremia, and some cases of retinoblastoma.

If the gene responsible for a disorder has been cloned and characterized, it may be possible to demonstrate the actual mutations responsible for the disease in a DNA sample obtained from the affected patient. Two categories of mutations have been observed to cause single gene defects: gross abnormalities (gene deletions, rearrangements, or insertions) and point mutations (a single DNA base pair change). Currently, molecular diagnosis based on the identification of the predisposing DNA mutation is possible in some patients affected with retinoblastoma, autosomal dominant retinitis pigmentosa, Kearns-Sayre syndrome, and Leber's hereditary optic neuropathy.

Retinoblastoma

Retinoblastoma is a cancer of the retina that appears usually in children younger than 4 years in both hereditary and nonhereditary forms. Approximately 40% of all patients have hereditary disease, and these children can pass on to their progeny a predisposition to retinoblastoma as an autosomal dominant disorder. Only 10% of the patients with hereditary retinoblastoma have a family history of the disease; the remaining 90% have new mutations of the germ cells (female eggs and male sperm). Children with new mutations can pass the disease on to their progeny, even though their parents could not pass the disease to the affected child or its siblings [94, 95]. Nonhereditary retinoblastoma is caused by somatic mutations of both copies of chromosome 13 in the region q14 in a single retinal cell. Patients with somatic mutations involving only the malignant retinal cell do not have the ability to pass the mutation on to subsequent generations.

The gene responsible for this cancer was first identified and cloned in 1986 [96–98]. This gene spans 200 kb on the long arm of chromosome 13 (band q14). Transcription of the retinoblastoma gene by RNA polymerase results in a 4.7-kb mRNA transcript [99–101]. The 4.7-kb mRNA codes for a 110-Kd nuclear phosphoprotein with DNA-binding activity [102]. This gene normally functions as a dominant suppressor of tumor formation, and alteration or inactivation of both homologous alleles (copies of the gene) is necessary for the development of retinoblastoma. Mutations in this gene have also been reported to be responsible for other types of tumors including osteosarcomas, various soft-tissue sarcomas, small-cell carcinomas of the lung, and carcinomas of the bladder and breast [103].

The cloning and characterization of the retinoblastoma gene makes it possible to use DNA analysis for diagnosis and genetic counseling of this condition. DNA analysis can be done either indirectly by genetic linkage to DNA markers (genetic linkage analysis) or by direct identification of the tumor-predisposing mutation in the retinoblastoma gene. The indirect approach using genetic markers requires that two or more family members be affected [99, 104]. The direct approach requires that a particular DNA mutation in the retinoblastoma gene can be recognized, either by direct DNA sequencing or by one of the other methods that can demonstrate a DNA sequence change [105]. Identification of a mutation in the retinoblastoma gene in an affected patient makes it possible to determine whether other family members at risk for the disease carry the same mutation.

DNA analysis of a pedigree affected with retinoblastoma can also identify families affected with hereditary retinoblastoma versus nonhereditary retinoblastoma and can identify a new germ-line mutation in an affected child [106].

Autosomal Dominant Retinitis Pigmentosa

Retinitis pigmentosa is a group of hereditary retinal degenerations that affect between 50,000 and 100,000 people in the United States. Affected patients typically develop night blindness and progressive loss of visual field, losing central vision by the age of 50 to 80 years. The disease is genetically heterogeneous and can be transmitted as an autosomal dominant, autosomal recessive, or X-linked trait [107]. In 1989, an RFLP from chromosome 3q was found to be tightly linked to the disease trait in one large family with autosomal dominant retinitis pigmentosa [108]. Since the gene coding for rhodopsin, the first protein involved in the visual transduction pathway, was located in the same region on chromosome 3q, Dryja and colleagues [109], using PCR and direct DNA sequencing, searched for mutations in the rhodopsin gene in patients affected with autosomal dominant retinitis pigmentosa. They identified a point mutation of the rhodopsin gene in codon 23, resulting in a nucleotide base change (cytosine to adenine). This single nucleotide substitution represents a point mutation that causes the amino acid proline in position 23 of the rhodopsin protein to be replaced by the amino acid histidine. The proline in this position of the protein molecule is normally highly conserved among populations of individuals and is probably critical for the proper tertiary structure of the protein molecule required for normal biological activity. This mutation was found in 17 of 148 unrelated patients with autosomal dominant retinitis pigmentosa and in none of 102 unaffected individuals.

Since this initial discovery, a number of other mutations in the gene coding for the rhodopsin molecule have been discovered in patients with autosomal dominant retinitis pigmentosa [110, 111]. In addition, recently a *null mutation* (a mutation that results in a premature protein termination codon so that a complete protein product is not synthesized) has been described in a patient with autosomal recessive retinitis pigmentosa [112]. Mutations in another protein, called *perpherin,* have also recently been described in patients with autosomal dominant retinitis pigmentosa [113]. Perpherin is an important structural component of the rod discs and, like rhodopsin, is a protein necessary for the proper function of the visual transduction pathway. These findings suggest that autosomal dominant retinitis pigmentosa is a genetically heterogeneous disorder—that is, mutations in more than one gene may be responsible for the disease.

Patients with autosomal dominant retinitis pigmentosa can have widely varying visual symptoms and findings. The clinical phenotypes of patients affected with various rhodopsin mutations is currently under investigation. It appears that some rhodopsin mutations may result in more severe disease than others. However, patients with the same rhodopsin mutation and belonging to the same affected pedigree can also demonstrate wide variation in the severity of the condition [114]. These results suggest that other factors may be important to the progression of this disease.

The abnormalities that have been identified in the gene for rhodopsin and perpherin in patients with autosomal dominant retinitis pigmentosa provide a basis for diagnostic DNA tests that can be used to identify individuals at risk for this disease. Patients found to have one of these mutations can be informed that with each pregnancy they have a 50% chance of having an affected child.

Mitochondrial DNA Disorders

Mutations in the genetic material of mitochondria have been described in patients with a range of neuro-ophthalmological and neuromuscular disorders. These include Leber's hereditary optic neuropathy, Kearns-Sayre syndrome, chronic external ophthalmoplegia, and other mitochondrial cytopathies [115]. Mitochondria are rod-shaped organelles found in the cytoplasm of most eukaryotic cells. They are called "the power plants" of aerobic cells because they contain the enzymes of the respiratory transport chain and are reponsible for providing the majority of the adenosine triphosphate (ATP) that is used by the body as energy necessary for biological processes [116]. In general, mitochondrial mutations have more of an effect in tissues with a high requirement for ATP, including the central nervous system, retina, type I skeletal muscle fibers, heart, and kidney [117].

Mitochondria contain their own genome consisting of a single circular chromosome that codes for 37 genes [3]. Mitochondrial inheritance is non-mendelian. Because mitochondria are found in the eggs and not sperm, an

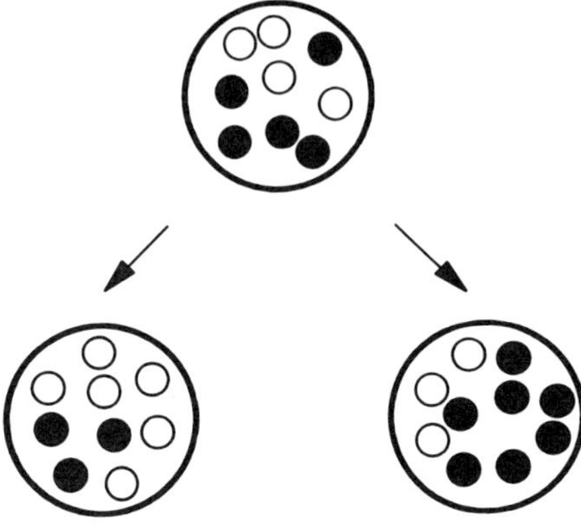

Figure 17 *Heteroplasmy as a result of random distribution of mutant mitochondria with cell division. Mutant mitochondria are represented by solid circles, and wild type mitochondria are shown as open circles.*

individual receives only maternal mitochondrial DNA; paternal mitochondrial DNA is never transmitted to offspring. Consequently, diseases caused by mitochondrial mutations are transmitted exclusively maternally. All the offspring of a woman affected with a mitochondrial disorder will be potential carriers of the mutant mitochondria [118].

Mutations of the mitochondrial chromosome give rise to heteroplasmy (different genetic species of mitochondria coexisting in the cytoplasm of the same cell). Human cells contain, with a few specialized exceptions, hundreds of mitochondria, and each mitochondrion contains several copies of its chromosome. After a single mutation event, a cell is therefore heteroplasmic, because it contains different genetic strains of mitochondria. When such heteroplasmic cells divide, different populations of cells are produced by variable segregation of the mitochondria. In some descendant lines, mutant mitochondria become the more frequent form, whereas in others the wild type population predominate (Fig 17) [119]. As a result of heteroplasmy, the clinical expression of mitochondrial mutations is variable and often unpredictable.

Three categories of mitochondrial mutations have been detected in human disease. In the first and most common type, DNA deletions result in a loss of a section of the mitochondria chromosome [120]. In the second type, segments of the mitochondrial genome duplicate, creating a larger-than-normal mitochondrial chromosome [121]. Deletions and duplications of mitochondrial DNA create large changes in the mitochondrial genome and generally result in severe forms of neuromuscular disease called *mitochondrial cytopathies.* These disorders comprise a spectrum of neuromuscular disease with overlapping clinical findings. Specific syndromes included in this group of disorders are mitochondrial myopathy, chronic progressive external ophthalmoplegia, mitochondrial encephalomyopathy, Kearns-Sayre disease, MELAS (*m*itochondrial myopathy, *e*ncephalopathy, *l*actic *a*cidosis, and *s*trokelike episodes), and MERRF (*m*itochondrial *e*pilepsy with *ragged red fibers*). Common features in this group of syndromes are defective mitochondria and neuromuscular impairment [122].

The third type of mutation responsible for mitochondrial DNA disorders is point mutations, which create a small change in the mitochondrial DNA and result in less severe disease than do DNA deletions and duplications. Point mutations represent the substitution of a single base pair of DNA and generally lead to a structural change and consequent functional change in a single protein. Point mutations in mitochondrial DNA have been described in patients with Leber's hereditary optic neuropathy [57].

Leber's hereditary optic neuropathy is an uncommon hereditary disorder presenting most often in male young adults, but it has been described in men and women at any age. The disease is characterized by a rapid onset of visual failure affecting both eyes within a few weeks of each other. In the acute stage, the optic discs are swollen and hyperemic and eventually become pale and atrophic [123]. Leber's hereditary optic neuropathy does not follow mendelian inheritance. Women pass the disease mainly to their sons, and the affected sons never pass the disease to their offspring [124].

In 1988, Wallace and colleagues [57] discovered a point mutation in mitochondrial DNA that was responsible for Leber's hereditary optic neuropathy in eleven independent pedigrees. The mutation of a single base at position 11778 of the mitochondrial chromosome, in the gene ND4, leads to the alteration of one amino acid of a subunit of the respiratory chain complex I, an enzyme necessary for ATP synthesis. Since this initial discovery, other mutations in mitochondrial DNA have been found in affected patients [125]. Interestingly, only point mutations in mitochondrial DNA have been found to be the cause of Leber's hereditary optic neuropathy, rather than the large deletions or gene duplications that cause mitochondrial cytopathies.

Mitochondrial DNA mutations can be sought in patients who may be at risk for Leber's hereditary optic neuropathy. In addition, patients who present with a constellation of symptoms that may be consistent with this disease diagnosis can be tested for mitochondrial DNA mutations to confirm the diagnosis [126].

■ Advances in Treatment

The first benefits from the application of molecular genetics to hereditary eye disease have been improved methods of diagnosis based on the genes and specific DNA mutations that are responsible for these conditions. Improved diagnosis alone will provide for better care of affected patients, because individuals at risk for hereditary ocular disease who are identified and treated at the earliest stages of the disease will have the best chance of a good visual outcome. The next step will be to realize new methods of treatment based on the specific molecular pathophysiology that has been discovered as a result of the characterization of the abnormal gene and resultant gene product. For example, if a specific gene can be found that is responsible for a particular disease, the characterization of that gene product will perhaps lead to novel therapy for the disease based on the specific activity of the normal protein. Ultimately, the characterization of the genes responsible for these conditions will be a first step toward gene therapy, which theoretically can involve the specific replacement, correction, or augmentation of a dysfunctional gene. Gene therapy is currently experimental, and the techniques required to place a particular gene into the relevant biological cell and to have that cell replicate properly and express the new gene have yet to be refined [127]. However, these ongoing studies hold enormous promise for the future treatment of all hereditary diseases, including many ocular disorders.

■ Conclusions

The novel techniques of molecular genetics are becoming increasingly important to our understanding of hereditary ocular disorders and are also reviewed excellently elsewhere [128–130]. In the next decade, ophthalmology as well as other disciplines in medicine should witness an explosion of information concerning the molecular basis of a variety of disorders. The knowledge gained from these studies will define the molecular pathophysiology of human genetic disease and lead to new methods of prevention, diagnosis, and treatment. It is possible that the techniques and concepts summarized in this chapter will no longer be applicable only to laboratory research but will become valuable clinical tools for the physician caring for these affected patients and their families.

■ References

1. Stephens JC, Cavanaugh ML, Gradie MI, et al. Mapping the human genome: current status. Science 1990;250:237–244
2. Watson JD, Crick FHC. Genetical implications of the structure of deoxyribonucleic acid. Nature 1953;171:964–967
3. Tzagoloff A, Myers AM. Genetics of mitochondrial biogenesis. Annu Rev Biochem 1986;55:249–285
4. Kunkel LM, Smith KD, Boyer SH, et al. Analysis of human Y-chromosome specific reiterated DNA in chromosomal variants. Proc Natl Acad Sci USA 1977;74: 1245–1249
5. Saiki RK, Gelfand DH, Stoffel S, et al. Primer directed enzymatic amplification of DNA with a thermostable DNA polymerase. Science 1988;239:487–491
6. Southern EM. Detection of specific sequences among DNA fragments separated by gel electrophoresis. J Mol Biol 1975;98:503–517
7. Roberts RJ. Restriction and modification enzymes and their recognition sequences. Nucleic Acids Res 1982;10:r117–r144

8. Sambrook J, Fritsch ER, Maniatis T. Molecular cloning: a laboratory manual, ed 2. Cold Spring Harbor, NY: Cold Spring Harbor Laboratory, 1989
9. Ausubel FM, Brent R, Kingston RE, et al, eds. Current protocols in molecular biology. New York: Wiley Interscience, 1987
10. Sanger F. Determination of nucleotide sequences in DNA. Science 1981;214:1205–1210
11. Yandell DW, Dryja TP. Detection of DNA sequence polymorphisms by enzymatic amplification and direct genomic sequencing. Am J Hum Genet 1989;45:547–555
12. Orita M, Suzuki Y, Sekiya T, Hayashi K. Rapid and sensitive detection of point mutations and DNA polymorphisms using the polymerase chain reaction. Genomics 1989;5:874–879
13. Myers RM, Larin Z, Maniatis T. Detection of single base substitutions by ribonuclease cleavage at mismatches in RNA:DNA duplexes. Science 1985;230:1242–1246
14. Nakamura T, et al. Variable number of tandem repeat (VNTR) markers for human gene mapping. Science 1987;235:1616
15. Weber JL, May PE. Abundant class of human DNA polymorphisms which can be typed using the polymerase chain reaction. Am J Hum Genet 1989;44:388–396
16. Ott J. A short guide to linkage analysis. In: Davies ED, ed. Human genetic diseases: a practical approach. Washington, DC: IRL Press, 1986:19–32
17. Morton NE. Segregation and linkage. In Burdette WJ, ed. Methodology in mammalian genetics. San Francisco: Holden-Day, 1962:17–52
18. Thompson EA, Dravits K, Hill S, Skolnick M. Linkage and the power of a pedigree structure. In: Morton NE, Chung CS, eds. Genetic epidemiology. New York: Academic, 1978:247–253
19. Weissenbach J, Gyapay G, Dib C, et al. Nature 1992;359:794–801
20. Muench KH. Medical genetics. New York: Elsevier, 1988:131–132
21. Derhaag PJFM, Linssen A, Broekema N, et al. A familial study of the inheritance of HLA-B27-positive acute anterior uveitis. Am J Ophthalmol 1988;105:603–606
22. Nakamura Y, Lathrop M, Leppert M, et al. Localization of the genetic defect in familial adenomatous polyposis within a small region of chromosome 5. Am J Hum Genet 1988;43:638–644
23. Ropers HH, Zuffardi O, Bianchi E, Tiepolo L. Agenesis of corpus callosum, ocular, and skeletal anomalies (X-linked dominant Aicardi's syndrome) in a girl with balanced X/3 translocation. Hum Genet 1982;61:364–368
24. Pillers DM, Towbin JA, Chamberlain JS, et al. Deletion mapping of Aland Island eye disease to Xp21 between DXS67 (B24) and Duchenne muscular dystrophy. Am J Hum Genet 1990;47:795–801
25. Barton DE, Kwon BS, Francke U. Human tyrosinase gene, mapped to chromosome 11 (q14-q21), defines second region of homology with mouse chromosome 7. Genomics 1988;3:17–24
26. Flinter FA, Abbs S, Bobrow M. Localization of the gene for classic Alport syndrome. Genomics 1989;4:335–338
27. Glaser T, Lewis WH, Gruns GAP, et al. The beta-subunit of follicle-stimulating hormone is deleted in patients with aniridia and Wilms' tumor, allowing a further definition of the WAGR locus. Nature 1986;321:882–887
28. Ferrell RE, Chakravarti A, Hittner HM, Riccardi VM. Autosomal dominant aniridia: probable linkage to acid phosphatase-1 on chromosome 2. Proc Natl Acad Sci USA 1980;77:1580–1582
29. Graham CA, Redmond RM, Nevin NC. X-linked clinical anophthalmos. Localization of the gene to Xq27-q28. Ophthalmic Paediatr Genet 1989;12:43–48
30. Ferrell RE, Hittner HM, Kretzer FL, Antoszyk JG. Anterior segment mesenchymal dysgenesis: probable linkage to the MNS blood group on chromosome 4. Am J Hum Genet 1982;34:245–249

31. Gatti RA, Berkel I, Boder E, et al. Localization of an ataxia-telangiectasia gene to chromosome 11q22-23. Nature 1988;336:577–580

32. Eiberg H, Gardiner RM, Mohr J. Batten disease (Spielmeyer-Sjogren disease) and haptoglobins (HP): indication of linkage and assignment to chromosome 16. Clin Genet 1989;36:217–218

33. Moross T, Vaithilingam SS, Styles S, Gardner HA. Autosomal dominant anterior polar cataracts associated with a familial 2;14 translocation. J Med Genet 1984;21:52–53

34. Conneally PM, Wilson AF, Merritt AD, et al. Confirmation of genetic heterogeneity in autosomal dominant forms of congenital cataracts from linkage studies. Cytogenet Cell Genet 1978;22:295–297

35. Cremers FPM, van de Pol DJR, van Kerlhoff LPM, et al. Cloning of a gene that is rearranged in patients with choroideremia. Nature 1990;347:674–677

36. Lewis RA, Nathans J, Holcomb JD, et al. Blue cone monochromacy: assignment of the locus to Xq28 and evidence for its molecular rearrangement. Am J Hum Genet 1987;41:A102

37. Nathans J. The genes for color vision. Sci Am 1989;260:42–49

38. Nathans J, Thomas D, Hogness DS. Molecular genetics of human color vision: the genes encoding blue, green and red pigments. Science 1986;232:193–202

39. Waarburg M, et al. Deletion mapping of a retinal cone-rod dystrophy: assignment to 18q211. Am J Med Genet 1991;39:288

40. Igbal MA, Chitayat D, Hahm SYE, Nitowsky HM. Linkage of gene for corneal dermoids with the DXS43 (Xp22.2-p22.1) locus. Am J Hum Genet 1987;41:A171

41. Garcia-Esquivel L, Garcia-Cruz D, Rivera H, et al. De novo del(7)(pter-p21.2::p15.2-qter) and craniosynostosis. Implications for critical segment assignment in the 7p2 monosomy syndrome. Ann Genet (Paris) 1986;29:36–38

42. Fain PR, Kimberling WJ, Ing PS, et al. Linkage analysis of reading disability with chromosome 15. Cytogenet Cell Genet 1985;40:625–628

43. Astrin KH, et al. Linkage between alpha-galactosidase A and DXS17, 87, 94, 101, 106 and 287. Cytogenet Cell Genet 1989;51:953–957

44. Friedman PA, Rao KW, Teplin SW, Aylsworth AS. Provisional deletion mapping of the focal dermal hypoplasia (FDH) gene to Xp22.31. Am J Hum Genet 1988;43:A50

45. Shih LY, Rosin I, Suslak L, et al. Localization of the structural gene for galactose-1-phosphate uridyl transferase to band p13 of chromosome 9 by gene dosage studies. Am J Hum Genet 1982;34:62A

46. McKusick VA. The morbid anatomy of the human genome: a review of gene mapping in clinical medicine. Baltimore: Williams & Wilkins, 1988

47. Burg J, Conzelmann E, Sandhoff K, et al. Mapping of the gene coding for the human G-M2 activator protein to chromosome 5. Am J Hum Genet 1985;49:41–45

48. Hodes ME, Gleiser S, De Rosa GP, et al. Trisomy 7 mosaicism and manifestations of Goldenhar syndrome with unilateral radial hypoplasia. J Craniofac Genet Dev Biol 1981;1:49–55

49. Eiberg H, Mohr J. Major genes of eye color and hair color linked to LU and SE. Clin Genet 1987;31:186–191

50. Mitchell GA, Brody LC, Looney J, et al. An initiation codon mutation in ornithine-delta-amino transferase causing gyrate atrophy of the choroid and retina. J Clin Invest 1988;81:630–633

51. Skovby F, Krassikoff N, Francke U. Assignment of the gene for cystathionine beta-synthase to human chromosome 21 in somatic cell hybrids. Hum Genet 1984;65:291–294

52. Schuchman EH, Astrin KH, Aula P, Desnick RJ. Regional assignment of the struc-

tural gene for human alpha-L-iduronidase. Proc Natl Acad Sci USA 1984;81: 1169–1173

53. Sefiani A, Abel L, Heuertz S, et al. The gene for incontinentia pigmenti is assigned to Xq28. Genomics 1989;4:427–429

54. Arias S, Rolo M, Gonzalez N. Terminal deletion of the short arm of chromosome 2, informative for acid phosphatase (*ASP1*), malate dehydrogenase (*MDH1*), and coloboma of iris loci. Cytogenet Cell Genet 1984;37:401–405

55. Zeviani M, Moraes CT, KiMauro S, et al. Deletions of mitochondrial DNA in Kearns-Sayre syndrome. Neurology 1988;38:1339–1346

56. Lyerla TA, Konola JT, Skiba MC, Raghavan S. Galactocerebrosidase activity in somatic cell hybrids derived from twitcher mouse/control human fibroblasts is associated with human chromosome 17. Am J Hum Genet 1989;44:198–207

57. Wallace DC, Singh G, Lott MT, et al. Mitochondrial DNA mutation associated with Leber's hereditary optic neuropathy. Science 1988;242:1427–1430

58. Reilly DS, Lewis RA, Nussbaum RL. Genetic and physical mapping of Xq24-q26 markers flanking the Lowe oculocerebrorenal syndrome. Genomics 1990;8:62–70

59. Ferrell RE, Hittner HM, Antoszyk JH. Linkage of atypical vitelliform macular dystrophy (*VMD-1*) to the soluble glutamate pyruvate transaminase (*GPT1*) locus. Am J Hum Genet 1983;38:78–84

60. Sykes B, Ogilvie D, Wordsworth P, et al. Consistent linkage of dominantly inherited osteogenesis imperfecta to the type I collagen loci COL1A1 and COL1A2. Am J Hum Genet 1990;46:293–307

61. Dietz HC, Puerita RE, Hall BD, et al. The Marfan syndrome locus: confirmation of assignment to chromosome 15 and identification of tightly linked markers at 15q15-21.3. Genomics 1991;9:355–361

62. Litjens T, Baker EG, Backmann KR, et al. Chromosomal localization of ARSB, the gene for human N-acetylgalactosamine-4-sulphatase. Hum Genet 1989;82:67–68

63. Chen JD, Mackey D, Fuller H, et al. X-linked megalocornea: close linkage to DXS87 and DXS94. Hum Genet 1989;83:292–294

64. Spranger JW. Beta-galactosidase and the Morquio syndrome. Am J Med Genet 1977;1:207–209

65. Nakamura Y, Larsson C, Julier C, et al. Localization of the genetic defect in multiple endocrine neoplasia type 1 within a small region of chromosome 11. Am J Hum Genet 1989;44:751–755

66. Simpson NE, Kidd KK, Goodfellow PJ, et al. Assignment of multiple endocrine neoplasia type IIA to chromosome 10 by linkage. Nature 1987;328:528–530

67. Jackson CE, Nocum RA, O'Neal LW, et al. Linkage between MEN 2B and chromosome 10 markers linked to MEN 2A. Am J Hum Genet 1988;43:A147

68. Schwartz M, Haim M, Skarsholm D. X-linked myopia: Bornholm eye disease: linkage to DNA markers on the distal part of Xq. Clin Genet 1990;38:281–286

69. Brunner HG, Kornelur RG, Coerwinkel-Driessen M, et al. Myotonic dystrophy is closely linked to the gene for muscle type creatine kinase (CKMM). Hum Genet 1989;81:308–310

70. Lewis RA, Nussbaum RL, Stambolian D. Mapping X-linked ophthalmic diseases: IV. Provisional assignment of the locus for X-linked congenital cataracts and microcornea (the Nance-Horan syndrome) to Xp22.2-p22.3. Ophthalmology 1990; 97:110–121

71. Cawthon RM, Weiss R, Xu G, et al. A major segment of the neurofibromatosis type 1 gene; cDNA sequence, genomic structure, and point mutations. Cell 1990; 62:193–201

72. Rouleau GA, Seizinger BR, Wertelecki W, et al. Flanking markers bracket the neurofibromatosis type 2 (NF2) gene on chromosome 22. Am J Hum Genet 1990;46:323–328

73. Fryburg JS, Bale SH, McBride OW, et al. Linkage study of the nevoid basal cell carcinoma syndrome (NBCCS). Cytogenet Cell Genet 1989;51:997
74. Konrad R, Wilson D. Assignment of the gene for acid lysosomal sphingomyelinase to human chromosome 17. Cytogenet Cell Genet 1987;46:641
75. Schnur RE, Nussbaum RL, Anson-Cartwright L, et al. Linkage analysis in X-linked ocular albinism. Genomics 1991;9:605–613
76. Kivlin JD, Lovrien EW, Bishop DT, Maumenee IH. Linkage analysis in dominant optic atrophy. Am J Hum Genet 1983;35:1190–1195
77. Woo SLC, et al. Regional mapping of the human phenylalanine hydroxylase gene and PKU locus to 12q21 qter. Am J Hum Genet 1984;36:210
78. Farrar GJ, McWilliam P, Bradley DG, et al. Autosomal dominant retinitis pigmentosa: linkage to rhodopsin and evidence for genetic heterogeneity. Genomics 1990;8:35–40
79. Sparkes RS, Sparkes MC, Wilson MG, et al. Regional assignment of the genes for human esterase D and retinoblastoma to chromosome band 13q14. Science 1980;208:1042–1044
80. Alitalo T, Kruse TA, de la Chapelle A. Refined localization of the gene causing X-linked juvenile retinoschisis. Genomics 1991;9:505–510
81. Ligutic I, Brecevic L, Petkovic I, et al. Interstitial deletion 4q and Rieger syndrome. Clin Genet 1981;20:323–327
82. Fox MF, Du Toit DL, Warnich L, Retief AE. Regional localization of alpha-galactosidase (*GLA*) to Xpter-q22 hexosaminidase B (*HEXB*) to 5q31-qter, and arylsulfatase B (*ARSB*) to 5 pter-q13. Cytogenet Cell Genet 1984;38:45–49
83. Robertson DA, Callen DF, Baker JG, et al. Chromosomal localization of the gene for human glucosamine-6-sulphatase to 12q14. Hum Genet 1988;79:175–178
84. Knowlton RG, Weaver EJ, Struyk AF, et al. Genetic linkage analysis of hereditary athro-ophthalmopathy (Stickler syndrome) and the type II procollagen gene. Am J Hum Genet 1989;45:681–688
85. Nakai H, Byers MG, Shows TB. Mapping HEXA to 15q23-24. Cytogenet Cell Genet 1987;46:667
86. Nathans J, Piantanida TP, Eddy RL, et al. Molecular genetics of inherited variation in human color vision. Science 1986;232:203–210
87. Haines JL, et al. Linkage heterogeneity in tuberous sclerosis. Cytogenet Cell Genet 1989;51:1010
88. Fryer AE, Connor JM, Povey S, et al. Evidence that the gene for tuberous sclerosis is on chromosome 9. Lancet 1987;1:659–660
89. Kimberling WJ, Weston MD, Moller C, et al. Localization of Usher syndrome type II to chromosome 1q. Genomics 1990;7:245–249
90. Vance JM, Small K, Stajich H. Linkage studies in Von Hippel Lindau disease. Cytogenet Cell Genet 1989;51:1097
91. Asher JH Jr, Morell R, Friedman TB. Waardenburg syndrome (WS): the analysis of a single family with a WS1 mutation showing linkage to RFLP markers on human chromosome 2q. Am J Hum Genet 1991;48:43–52
92. Bonne-Tamir B, Farrer LA, Frydman M, Kanaaneh H. Evidence for linkage between Wilson disease and esterase D in three kindreds: detection of linkage for an autosomal recessive disorder by the family study methods. Genet Epidemiol 1986;3:201–209
93. Naritomi K, Hyakuna N, Suzuki Y, et al. Zellweger syndrome and microdeletion of the proximal long arm of chromosome 7. Hum Genet 1988;80:201–202
94. Knudson AG Jr. Mutation and cancer: statistical study of retinoblastoma. Proc Natl Acad Sci USA 1971;68:820–823
95. Brookstein R, Lee EYHP, To H, et al. Human retinoblastoma susceptibility gene: genomic organization and analysis of heterozygous intragenic deletion mutants. Proc Natl Acad Sci USA 1983;85:2210–2214

96. Friend SH, Bernards R, Rogelj S, et al. A human DNA segment with properties of the gene that predisposes to retinoblastoma and osteosarcoma. Nature 1986; 323:643–646

97. Fung YKT, Murphree AL, T'Ang A, et al. Structural evidence for the authenticity of the human retinoblastoma gene. Science 1987;236:1657–1661

98. Lee WH, Bookstein R, Hong F, et al. Human retinoblastoma susceptibility gene: cloning, identification, and sequence. Science 1987;235:1394–1399

99. Wiggs JL, Nordenskjold M, Yandell D, et al. Prediction of the risk of hereditary retinoblastoma, using DNA polymorphisms within the retinoblastoma gene. N Engl J Med 1988;318:151–157

100. Hong FD, Huang HJS, To H, et al. Structure of the human retinoblastoma gene. Proc Natl Acad Sci USA 1989;86:5502–5506

101. McGee TL, Yandell DW, Dryja TP. Structure and partial genomic sequence of the human retinoblastoma susceptibility gene. Gene 1989;80:119–128

102. DeCaprio JA, Ludlow JW, Figge J, et al. SV40 large T antigen forms a specific complex with the product of the retinoblastoma susceptibility gene. Cell 1988; 54:275–283

103. Horowitz JM, Yandell DW, Park SH, et al. Point mutational inactivation of the retinoblastoma antioncogene. Science 1989;243:937–940

104. Wiggs JL, Dryja TP. Predicting the risk of hereditary retinoblastoma. Am J Ophthalmol 1988;106:346–351

105. Yandell DW, Campbell TA, Dayton SH, et al. Oncogenic point mutations in the human retinoblastoma gene: their application to genetic counseling. N Engl J Med 1989;321:1689–1695

106. Yandell DW, Dryja TP. Direct genomic sequencing of alleles at the human retinoblastoma locus: application to cancer diagnosis and genetic counseling. In: Cancer Cells 7/Molecular Diagnostics of Human Cancer. Cold Spring Harbor, NY: Cold Spring Harbor Laboratory, 1989:223–227

107. Boughman JA, Conneally PM, Nance WE. Population genetic studies of retinitis pigmentosa. Am J Hum Genet 1980;32:223–235

108. McWilliam P, Farrar GJ, Kenna P, et al. Autosomal dominant retinitis pigmentosa (ADRP): localization of an ADRP gene to the long arm of chromosome 3. Genomics 1989;5:619–622

109. Dryja TP, McGee TL, Reichel E, et al. A point mutation of the rhodopsin gene in one form of retinitis pigmentosa. Nature 1990;343:364–366

110. Dryja TP, McGee TL, Hahn LB, et al. Mutations within the rhodopsin gene in patients with autosomal dominant retinitis pigmentosa. N Engl J Med 1990; 323:1302–1307

111. Dryja TP, Hahn LB, Cowley GS, et al. Mutation spectrum of the rhodopsin gene among patients with autosomal dominant retinitis pigmentosa. Proc Natl Acad Sci USA 1991;88:9370–9374

112. Rosenfeld PJ, et al. A *null* mutation in the rhodopsin gene causes rod photoreceptor dysfunction and autosomal recessive retinitis pigmentosa. Nature Genetics 1992;1:209–213

113. Kajiwara K, Hahn LB, Mukai S, et al. Mutations in the human retinal degeneration slow gene in autosomal dominant retinitis pigmentosa. Nature 1991;354: 480–483

114. Berson EL, Rosner B, Sandberg MA, Dryja TP. Ocular findings in patients with autosomal dominant retinitis pigmentosa and a rhodopsin gene defect (pro-23-his). Arch Ophthalmol 1991;109:92–101

115. Morris MA. Mitochondrial mutations in neuro-ophthalmological diseases: a review. J Clin Neuro-ophthalmol 1990;10:159–166

116. Lehninger AL. The mitochondrion. New York: WA Benjamin, 1964:7

117. Wallace DC, Zheng X, Lott MT, et al. Familial mitochondrial encephalomyopathy

(MERRF): genetic, pathophysiological, and biochemical characterization of a mitochondrial DNA disease. Cell 1988;55:601–610

118. Giles RE, Blanc H, Cann HM, Wallace DC. Maternal inheritance of human mitochondrial DNA. Proc Natl Acad Sci USA 1980;77:6715–6719

119. Linnane AW, Haslam JM, Lukins HB, Nagley P. The biogenesis of mitochondria in microorganisms. Annu Rev Microbiol 1972;26:163–198

120. Moraes CT, DiMauro S, Zeviani M, et al. Mitochondrial DNA deletions in progressive external ophthalmoplegia and Kearns-Sayre syndrome. N Engl J Med 1989; 320:1293–1299

121. Poulton J, Deadman ME, Gardiner RM. Tandem direct duplications of mitochondrial DNA in mitochondrial myopathy: analysis of nucleotide sequence and tissue distribution. Nucleic Acids Res 1989;17:10223–10229

122. Rutledge SL, Johns DR, Hurko O. Mitochondrial DNA analysis in a mitochondrial cytopathy overlap syndrome. Am J Hum Genet 1989;45:A216

123. Van Senus AHC. Leber's disease in the Netherlands. Doc Ophthalmol 1963; 17:1–162

124. Seedorff T. The inheritance of Leber's disease: a genealogical follow-up study. Acta Ophthalmol (Copenh) 1985;63:135–145

125. Holt IJ, Miller DH, Harding AE. Genetic heterogeneity and mitochondrial DNA heteroplasmy in Leber's hereditary optic neuropathy. J Med Genet 1989;26: 739–743

126. Hotta Y, Hoyakawa M, Saito K, et al. Diagnosis of Leber's optic neuropathy by means of polymerase chain reaction amplification. Am J Ophthalmol 1989; 108:601–602

127. Friedmann T. Progress toward human gene therapy. Science 1989;244:1275–1281

128. Musarella MA. Gene mapping of ocular diseases. Surv Ophthalmol 1992;36: 285–312

129. Jay B, Jay M. Molecular genetics in clinical ophthalmology. In: Davidson SI, Jany B, eds. Recent advances in ophthalmology, vol 8. New York: Churchill Livingstone, 1992:185–206

130. Petrash JM. Applications of molecular biological techniques to the understanding of visual system disorders. Am J Ophthalmol 1992;113:573–582

Genetic Influences on Differentiation, Mitosis, and Dystrophies of the Corneal Endothelium

Eric A. Sieck, M.D.

Nancy C. Joyce, Ph.D.

The corneal endothelium plays an important role in vision. Its barrier and pump functions are integral parts of a system that provides a clear yet strong window to the world. The maintenance of a clear cornea is a prerequisite for sharp visual acuity, which in lower animals is equivalent to survival and in humans is a major quality-of-life concern. Alterations in function of the corneal endothelium can cause loss of clarity. Many factors in corneal health and disease are genetically determined. Recent advances in our understanding of the corneal endothelium include (1) its differentiation into this unique tissue and then its transformation from a mitotically active cell line to the amitotic adult form, (2) recent evidence of a proliferative capacity and its manipulation, and (3) the hereditary pattern analysis of the endothelial dystrophies.

Background

Embryological Development of Corneal Endothelium

To understand the natural history of the corneal endothelium, it is important to understand its origin. Early theories posited that the corneal endothelium was derived from mesoderm. More recent studies show that mesoderm forms primary mesenchyme and plays an insignificant role in corneal differentiation. Migrating neural crest cells form secondary mesenchyme and become the corneal stroma, endothelium, and anterior chamber structures. The embryological source of the corneal endothelium in the chick embryo was shown by Johnston and colleagues [1] to be neural crest. Neural crest cells marked by [³H]thymidine or heterotopic transplantation (i.e., quail neural crest cells) were implanted in chicken embryos. Following these labels through differentiation proved that the origin of the corneal endothelium was neural crest (Table 1) [1].

This developmental model parallels other species, including humans. The neural crest cells arise from the summit of the neural folds and migrate anteriorly. They fill the rim of the optic cup and are positioned to develop into various ocular structures.

Additional studies by Hay [2] and Meier [3] have illustrated the developmental sequence. Starting at the sixth week, three waves of neural crest cells migrate centripetally from the optic rim. After the surface ectoderm separates from the lens vesicle, mesenchyme insinuates itself between the separating basement membranes of the corneal epithelium and lens. The first wave forms the corneal endothelium and trabecular meshwork. The second is anterior to the first and becomes the keratocytes, which synthesize the collagen of the corneal stroma. The third wave differentiates into the iris stroma.

Endothelial development continues during fetal life, evolving from a double layer to a monolayer of densely packed hexagonal cells. The endothelium produces a thick basement membrane, Descemet's membrane. This structure first appears at stage 35 in the chicken embryo and approximately the fourth month of gestation in the human embryo. The fetal corneal endothelium secretes a banded basement membrane. The anterior banded zone is approximately 2 to 4 μm thick and does not increase during life. At birth a putative terminal differentiation occurs. This is evident in the change to secretion of a nonbanded basement membrane and a dramatic decrease in cell density. The posterior nonbanded zone of Descemet's membrane is laid down throughout life. This is a record of

Table 1 *Neural Crest Migration*

Chick Embryo Stage	Migration
9	Markers implanted
10	Emigration from neural folds
12	Immigration to optic vesicle
14	Positioned at rim of optic cup
17	Insinuation between surface and lens ectoderm
22	Separation of basement membranes
26	Confluent layer on posterior corneal surface
28	Influx of primitive keratocytes

Source: Data from MC Johnston et al, Origins of avian ocular and periocular tissues. Exp Eye Res 1979;29:27–43.

endothelial differentiation and is altered in certain disorders. The growth of the corneal endothelium is not in proportion to the growth of the cornea. The number of cells per square millimeter greatly diminishes before birth. This phenomenon slows but continues throughout life.

The neural crest origin of the corneal endothelium differs from that of the vascular endothelium, which is derived from mesoderm. The pluripotential nature of neural crest cells explains the ability of the corneal endothelium, in some disease states, to assume the characteristics of other cell types. Normal endothelial cells contain gap and apical tight junctions and many mitochondria and secrete a thick basement membrane. In some disease conditions, this cell type is transformed into epitheliallike cells with desmosomal attachments, cytoplasmic keratin, and a thin basement membrane, or into fibroblastlike cells with cytoplasmic filaments and rough endoplasmic reticulum that secrete fibrillar collagens [4].

Classification of Developmental Disorders

Bahn and colleagues [5] have organized the observations of neural crest differentiation and clinical appearance in corneal endothelial disorders into five categories (Table 2). The first category relates to deficient neural crest formation and is exemplified by brain-eye-face malformations. The second set of conditions are the result of abnormal crest cell migration and include congenital glaucoma, anterior dysgenesis syndromes, and sclerocornea. In the third group, there is abnormal crest cell proliferation, which encompasses the spectrum of the iridocorneal endothelial (ICE) syndromes. The fourth set involves abnormal crest cell terminal differentiation and includes congenital hereditary endothelial dystrophy, posterior polymorphic dystrophy, and Fuchs' dystrophy. Finally, the fifth group comprises acquired abnormalities such as metaplasia, abiatrophy, and proliferation.

Table 2 *Classification of Corneal Endothelial Disorders*

Cell Abnormality	Disorder
Deficient neural crest formation	Brain-eye-face malformations
Abnormal crest cell migration	Congenital glaucoma; anterior dysgenesis syndromes; sclerocornea
Abnormal crest cell proliferation	Iridocorneal endothelial syndromes
Abnormal crest cell terminal differentiation	Congenital hereditary endothelial dystrophy; posterior polymorphic dystrophy; Fuchs' dystrophy
Acquired abnormalities	Metaplasia; abiatrophy; proliferation

Source: Adapted from CF Bahn et al, Classification of corneal endothelial disorders based on neural crest origin. Ophthalmology 1984;91:558–563.

Natural History

The infant corneal endothelium is a confluent monolayer of polygonal cells. The average cell density is 6,160/mm^2 [5]. In cross-section, the cells are cuboidal. They contain a central nucleus and the organelles necessary for active transport. Gap junctions characterize the intercellular complexes. This arrangement is optimal for the physiological functions of partial barrier and deturgescent pump.

Aging changes in the human corneal endothelium result in gradual cell loss, and these cells are not replaced. The cell density per square millimeter slowly decreases to 1,000 to 3,500 at age 50 and 900 to 2,000 at age 80. As cells are lost, the remaining cells increase in size and move to close empty areas, resulting in variations of cell size and shape (i.e., polymegathism and polymorphism). Cells are constantly rearranging and enlarging. The shapes formed obey the principle of minimizing cell surface tension [6]. There did not appear to be any component of cell division in replacing lost cells in the normal human [7]. The slow loss of cells is compensated for by a large functional reserve of eight to nine times the pumping capacity. It was suggested that this compensatory mechanism could allow normal humans to live several hundred years with clear corneas [8].

Corneal injury results in an acceleration of endothelial cell loss. Traditional explanations of human corneal wound healing have allowed only for migration and hypertrophy. Cats and primates also have limited mitotic responses, but other species utilize cell division as a predominant healing factor. In humans, migration and hypertrophy have limits. Cellular densities of 300 to 400 cells/mm^2 approach the threshold at which the monolayer loses its integrity, resulting in corneal edema. This is seen clinically after trauma or with a dystrophy. Cell loss from injury varies with the extent of insult. Estimates of cell loss after various surgical procedures range from 6% to 60%, depending on the technique and procedure. This obviously stresses a nonproliferative wound-healing system and can accelerate decompensation. Preexisting endothelial disorders will compound this problem. At present, the only technique to restore endothelial density and corneal clarity is to transplant a new population of corneal endothelial cells on the posterior surface of a clear, penetrating keratoplasty.

■ Advances in the Regulation of Mitosis

Wound Healing

The traditional teaching was that the human corneal endothelium was an end cell line, incapable of cell division. Early studies showed that wounded organ-culture cells healed by migration and elongation. No mitotic figures were seen [9]. The human corneal endothelium was believed to have poor regenerative capacity. Some authors advanced theories of a central cilium that connected the centrioles and thereby prevented mitotic activity. Many observers noted cell spreading and enlargement to compensate for cell injury. The presence of multinucleate cells was explained as resulting from amitotic nuclear division [10] or coalescence of neighboring cells [11]. Other researchers began to see the possibility of endothelial cell proliferation. Cultures were closely scrutinized and cellular activity carefully monitored.

Evidence in vitro and in vivo of cell division as a healing mechanism of corneal endothelium was well demonstrated by Treffers [12]. He studied 85 organ-cultured, wounded human corneas by silver stain, nuclear stain, and tritiated thymidine incorporation. Cell migration into the wounded area occurred within 48 hours. Mitotic figures were most numerous at 72 hours. Autoradiography demonstrated DNA synthesis with [^{3}H]thymidine. The ability to stimulate synthesis of DNA occurred despite donor age. An 86-year-old cornea with evidence of endothelial dystrophy was able to synthesize DNA. This study also included 2 in vitro wounds. Eyes scheduled for enucleation because of malignancy underwent a central corneal freeze injury. The corneas were retrieved at surgery and studied in the organ-culture system; both showed DNA synthesis and mitotic figures. A similar situation and technique was used on 5 corneas at the University of Oslo [13] with findings equivalent to those of Treffers [12]: There was DNA synthesis and mitosis.

Improvements in specular microscopy added more information about the role of mitosis in vivo. Laing and co-workers [14] reported the presence of mitotic figures after a graft rejection. The eye was followed with serial specular microscopical photographs for 8 months. The entire sequence was later reviewed and provided surprising evidence. Mitotic figures were seen early in the course. Later photographs showed an increased number of smaller cells. The increase in cell density and reduction in cell area were statistically significant and proved that mitosis had occurred in vivo in this situation.

Growth Factors

The explosion of information surrounding growth factors began when Cohen [15] isolated a low-molecular-weight protein from mouse salivary glands. This substance had a profound effect on the development of newborn mice, causing accelerated opening of the eyes and earlier eruption of the incisors. It became known as epidermal growth factor (EGF) [16], and its effect on other tissues was profound: It stimulated cell proliferation. Many other growth factors have since been identified, including fibroblast growth factor (FGF), mesodermal growth factor (MGF), transforming growth factor beta (TGF-β_1), platelet-derived growth factor

(PDGF), nerve growth factor (NGF), and insulinlike growth factor (IGF). These substances are often mitogenic. The normal physiological need for growth factors is not completely understood.

The stimulating effect of certain growth factors on corneal endothelial cells in culture is well documented for many species. An early and complete report by Gospodarowicz and associates [17] demonstrated increased proliferation of bovine corneal endothelial cells in vitro with several growth factors. Both FGF and EGF reduced the doubling time from 48 hours to 20 to 24 hours. Autoradiography was used with [³H]thymidine to prove an increase in DNA synthesis. This effect was also seen with serum used in culture media and led to the presumption that growth factors are present in serum.

Human corneal endothelium also responds to growth factor stimulation. Fabricant and colleagues [18] demonstrated the presence of EGF receptors on the human corneal endothelium. Nayak and Binder [19] cultured human corneal endothelium from corneoscleral rims with the aid of growth factors.

Organ-culture studies have also shown stimulatory effects of growth factors. Recombinant EGF was used in vitro in the serum-free organ culture of 87 human corneas [20]. After preliminary studies suggested the optimum time course, 25 corneas were cultured and then examined histologically. EGF resulted in a 50% increase in the number of mitotic figures. Cells were seen in all phases of division. Donor age ranged from 26 to 76 years. The most convincing evidence was presented when both corneas from the same donor were cultured, one with and one without EGF in the culture medium. The EGF resulted in a 50% increase of mitotic figures in *all* of these specimens.

Wilson and Lloyd [21] recently showed that cultured human corneal endothelial cells produce messenger RNA (mRNA) for EGF, EGF receptors, bFGF, TGF-β_1, and interleukin 1 (IL-1) alpha. The production of both EGF and EGF receptors in these cells suggests an autocrine role, though this relationship is not completely understood.

The pharmacological application of growth factors on the corneal endothelium is intriguing. A primate study involved injecting EGF into the anterior chamber at the time of penetrating keratoplasty [22]. Twelve animals underwent corneal autograft with denuding of the central endothelium at the time of surgery. Six of the monkeys were treated with EGF irrigation of the anterior chamber at the end of the procedure, and they received another intracameral injection of EGF 3 weeks later. At 10 weeks, the corneal buttons were removed for histological examination. The cell densities for untreated monkeys were 1,000 cells/mm^2 and, for EGF-treated monkeys, 1,200 cells/mm^2. Comparing the mean repopulation indexes, 20.5% in controls and 34.2% with EGF, a 67% greater repopulation occurred in the presence of EGF.

Senescence

The human corneal endothelium is not senescent during adult life. Senescence is a phenomenon seen in culture; it is characterized by morphological changes not seen in vivo. Techniques for mass cell culture of human endothelium have evolved from the first successful report. Baum and associates [23] successfully cultured human endothelium from donors younger than 20 years. Older donors and multiple passages exhibited slowed growth and morphological changes. The oldest culture in that study was six passages over approximately 15 months. Since that report in 1979, many technical advances have occurred. Growth factors have pushed long-term cultures to twenty generations [24]. All long-term cultures eventually become senescent. Senescence is characterized by morphological changes in which cells become enlarged and multinucleate and contain many vacuoles [25]. Cells actively growing in culture show a doubling time of 36 to 57 hours. After approximately thirty population doublings, the morphology changes, doubling time increases to 140 to 160 hours, and cell densities decrease [26].

The phenomenon of senescence is seen in other cell lines. It appears to be a genetically programmed process. In cell fusion experiments, senescent cells are fused either to proliferating cells of the same type [27] or to immortal cell lines [28]. The senescent cell is dominant and stops the active cell from growing. It has been suggested that there is an inhibiting factor in the cytoplasm of the senescent cells [29]. Microinjections of poly(A)-positive RNA from senescent cells inhibits rapidly dividing cells. Senescent vascular endothelial cells (that did not respond to exogenous growth factors) were shown to produce IL-1 alpha mRNA. When the antisense oligonucleotide complementary to the IL-1 alpha mRNA was added to the growth medium of presenescent cells, there was an extension of proliferation [30].

IL-1 alpha inhibits the proliferation of vascular endothelial cells. Conversely, it stimulates fibroblasts. Wilson and Lloyd [21] showed a decrease in EGF, TGF-β_1, and IL-1 alpha mRNA in senescent corneal endothelial cells. In this case, IL-1 alpha may be responsible for the limited mitotic response of adult human corneal endothelium [21]. This is an interesting explanation of the usual limited proliferative state of adult human corneal endothelium.

■ Hereditary Dystrophies of the Corneal Endothelium

Fuchs' Dystrophy

Fuchs' dystrophy, also known as *late hereditary endothelial dystrophy* and *adult-onset endothelial dystrophy*, is the most common of the endothelial dys-

Table 3 *Inherited Corneal Dystrophies*

Name	Inheritance Pattern	Age of Onset
Fuchs' dystrophy	Polygenic	Middle age
CHED	AD	First 1–2 years
CHED	AR	Congenital
PPD	AD	Congenital, early years

CHED = congenital hereditary endothelial dystrophy; PPD = posterior polymorphic dystrophy; AD = autosomal dominant; AR = autosomal recessive.

trophies. It was first described in 1910 by Ernst Fuchs [31]. His initial description was made without the aid of a biomicroscope. The condition he called *dystrophia epithelialis corneae* was characterized by epithelial edema, stromal clouding, and decreased corneal sensation. We now know that these observations are accurate and result from corneal endothelial dysfunction. The exact mechanism of failure or reason for cellular attrition is not known.

Symptoms of Fuchs' dystrophy typically begin in the fifth or sixth decade of life (Table 3). The condition is bilateral, although it can be very asymmetrical. Women are affected two and a half times more often than men. The condition involves loss of corneal endothelial pump and barrier functions, leading to corneal edema. It is a slowly progressive process, evolving over many years. Visual acuity worsens as the cornea becomes edematous. In later stages, bullous changes occur in the epithelium, often associated with pain. No effective medical therapy is available to reverse this process. Late stages may require surgical intervention to improve vision or alleviate pain.

Clinically, the dystrophy is characterized by guttae, excrescences on Descemet's membrane that give the endothelium a peau d'orange appearance. Guttae and pseudoguttae may be seen in various conditions. Confluent and bilateral guttae are diagnostic of Fuchs' dystrophy. They occur centrally and may become pigmented. Histologically, the guttae are discrete clumps of collagenous tissue on Descemet's membrane. They may protrude from or be buried in the membrane. By electron microscopy, the anterior banded zone is normal, the posterior nonbanded zone is thin, and a posterior collagenous layer may be present. The endothelium is markedly attenuated. The metabolic defect is not conclusively defined.

The hereditary pattern in Fuchs' dystrophy is complex. Some observers classified this entity as autosomal dominant. Pedigrees suggesting true mendelian autosomal dominant inheritance [32] and autosomal dominant mutation [33] have been reported. Careful evaluation of many families helped delineate some associations but did not fully describe the inheritance. In a study of 64 families comprising 228 relatives with endothelial dystrophy, Krachmer and co-workers [34] found that 38% of relatives older than 40 years had confluent guttae. Women were affected two and a half times more frequently and more severely than men, the frequency and severity increasing with age. There was no association between edema in the parent and in the offspring. There was a strong family tendency, 1 family having three generations affected and 16 families having two generations affected.

An additional statistical study of these families by Krachmer and colleagues [35] moved further toward an explanation. The mendelian autosomal dominant pattern cannot account for the gender difference. Sex-linked dominant conditions affect male subjects more severely, but Fuchs' dystrophy affects female individuals more frequently and severely. Possible explanations are that the disease affects women at an earlier age or with a higher penetrance, but Krachmer's data did not substantiate a difference in the age of onset or the penetrance between the sexes. Rigorous statistical analysis excludes a dominant inheritance pattern. Krachmer concluded that the significantly higher incidence in related persons implies that this is an inherited condition, of either polygenic inheritance or genetic heterogeneity, alone or in combination with an environmental factor [35].

Congenital Hereditary Endothelial Dystrophy

Congenital hereditary endothelial dystrophy (CHED) was first described by Maumenee in 1960 [36]. It is characterized by diffuse and symmetrical corneal edema, and it varies in severity from mild haze to opacification. Histologically, there is evidence of epithelial and stromal edema. Descemet's membrane is uniform with no guttae. The anterior banded zone is always present and of normal thickness. This represents normal endothelial differentiation to a point late in gestation. The posterior non-banded zone is thin and has a multilaminar appearance, suggesting the onset of the dystrophy at the putative terminal differentiation, shortly before birth. The endothelial cell layer is thin and atrophic. This condition exists in two forms, autosomal dominant and autosomal recessive, basically differentiated by the time of onset (see Table 3).

In the recessive form, corneal clouding, usually severe, is noted at birth or shortly thereafter. Nystagmus is frequently observed, but the infant is not photophobic. There is little or no progression over time [37]. The dominant form shows slow progression. The corneal clouding develops after 2 years of age or even later, there is wide variation in the severity of the opacity, and the patient is symptomatic, with photophobia and epiphora. Nystagmus is infrequently seen. A review of patients at Moorfields Eye Hospital in London identified 23 CHED patients from 1971 to 1986 [38]. Seventeen of the 23 were the recessive type. Fourteen of the recessive cases and only 1 of the dominant cases presented before 1 year of age. Harboyan and colleagues [39] described a pedigree of patients similar to recessive CHED and associated with sensorineural hearing loss. Other authors have pointed out the wide variation in clinical involvement [40].

Some affected relatives may have no symptoms and very subtle signs. It is prudent to examine all family members to counsel CHED patients accurately on the potential for affected offspring.

Posterior Polymorphic Dystrophy

Posterior polymorphic dystrophy (PPD) was first described by Leonhard Koeppe [41] in 1916. He originally called this condition *keratitis bullosa interna*. PPD is bilateral, but it can be very asymmetrical, often with overlooked signs in the less affected eye. Typically, there is little or no progression. Only rarely is there loss of visual acuity from corneal edema. The quantity and quality of the endothelial changes vary greatly. The polymorphic opacities can appear vesicular, as isolated lesions, or grouped into linear arrangements. Most cases are dominantly inherited (see Table 3) [42], though there may also be a recessive form of PPD [43].

Histologically, Descemet's membrane shows multilaminar thickening. Corresponding to the vesicular changes are nodules up to 20 μm in diameter. The endothelium is thinned [44]. On electron microscopy, the affected endothelium resembles epithelium [45]. The cells contain microvilli, vacuoles, keratofibrils, and desmosomes. Some cells assume a fibroblastic appearance.

■ References

1. Johnston MC, Noden DM, Hazelton RD, et al. Origins of avian ocular and periocular tissues. Exp Eye Res 1979;29:27–43
2. Hay ED. Development of the vertebrate cornea. Int Rev Cytol 1979;63:263–322
3. Meier S. The distribution of cranial neural crest cells during ocular morphogenesis. Prog Clin Biol Res 1982;82:1–15
4. Rodrigues MM, Waring GO, Laibson PR, et al. Endothelial alterations in congenital corneal dystrophies. Am J Ophthalmol 1975;80:678–689
5. Bahn CF, Falls HF, Varley GA, et al. Classification of corneal endothelial disorders based on neural crest origin. Ophthalmology 1984;91:558–563
6. Matsuda M, Suda T, Manabe R. Serial alterations in endothelial cell shape and pattern after intraocular surgery. Am J Ophthalmol 1984;98:313–319
7. Kaufman HE, Capella JA, Robbins JE. The human corneal endothelium. Am J Ophthalmol 1966;61:835–841
8. Mishima S. Clinical investigations on the corneal endothelium. Ophthalmology 1982;89:525–530
9. Doughman DJ, Van Horn D, Rodman WP, et al. Human corneal endothelial layer repair during organ culture. Arch Ophthalmol 1976;94:1791–1796
10. Renard G, Pouliquen Y, Hirsch M. Regeneration of the human corneal endothelium. Graefes Arch Clin Exp Ophthalmol 1981;215:341–348
11. Laing RA, Neubauer L, Leibowitz HM, Oak SS. Coalescence of endothelial cells in the traumatized cornea: II. Clinical observations. Arch Ophthalmol 1983;101:1712–1715
12. Treffers WF. Human corneal endothelial wound repair, in vitro and in vivo. Ophthalmology 1982;89:605–613

13. Olsen EG, Davanger M. The healing of human corneal endothelium: an in vitro study. Acta Ophthalmol (Copenh) 1984;62:885–892
14. Laing RA, Neubauer L, Oak SS, et al. Evidence for mitosis in the adult corneal endothelium. Ophthalmology 1984;91:1129–1134
15. Cohen S. Isolation of a mouse submaxillary gland protein accelerating incisor eruption and eyelid opening in the newborn animal. J Biol Chem 1962;237:1555–1562
16. Savage CR Jr, Cohen S. Epidermal growth factor and a new derivative: rapid isolation procedures and biological and chemical characterization. J Biol Chem 1972; 247:7609–7611
17. Gospodarowicz D, Mescher AL, Birdwell CR. Stimulation of corneal endothelial cell proliferations in vitro by fibroblast and epidermal growth factors. Exp Eye Res 1977;25:75–89
18. Fabricant RN, Alpar AJ, Centifanto YM, Kaufman HE. Epidermal growth factor receptors on corneal endothelium. Arch Ophthalmol 1981;99:305–308
19. Nayak SK, Binder PS. The growth of endothelium from human corneal rims in tissue culture. Invest Ophthalmol Vis Sci 1984;25:1213–1216
20. Couch JM, Cullen P, Casey TA, Fabre JW. Mitotic activity of corneal endothelial cells in organ culture with recombinant human epidermal growth factor. Ophthalmology 1987;94:1–6
21. Wilson SE, Lloyd SA. Epidermal growth factor and its receptor, basic fibroblast growth factor, transforming growth factor beta-1, and interleukin-1 alpha messenger RNA production in human corneal endothelial cells. Invest Ophthalmol Vis Sci 1991;32:2747–2756
22. Frabricant R, Salisbury JD, Berkowitz RA, Kaufman HE. Regenerative effects of epidermal growth factor after penetrating keratoplasty in primates. Arch Ophthalmol 1982;100:994–995
23. Baum JL, Niedra R, Davis C, Yue BYJT. Mass culture of human corneal endothelial cells. Arch Ophthalmol 1979;97:1136–1140
24. Engelmann K, Bohnke M, Friedl P. Isolation and long-term cultivation of human corneal endothelial cells. Invest Ophthalmol Vis Sci 1988;29:1656–1662
25. Yue BYJT, Sugar J, Gilboy JE, Elvart JL. Growth of human corneal endothelial cells in culture. Invest Ophthalmol Vis Sci 1989;30:248–253
26. Engelmann K, Bohnke M, Friedl P. Life span of human corneal endothelial cells in long-term cultures. Ophthalmic Res 1989;21:303–308
27. Norwood TH, Pendergrass WR, Sprague CA, Martin GM. Dominance of the senescent phenotype in the heterokaryons between replicative and post-replicative human fibroblast-like cells. Proc Natl Acad Sci USA 1974;71:2231–2235
28. Stein GH, Yanishevsky RM. Entry into S phase is inhibited in two immortal cell lines fused to senescent human diploid cells. Exp Cell Res 1979;120:155–165
29. Lumpkin CK Jr, McClung JK, Smith JR. Entry into S phase is inhibited in human fibroblasts by rat liver poly(A)+ RNA. Exp Cell Res 1985;160:544–549
30. Maier JAM, Voulalas P, Roeder D, Maciag T. Extension of the life-span of human endothelial cells by an interleukin-1 alpha antisense oligomer. Science 1990;249: 1570–1574
31. Fuchs E. Dystrophia epithelialis corneae. Albrecht von Graefes Arch Klin Exp Ophthalmol 1910;76:478–508
32. Magovern M, Beauchamp GR, McTigue JW, et al. Inheritance of Fuchs' combined dystrophy. Ophthalmology 1979;86:1897–1920
33. Cross HE, Maumenee AE, Cantolino SJ. Inheritance of Fuchs' endothelial dystrophy. Arch Ophthalmol 1971;85:268–272
34. Krachmer JH, Purcell JJ Jr, Young CW, Bucher KD. Corneal endothelial dystrophy: a study of 64 families. Arch Ophthalmol 1978;96:2036–2039
35. Krachmer JH, Bucher KD, Purcell JJ Jr, Young CW. Inheritance of endothelial dystrophy of the cornea. Ophthalmologica 1980;181:301–313

36. Maumenee AE. Congenital hereditary corneal dystrophy. Am J Ophthalmol 1960; 50:1114–1124
37. Judisch GF, Maumenee IH. Clinical differentiation of recessive congenital hereditary endothelial dystrophy and dominant hereditary endothelial dystrophy. Am J Ophthalmol 1978;85:606–612
38. Kirkness CM, McCartney A, Rice NSC, et al. Congenital hereditary corneal oedema of Maumenee: its clinical features, management, and pathology. Br J Ophthalmol 1987;71:130–144
39. Harboyan G, Mamo J, der Kaloustian V, Karam F. Congenital corneal dystrophy: progressive sensorineural deafness in a family. Arch Ophthalmol 1971;85:27–32
40. Levenson JE, Chandler JW, Kaufman HE. Affected asymptomatic relatives in congenital hereditary endothelial dystrophy. Am J Ophthalmol 1973;76:967–971
41. Koeppe L. Klinische Beobachtungen mit der Nernstspaltlampe und dem Hornhautmikroskop. Albrecht von Graefes Arch Klin Exp Ophthalmol 1916;91:363–379
42. Grayson M. The nature of hereditary deep polymorphous dystrophy of the cornea: its association with iris and anterior chamber dysgenesis. Trans Am Ophthalmol Soc 1974;72:516–559
43. Cibis GW, Krachmer JH, Phelps CD, Weingeist TA. The clinical spectrum of posterior polymorphous dystrophy. Arch Ophthalmol 1977;95:1529–1537
44. Morgan G, Patterson A. Pathology of posterior polymorphous degeneration of the cornea. Br J Ophthalmol 1967;51:433–437
45. Boruchoff SA, Kuwabara T. Electron microscopy of posterior polymorphous degeneration. Am J Ophthalmol 1971;72:879–887

Application of Genotypical Analysis in Orbital Lymphoid Disease

William L. White, M.D.
Judith A. Ferry, M.D.

Based on clinical information and light-microscopical analysis, the prediction of ultimate outcome for patients with orbital lymphoid tumors is difficult. In one large clinicopathological series, 60% of patients with an initial diagnosis of orbital malignant lymphoma developed systemic disease, but a 15% incidence of systemic disease was seen in those with orbital lymphoid tumors diagnosed as benign [1]. These data generally confirm the predictions of clinical behavior based on light-microscopical analysis, but the basic system left room for improvement.

Application of immunohistochemical techniques increased the ability to classify orbital lymphoid tumors by identifying specific cytoplasmic products or cell surface receptors. For instance, specific immunoglobulin heavy (G, M, A, etc.) and light (κ, λ) chains may be identified, along with other lymphocyte-associated antigens. Approximately 75% of histologically indeterminate tumors are found to be monotypic on immunophenotypical analysis and thus probably represent neoplasia rather than a reactive process [2, 3]. For a lesion to be identified reliably as monoclonal, however, these cells must constitute approximately 20% to 25% of the total lymphocytes present. Hence, reliable identification may be confounded, as small monoclonal proliferations could easily be missed and thus possibly lead to inappropriate treatment. Furthermore, the classification of these lesions as benign or malignant utilizing immunophenotypical analysis is not always helpful in predicting the occurrence of extraorbital disease [4].

Electron-microscopical analysis has also been shown to be an asset in indirectly identifying monoclonal proliferations and has enjoyed reason-

The opinions and assertions contained herein are the private views of the authors and are not to be construed as reflecting the views of the U.S. Department of the Army or Defense.

able success in predicting clinical outcome [5]. In one study with limited follow-up, none of the suspected benign lesions identified were associated with extraorbital disease, whereas 50% of the malignant cases were [5]. One primary limitation of this technique is the *indirect* nature of the analysis, which depends on careful scrutiny of cytological detail of the electron-microscopical preparations. The analysis is also somewhat subjective and the results may be difficult to reproduce.

These methods represented the best that were available to apply to patients with orbital lymphoid disease and, when employed together, they were capable of predicting clinical outcome with a moderate degree of accuracy. The application of molecular genetic techniques to the analysis of lymphoid tumors represented a significant opportunity to advance our understanding of these lesions.

■ Historical Perspective

Southern [6], in 1975, described a technique that allowed analysis of the structure of specific genes in eukaryotes, which was further elaborated by Watson and co-workers [7]. The major advance in Southern's work was the *direct* nature of the analysis, thus eliminating prior gene cloning in bacteria. Arnold and colleagues [8] subsequently described the application of this method to human lymphoid neoplasms as we currently utilize it.

■ Method

For investigating lymphoid tumors, the Southern blotting technique includes the following steps (see Figure):

1. Double-stranded DNA is extracted from lymphocyte suspensions by cell lysis.
2. Restriction endonucleases are then applied to the DNA to cleave it into several pieces. Restriction endonucleases reliably cut double-stranded DNA at a specific base pair sequence. The frequently used abbreviations for these enzymes identify their source. For instance, *Eco*RI is derived from *Escherichia coli*, and *Hind*III comes from *Hemophilus influenzae.*
3. The resultant fragments are electrophoresed on agarose gel slabs, which separates them based on their size and charge.
4. The fragments are then denatured, which breaks them into single-stranded pieces of DNA. This is necessary in order for the sequences to be recognized by the probes in step 6.
5. The single-stranded DNA fragments are transferred to nitrocellulose filter.

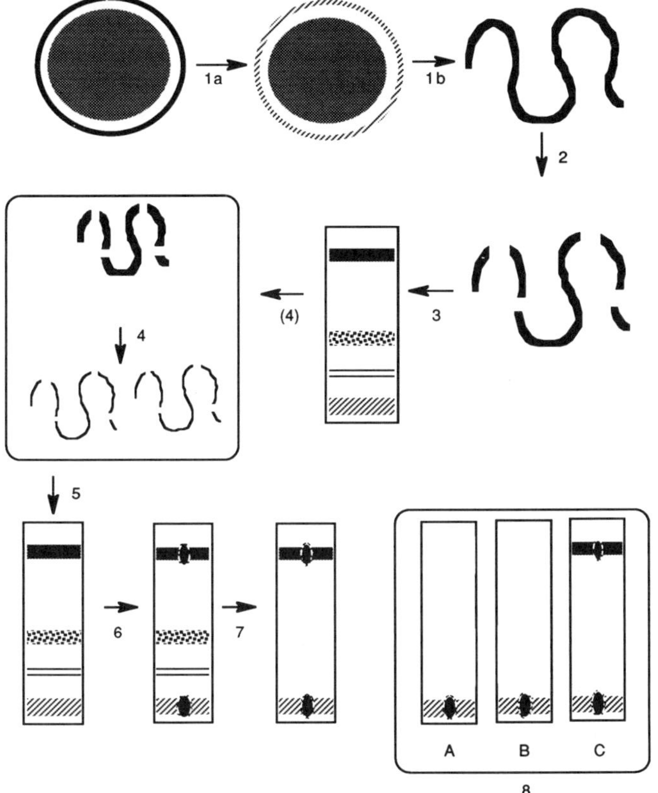

Steps in the Southern blot technique for lymphoid tumors (see text for details).

6. The fragments are then incubated with ^{32}P-labeled DNA probes, which are single-stranded nucleic acid segments that will hybridize (bind to) specific base sequences from the original specimen. Probes are used for regions known to encode for the κ or λ light chains, the immunoglobulin heavy-chain region, and the T-cell receptor β chain.

7. Autoradiography is utilized to identify the ^{32}P-labeled material. This yields a blot that varies in intensity depending on the amount of labeled material present in a given electrophoretic band.

8. Each assessment is performed side by side with a suspension of fibroblasts, which serve as a control. The fibroblasts (8A in figure) contain DNA with genes for immunoglobulin and the T-cell receptor β chain in the germ-line configuration. The electrophoretic location of the germ-line DNA containing the probed region is thus identified. In nonneoplastic lymphocyte populations, each cell will have rearranged its DNA in a different way, and the most frequently encountered fragment will again be a germ-line band (8B in figure). Monoclonal lymphocytes, however, have genetic material repetitively reorganized in the same way and electrophorese to a location different from the germ-line DNA (8C in figure). Thus, the non-germ-line, rearranged bands are identified.

The basis for the application of this technique to orbital lymphoid tumors is the identical rearrangement of DNA that occurs in a neoplastic process. From the finite number of nucleotide sequences present in a B-lymphocyte, it is estimated that 20 billion different antibody molecules may be produced. When enough cells have the same rearranged DNA sequences, that DNA segment can be recognized with this technique.

■ Early Investigational Results

Neri and co-authors [9] reported their experience in 1987 investigating ocular adnexal lymphoid tumors in 18 patients by light-microscopical, immunohistological, and molecular genetic analysis. In classifying the proliferations by using the first two methods, all but 5 of the lesions were found to express monotypic immunoglobulin and were diagnosed as B-cell lymphomas. Southern blot analysis confirmed that all of the malignant lymphomas were monoclonal proliferations, as non-germ-line bands were seen. Of the remaining 5 cases that were diagnosed as reactive lymphoid hyperplasias based on light microscopy and immunological analysis, 3 were found to contain non-germ-line bands on genotypical analysis and thus contained monoclonal proliferations of B cells.

Two patients had bilateral lymphoid lesions in the study by Neri and colleagues [9]. The molecular genetic "fingerprints" of each set of lesions showed that they were both derived from the same lymphocytic clone of cells.

Although the application of this technique should improve the ability to predict clinical outcome, its limitations in this specific disease process were also illuminated in Neri's report. One of the 2 patients with a polyclonal lesion on molecular genetic analysis developed a monoclonal proliferation in the contralateral orbit 43 months later. The authors proposed that many lesions interpreted as benign extranodal pseudolymphomas likely contain clonal populations of B cells. They also concluded that their observations lend support to the hypothesis that monoclonal B-cell lymphomas arise within so-called benign extranodal pseudolymphomas [9].

These investigators advised caution against concluding that clonality relates directly to clinically malignant behavior and cite the observation that nodal, small (well-differentiated) lymphocytic lymphomas routinely exhibit clonal rearrangements but are often clinically indolent and slowly progressive [9]. Molecular genetic analysis thus did not obviate the need for diligent light-microscopical and immunohistological techniques; it merely added a more sensitive method of identifying clonal populations. Neri's group [9] found the technique useful, accurate, and objective and recommended its use in lesions that are indeterminate by morphological and immunophenotypical analysis.

Probably the best-known paper in the ophthalmic literature concerning the molecular genetic analysis of lymphoid tumors was presented as the 1986 Wendell Hughes Lecture by Jakobiec [10], in which he described 5 patients with orbital lymphoid disease, only 2 of whom had lesions that were monotypic based on immunophenotypical analysis. All 5 patients had monoclonal populations of lymphocytes on molecular genetic analysis.

McNally and co-authors [11] reported their experience with 17 patients with bilateral ocular adnexal lymphoid neoplasms. Each pair of 3 simultaneous bilateral lesions in a given patient exhibited identical Southern blotting patterns. They examined 1 case each of benign follicular hyperplasia, intermediate lymphocytic lymphoma, and follicular and diffuse small cleaved-cell lymphoma. In the first case, the lesions contained germ-line DNA bilaterally, thereby enforcing the benign diagnosis. The latter 2 had identical rearrangement patterns bilaterally, indicating that in each patient the tumors were from the same progenitor B cell.

■ Insights from Nonocular Lymphoid Tumors

The discovery of benign clonal lymphoid proliferations provides support for the argument that not all lesions with clonal gene rearrangements will exhibit biologically malignant behavior [12]. Such clonal proliferations are seen in posttransplant immunosuppression, congenital immunodeficiency, acquired immunodeficiency syndrome, and angioimmunoblastic lymphadenopathy. A somewhat unusual situation exists with respect to immunosuppression after organ transplantation. B lymphocytes may become infected by the Epstein-Barr virus and, in some instances, proliferate in an uncontrolled manner. Genotypical analysis of such lesions may reveal the presence of clonal populations of B cells. The situation is further clouded in that some of these cases progress to frank malignant lymphoma, whereas in others the monoclonal population regresses after the immunosuppressive agents are withdrawn.

Another unique advantage of molecular genetic analysis of lymphoid lesions stems from the sensitivity of the technique: It allows both the detection of very small populations of neoplastic cells during staging and the detection of a very early relapse following therapy. Genotypical analysis can determine also whether a second lymphoid malignancy in a patient with a prior history of lymphoma is related to the original tumor. This is possible because the Southern blot of a monotypic lesion is, in essence, a fingerprint of the tumor. A recurrence will generally have rearranged bands in the same position as the original tumor.

The question has been asked whether 2 neoplasms with different clonal antigen receptor gene rearrangements appearing in a single patient are in fact unrelated. In the case of nonorbital B-cell lymphomas, the answer usually appears to be no. Because these cell populations undergo secondary restructuring by heavy-chain gene switching, DNA deletion, and point mutation, it is easy to visualize that this genetic restructuring would lead to restriction fragment size changes. In one study of patients with follicular B-cell lymphoma, 6 of 16 patients were found to have alteration in the immunoglobulin genes over the course of the disease [13]. However, there have been no reports of such studies for orbital lesions.

It has also been recognized that for some nonocular lymphomas, clinically and histologically malignant lymphomas may rarely have DNA still in the germ-line configuration [14]. No data are available on this issue as it relates to ocular proliferations, but the implications for nonocular disease are clearly that genotypical analysis cannot be used as the absolute standard in lymphoma diagnosis and must not be used in lieu of other more traditional methods of analysis.

■ Genotyping Versus Immunophenotyping

Two recent reports have contrasted genotyping and immunophenotyping of lymphoid neoplasms in general [15, 16]. The investigation by Sun and colleagues [15] included 51 specimens of varying sources including bone marrow, body fluids, and solid tissue samples. The two techniques yielded basically compatible information, with the exception of one B-cell lymphoma that was found to be clonal on molecular genetic analysis but not on phenotypical analysis. Sun's group [15] found that in vitro they could identify a monoclonal tumor population of 2% when mixed with 98% normal cells, but they believed that a 5% level was necessary to make the finding with confidence.

In these authors' institutions, immunophenotyping by flow cytometry takes approximately 2 days and *must* be done with fresh tissue to obtain reliable results, whereas genotypical analysis can be done on fresh or frozen samples but requires 14 days. The authors recommended that routine laboratory analysis (i.e., light microscopy, immunoperoxidase studies) be done on all lymphoid lesions, withholding genotypical studies for situations wherein there is ambiguity or a need to determine whether a lesion is a new primary tumor or a recurrence.

One of Sun's specimens had been frozen for 7 months before being analyzed genotypically, with satisfactory results being obtained [15]. Another specimen was stored inadvertently at 4°C for 4 months and also yielded satisfactory genotypical analysis results. These cases confirm the flexibility of the Southern blotting technique.

Wu and colleagues [16] examined 37 separate well-characterized lymphoid proliferations of various types. They modified previous techniques using fresh frozen cryostat sections and were able to complete the genotypical analysis in 6 to 8 days with no apparent loss of information or sacrifice in sensitivity. Although the technique remained relatively expensive and labor-intensive, the halving of the time for analysis represented an important improvement for cases where the clinical setting required prompt results. Nevertheless, these investigators likewise recommend that genotypical analysis of lymphoid lesions be withheld unless necessary to answer a specific diagnostic query. They cite labor intensiveness, cost of analysis, and the still relatively lengthy processing time as reasons for their recommended restriction.

■ Conclusion

Genotypical analysis of orbital lymphoid tumors can reliably identify the presence or absence of lymphocyte clones in a specimen. Currently, however, this sensitive examination process appears to be indicated only when a specific diagnostic question needs to be answered, such as in the instance of indeterminate lesions. The analysis can also be useful when trying to determine whether a tumor represents recurrence of disease or a second primary lesion [9, 15, 16]. It may be beneficial as well in examining small specimens, for which routine immunophenotypical analysis can be difficult. If genotypical analysis is required, it is appropriate to make arrangements with the pathologist prior to surgery to ensure proper tissue handling and transport.

■ References

1. Knowles DM II, Jakobiec FA. Orbital lymphoid neoplasms: a clinicopathologic study of 60 patients. Cancer 1980;46:576–589
2. Harris NL, Pilch BZ, Bhan AK, et al. Immunohistologic diagnosis of orbital lymphoid infiltrates. Am J Surg Pathol 1984;8:83–91
3. Medeiros LJ, Harris NL. Lymphoid infiltrates of the orbit and conjunctiva: a morphologic and immunophenotypic study of 99 cases. Am J Surg Pathol 1989; 13:459–471
4. Knowles DM, Jakobiec FA, McNally L, Burke JS. Lymphoid hyperplasia and malignant lymphoma occurring in the ocular adnexa (orbit, conjunctiva, and eyelids): a prospective multiparametric analysis of 108 cases during 1977 to 1987. Hum Pathol 1990;21:959–973
5. Jakobiec FA, Iwamoto T, Knowles DM II. Ocular adnexal lymphoid tumors: correlative ultrastructural and immunologic marker studies. Arch Ophthalmol 1982; 100:84–98

6. Southern EM. Detection of specific sequences among DNA fragments separated by gel electrophoresis. J Mol Biol 1975;98:503–517

7. Watson JD, Tooze J, Kurtz DT. Recombinant DNA: a short course. New York: Freeman, 1983:83–84

8. Arnold A, Cossman J, Bakhshi A, et al. Immunoglobulin-gene rearrangements as unique clonal markers in human lymphoid neoplasms. N Engl J Med 1983;309: 1593–1599

9. Neri A, Jakobiec FA, Pelicci PG, et al. Immunoglobulin and T-cell receptor β chain gene rearrangement analysis of ocular adnexal lymphoid neoplasms: clinical and biologic implications. Blood 1987;70:1519–1529

10. Jakobiec FA, Neri A, Knowles DM II. Genotypic monoclonality in immunophenotypically polyclonal orbital lymphoid tumors: a model of tumor progression in the lymphoid system. Ophthalmology 1987;94:980–994

11. McNally L, Jakobiec FA, Knowles DM II. Clinical, morphologic, immunophenotypic and molecular genetic analysis of bilateral ocular adnexal lymphoid neoplasms in 17 patients. Am J Ophthalmol 1987;103:555–568

12. Cossman J, Uppenkamp M, Sundeen J, et al. Molecular genetics and the diagnosis of lymphoma. Arch Pathol Lab Med 1988;112:117–127

13. Raffeld M, Wright JJ, Lipford E, et al. Clonal evolution of t(14;18) follicular lymphomas demonstrated by immunoglobulin genes and the 18q21 major breakpoint region. Cancer Res 1987;47:2537–2542

14. Kneba M, Bolz I, Bergholz M, et al. Clinical characteristics of high-grade lymphomas with immune genes in germline configuration. Cancer 1991;67:603–609

15. Sun T, Eisenberg A, Benn P, et al. Comparison of phenotyping and genotyping of lymphoid neoplasms. J Clin Lab Anal 1989;3:156–162

16. Wu AM, Winberg CD, Sheibani K, et al. Genotype and phenotype: a practical approach to the immunogenetic analysis of lymphoproliferative disorders. Hum Pathol 1990;21:1132–1141

Genetics of Retinoblastoma

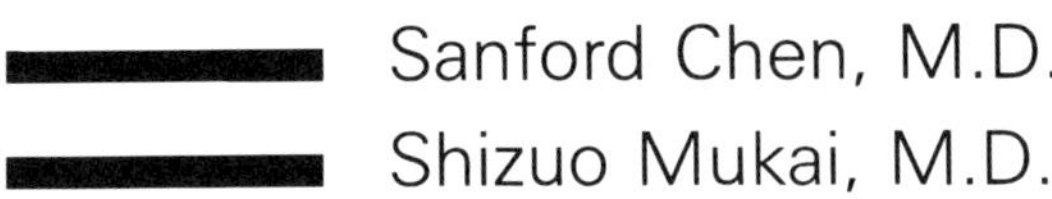

Sanford Chen, M.D.

Shizuo Mukai, M.D.

Retinoblastoma is a cancer of the retina first described in 1809 [1]. It is the most common primary intraocular malignancy in children and, after uveal melanoma, the second most common primary intraocular cancer in the general population. Left untreated, the disease is uniformly fatal. However, with early detection and currently available treatment modalities, the cure rate is well over 90% [2].

The incidence of retinoblastoma is reported to be between 1 in 15,000 and 1 in 34,000 live births [3, 4]. This number remains remarkably constant from study to study, suggesting a minor role of environmental influences in the pathogenesis of retinoblastoma. There are 200 to 300 new cases reported annually in the United States [3].

Fifty percent of all cases of retinoblastoma in the United States present with leukocoria, 20% present with strabismus, and 10% with signs suggestive of inflammation (i.e., red, painful eye). Atypical manifestations include heterochromia, hyphema, retinal detachment, proptosis, and glaucoma [5, 6]. On average, bilateral retinoblastoma is diagnosed at approximately 13 months of age and unilateral cases at 24 months of age. Almost 90% of all retinoblastoma cases are diagnosed before the child reaches the age of 5 years [7].

Recent advances in molecular genetics have led to the isolation of the gene that, when inactivated, leads to retinoblastoma formation [8–10]. This chapter will review the molecular genetics of the retinoblastoma gene and the diagnostic tests that have been developed as a result of these studies.

■ Heredity

In 60% to 70% of retinoblastoma patients, the disease is sporadic and not heritable (Fig 1). The remaining 30% to 40% of patients have heredi-

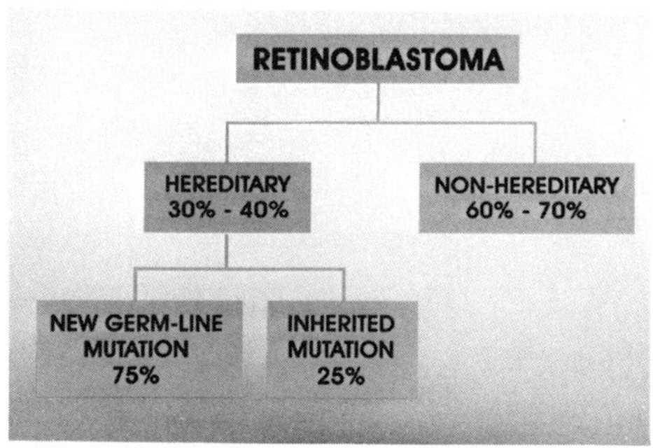

Figure 1 *Hereditary pattern of retino-blastoma.*

tary disease and can pass on the predisposition to retinoblastoma to their children in an autosomal dominant fashion (and, therefore, to one-half of the offspring) [4].

Of the patients with hereditary disease, 25% have a positive family history and have inherited from a carrier parent the mutation predisposing to retinoblastoma. The remaining 75% of hereditary cases are tumors caused either by new germ-line mutations that are heritable but not present in either parent or by inheritance from an asymptomatic carrier parent. Retinoblastoma does not develop in approximately 10% of individuals who carry the heritable mutation [4].

■ Retinoblastoma Gene

The gene in which inactivating mutations cause retinoblastoma was first identified and cloned in 1986 [8] and later confirmed in other laboratories [9, 10]; it is referred to as the *retinoblastoma gene*. The gene consists of 27 exons (coding sequence of gene) ranging in size from 31 base pairs to 1,873 base pairs. It is spread over a genomic locus of approximately 200 kilobases and is located on the q14 band of the human chromosome 13 (13q14) (Fig 2) [11]. The gene codes for a 4.7-kilobase messenger RNA (mRNA) transcript that represents 928 amino acids. It codes for a 105- to 114-kilodalton nuclear phosphoprotein with DNA-binding activity [12]. This gene product is present in all normal adult tissue. Although the precise physiological role of it is not known, the protein appears to be a member of a transcription factor complex and may regulate the expression of other genes important in progression through the cell cycle [13–15].

It appears that the absence of a functional retinoblastoma gene product leads to retinoblastoma tumorigenesis. For this to take place, both copies of the homologous retinoblastoma gene must be inactivated. This is the "two-hit" hypothesis of retinoblastoma formation.

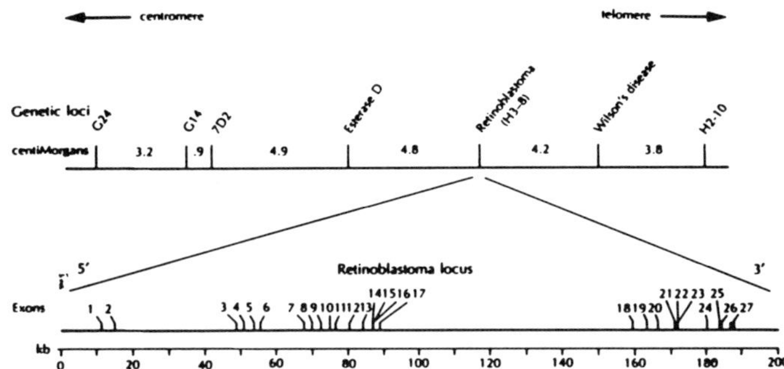

Figure 2 *Schematic map of the retinoblastoma gene and its neighbors. (Reprinted with permission from TP Dryja, Genetics of retinoblastoma. Curr Opin Pediatr 1989;1:413–420.)*

■ Knudson's Two-Hit Hypothesis

In 1971, Knudson [16, 17] postulated the two-hit theory of retinoblastoma tumorigenesis, based on statistical analysis of the clinical differences in hereditary versus nonhereditary retinoblastoma. He predicted that two genetic events are necessary for retinoblastoma to occur.

The mutation rate of the retinoblastoma gene is 10^{-7} per year. It has been calculated that the development of each human retina requires 10^8 cellular divisions. It is likely, then, that at least one cell in every human retina will have one of its retinoblastoma genes inactivated by a mutation during normal retinal development. This, however, is not sufficient to cause retinoblastoma since the homologous retinoblastoma gene is usually normal. If, on the other hand, the individual carries a mutation that has already inactivated one copy of the retinoblastoma gene, the inactivation of the homologous gene will result in tumor formation. In hereditary retinoblastoma, each retinal precursor cell has already inherited a mutation inactivating one retinoblastoma gene (Fig 3). The high probability of the second mutation inactivating the remaining normal retinoblastoma gene causes bilateral and multifocal disease in the hereditary cases [18]. In contrast, somatic retinoblastoma results from sequential somatic inactivation of both genes in a single retinal cell in a patient who has inherited both normal genes (see Fig 3). Because the probability of this happening in more than one cell is exceedingly rare, these cases are always unilateral [18].

■ Genetic Counseling

The key to genetic counseling in retinoblastoma is identification of those individuals that carry the heritable germ-line first mutation that has

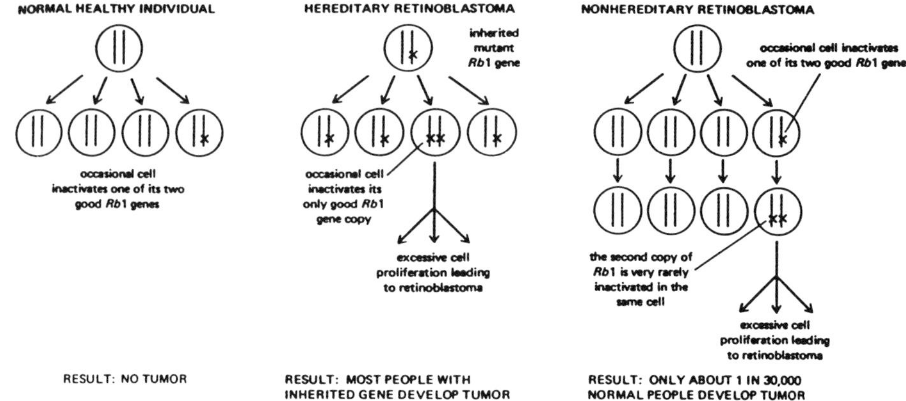

Figure 3 *The Knudson two-hit hypothesis. (Reprinted with permission from B Alberts et al, Molecular biology of the cell, ed 2. New York: Garland Publishing, 1989:1213.)*

already inactivated one copy of the retinoblastoma gene in all of their cells. Such an individual has approximately a 90% chance of developing retinoblastoma and a 50% chance of passing the predisposition to his or her children. We will review some of the ingenious ways currently being used to detect the tumor-predisposing mutations.

The distinction between hereditary and nonhereditary retinoblastoma is a critical issue in genetic counseling. Clinical features of patients with retinoblastoma can often be used to identify patients with hereditary disease (Fig 4). For example, all bilateral or multifocal cases carry heritable mutations. Likewise, all unifocal cases with a positive family history of retinoblastoma or a second malignancy associated with retinoblastoma (i.e., osteosarcoma) carry heritable mutations. Of the unilateral or unifocal cases with negative family history, 85% to 95% are nonhereditary. The remainder (5%–15%) are the result of germ-line mutations and are therefore hereditary [4].

Karyotyping

Cytogenetic analysis using high-resolution chromosome banding techniques is able to detect only a small proportion (3%–5%) of microscopically visible deletions of one chromosome 13 homologue in the patient's constitutional cells [19]. Human chromosome 13 contains approximately 100 million base pairs of DNA. To detect a visible deletion, 2 million to 5 million base pairs must be missing or, in other words, approximately 2% to 5% of the entire chromosome 13.

As stated before, the retinoblastoma gene is spread over a genomic locus of approximately 200,000 base pairs or nearly one-tenth of the DNA necessary for a microscopically visible chromosomal deletion. This is the reason so few patients with retinoblastoma can be identified by karyotyp-

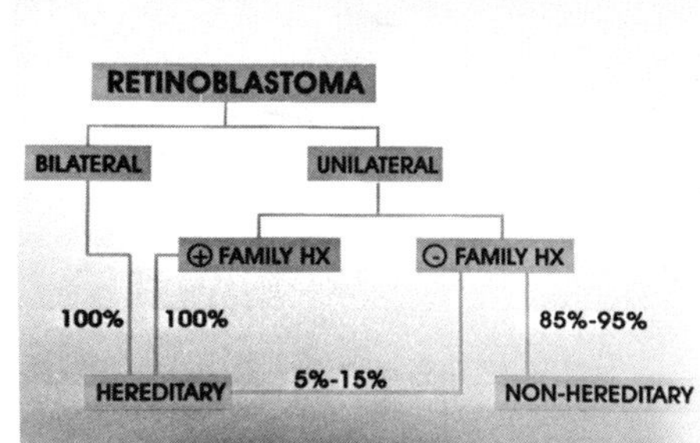

Figure 4 *Clinical characteristics of retinoblastoma.*

ing. In practice, this technique is limited to the study of lesions that create gross structural changes in the chromosome, including larger deletions and chromosomal rearrangements.

Esterase D

Esterase D is an enzymatic polymorphism originally described by Hopkinson and colleagues [20] in 1973. The esterase D locus was assigned to chromosome 13 [21] and linked to the retinoblastoma locus [22]. There are two common alleles of esterase D and 19 rarer alleles. These alleles are codominant, and each allele contributes one-half of the total enzyme activity.

Squire and co-workers [23] successfully identified and cloned the esterase D gene in 1986. This gene is expressed in virtually all cells and codes for mRNA of 1.2 kilobases. It lies approximately 5 million base pairs proximal to the retinoblastoma gene on 13q14 [24]. Linkage with the retinoblastoma gene is very tight (5 centimorgans).

Esterase D can be used as a marker for retinoblastoma mutation in either of two ways. The measurement of decreased enzymatic activity or detection of loss of alleles at the genetic level indicates a deletion involving the esterase D locus. Since the retinoblastoma locus is in close proximity to the esterase D locus, there is high likelihood that such deletions involve the retinoblastoma locus [22, 25, 26]. Sparkes and associates [22] studied several patients with retinoblastoma and karyotypically detectable deletions of the long arm of chromosome 13. They found that, in addition to the chromosomal deletion, there was a 50% decrease in esterase D activity. This test may be more sensitive than cytogenetic analysis in detecting mutations, but the deletion would still have to be at least 5 million base pairs in size, the estimated distance between the esterase D and retinoblastoma loci.

In cases of familial retinoblastoma, the polymorphisms of esterase D can be used as a linked genetic marker informative for esterase D [23, 27, 28]. Since the esterase D locus is located close to the retinoblastoma locus on chromosome 13, an allele of esterase D is usually inherited with the same allele of the retinoblastoma gene in a given kindred. In this way, the esterase D allele can be used as a genetic marker for the disease in such a family.

Southern Blot Analysis

Cloning of the retinoblastoma gene made available DNA probes from within the retinoblastoma gene and opened the door for new approaches to molecular genetic diagnosis of retinoblastoma. Southern blotting is one such technique and can be used to determine the difference in the number of copies or the size of the gene [29].

Genomic DNA is isolated and digested with restriction enzymes to create multiple DNA fragments. These restriction fragments are then separated by agarose gel electrophoresis. Following this, they are denatured, and the resulting single-stranded DNA fragments are transferred to a nitrocellulose or a nylon filter. The filter is then hybridized with a radiolabeled cDNA probe, and the position of the complementary nucleic acid fragment is detected by autoradiography. This analysis can detect deletions in the range of a few hundred base pairs, in contrast to karyotyping, which detects deletions of a few million base pairs. Unfortunately, deletions and rearrangements detectable by Southern blot analysis still constitute only approximately 20% of the mutations causing a predisposition to retinoblastoma [30, 31].

DNA Sequence Polymorphisms

The human genome contains naturally occurring variations in the DNA sequence; these variations can be used as genetic markers similar to esterase D. Restriction enzymes recognize specific sequences of DNA and cut at that site. When genomic DNA is cut with restriction enzymes, a variation in the DNA sequence can produce a variation in the sizes of fragments generated. DNA probes that recognize DNA at or near the site of the fragment variation can reveal restriction fragment length polymorphisms (RFLPs) [32]. These markers can be extremely valuable in following the inheritance of the allele carrying the disease-producing mutation in a given family with retinoblastoma.

Another type of DNA polymorphism is due to variation in the number of tandem repeats of a short DNA sequence (VNTRs) [33]. Many cases of VNTRs can be detected by Southern blot analysis. The length of the restriction fragment detected by the probe homologous to the repeated DNA sequence is a function of the number of copies of the tandem repeats present within the fragment. Other VNTRs can be detected by primer-directed amplification of the repeated sequence by polymerase chain reaction (PCR) [34, 35]. VNTRs produce a wide variety of repeated sequences and therefore are highly polymorphic. There are at least seven known

DNA sequence polymorphisms (two of these result from VNTRs) within the retinoblastoma gene [30, 34, 36].

For linkage analysis using RFLP and VNTR markers to be informative in a given family requires that two or more family members be affected and also that parents be heterozygous at the linked-marker locus. This allows one to mark the disease allele with a specific marker allele in a given kindred. Since the initial mutation leading to tumor formation is different in each family, separate genetic analysis must be performed for each pedigree. Linkage analysis using DNA polymorphism is therefore very helpful in indirectly identifying unaffected family members who carry or do not carry the disease-predisposing mutation. Using markers from within the retinoblastoma gene, linkage analysis is useful in approximately 95% of the retinoblastoma families and has an accuracy exceeding 95% [31].

Polymerase Chain Reaction, Single-Strand Conformation Polymorphism Analysis, and DNA Sequence Analysis

Approximately 80% of the retinoblastoma-causing mutations are too small to be detected by the methods just described. Most tumor-predisposing mutations result from small DNA abnormalities that ultimately require DNA sequence analysis for detection. The current strategy for detecting these mutations involves screening the retinoblastoma gene exon by exon, using exon-specific PCR amplification [35]. This method allows one to obtain multiple copies of desired DNA sequences rapidly. The next step is screening for mutations within the amplified fragments by using the single-strand conformation polymorphism (SSCP) analysis [37, 38]. This is a sensitive technique that detects more than 90% of the mutations, including point mutations. Finally, after the exon with the abnormal SSCP band is localized, direct DNA sequence analysis is used to identify exactly the mutation in the DNA sequence. This technique allows the identification of mutations as small as a single base pair change in the retinoblastoma gene [39].

■ Conclusion

Retinoblastoma is a devastating intraocular malignancy mostly involving children younger than 5 years. Hereditary cases are estimated to occur approximately 40% of the time. It is important to the individual and the family to determine whether they are at risk for developing retinoblastoma. With currently available molecular genetic diagnostic techniques, we are able to predict in many families with retinoblastoma, with a high degree of certainty, which individuals are at increased risk. Future work will be directed toward increasing the sensitivity and the accuracy of this prediction.

■ References

1. Virchow R. Die Krankhaften Geschwultste, vol 2. Berlin: August Hirschwald, 1864:15
2. Devesa SS. The incidence of retinoblastoma. Am J Ophthalmol 1975;80:263–265
3. Pendergrass TW, Davis S. Incidence of retinoblastoma in the United States. Arch Ophthalmol 1980;98:1204–1210
4. Vogel F. Genetics of retinoblastoma. Hum Genet 1979;52:1–54
5. Shields JA, Augsburger JJ. Current approaches to the diagnosis and management of retinoblastoma. Surv Ophthalmol 1981;25:347–372
6. Binder PS. Unusual manifestations of retinoblastoma. Am J Ophthalmol 1974; 77:674–679
7. Rubenfeld M, Abramson DH, Ellsworth RM, Kitchin FD. Unilateral vs. bilateral retinoblastoma: correlations between age at diagnosis and stage of ocular disease. Ophthalmology 1986;93:1016–1019
8. Friend SH, Bernards R, Rogelj S, et al. A human DNA segment with properties of the gene that predisposes to retinoblastoma and osteosarcoma. Nature 1986;323: 643–646
9. Lee WH, Bookstein R, Hong F, et al. Human retinoblastoma susceptibility gene: cloning, identification, and sequence. Science 1987;235:1394–1399
10. Fung YKT, Murphree AL, T'Ang A, et al. Structural evidence for the authenticity of the human retinoblastoma gene. Science 1987;236:1657–1661
11. Dryja TP. Genetics of retinoblastoma. Curr Opin Pediatr 1989;1:413–420
12. Lee WH, Shew JY, Hong FD, et al. The retinoblastoma susceptibility gene encodes a nuclear phosphoprotein associated with DNA binding activity. Nature 1987; 329:642–645
13. DeCaprio JA, Ludlow JW, Lynch D, et al. The product of the retinoblastoma susceptibility gene has properties of a cell cycle regulatory element. Cell 1989;58: 1085–1095
14. Buchkovich K, Duffy LA, Harlow E. The retinoblastoma protein is phosphorylated during specific phases of the cell cycle. Cell 1989;58:1097–1105
15. Chen PL, Scully P, Shew JY, et al. Phosphorylation of the retinoblastoma gene product is modulated during the cell cycle and cellular differentiation. Cell 1989;58:1193–1198
16. Hethcote HW, Knudson AG Jr. Model for the incidence of embryonal cancers: application to retinoblastoma. Proc Natl Acad Sci USA 1978;75:2453–2457
17. Knudson AG Jr. Mutation and cancer: statistical study of retinoblastoma. Proc Natl Acad Sci USA 1971;68:820–823
18. Alberts B, Bray D, Lewis J, et al. Molecular biology of the cell, ed 2. New York: Garland Publishing, 1989:1213
19. Ejima Y, Sasaki MS, Kaneko A, Tanooka H. Types, rates, origin and expressivity of chromosome mutations involving 13q14 in retinoblastoma patients. Hum Genet 1988;79:118–123
20. Hopkinson DA, Mestriner MA, Cortner J, et al. Esterase D. A new human polymorphism. Ann Hum Genet 1973;37:119
21. Sparkes RS, Sparkes MC, Wilson MG, et al. Regional assignment of genes for human esterase D and retinoblastoma to chromosome band 13q14. Science 1980;208: 1042–1044

22. Sparkes RS, Murphree AL, Lingua RW, et al. Gene for hereditary retinoblastoma assigned to human chromosome 13 by linkage to esterase D. Science 1983; 219:971–973

23. Squire J, Dryja TP, Dunn J, et al. Cloning of the esterase D gene: a polymorphic gene probe closely linked to the retinoblastoma locus on chromosome 13. Proc Natl Acad Sci USA 1986;83:6573–6577

24. Mitchell CD, Cowell JK. Molecular evidence that the esterase-D gene lies proximal to the retinoblastoma susceptibility locus in chromosome region 13q14. Hum Genet 1988;81:57–60

25. Schmickel RD. Chromosomal deletions and enzyme deficiencies. J Pediatr 1986; 108:244–246

26. Cowell JK, Thompson E, Rutland P. The need to screen all retinoblastoma patients for esterase D activity: detection of submicroscopic chromosome deletions. Arch Dis Child 1987;62:8–11

27. Mukai S, Rapaport JM, Shields JA, et al. Linkage of genes for human esterase D and hereditary retinoblastoma. Am J Ophthalmol 1984;97:681–685

28. Halloran SL, Boughman JA, Dryja TP, et al. Accuracy of detection of the retinoblastoma gene by esterase D linkage. Arch Ophthalmol 1985;103:1329–1331

29. Southern EM. Detection of specific sequences among DNA fragments separated by gel electrophoresis. J Mol Biol 1975;98:503–517

30. Wiggs J, Nordenskjold M, Yandell D, et al. Prediction of the risk of hereditary retinoblastoma, using DNA polymorphisms within the retinoblastoma gene. N Engl J Med 1988;318:151–157

31. Wiggs JL, Dryja TP. Predicting the risk of hereditary retinoblastoma. Am J Ophthalmol 1988;106:346–351

32. Botstein D, White RL, Skolnick M, Davies RW. Construction of a genetic linkage map in man using restriction fragment length polymorphisms. Am J Hum Genet 1980;32:314–331

33. Nakamura Y, Leppert M, O'Connell P, et al. Variable number of tandem repeat (VNTR) markers for human gene mapping. Science 1987;235:1616–1622

34. Yandell DW, Dryja TP. Detection of DNA sequence polymorphisms by enzymatic amplification and direct genomic sequencing. Am J Hum Genet 1989;45:547–555

35. Saiki RK, Gelfand DH, Stoffel S, et al. Primer-directed enzymatic amplification of DNA with a thermostable DNA polymerase. Science 1988;239:487–491

36. Bookstein R, Lee EYH, To H, et al. Human retinoblastoma susceptibility gene: genomic organization and analysis of heterozygous intragenic deletion mutants. Proc Natl Acad Sci USA 1988;85:2210–2214

37. Orita M, Iwahana H, Kanazawa H, et al. Detection of polymorphisms of human DNA by gel electrophoresis as single-strand conformation polymorphisms. Proc Natl Acad Sci USA 1989;86:2766–2770

38. Orita M, Suzuki Y, Sekiya T, Hayashi K. Rapid and sensitive detection of point mutations and DNA polymorphisms using the polymerase-chain-reaction. Genomics 1989;5:874–879

39. Yandell DW, Campbell TA, Dayton SH, et al. Oncogenic point mutations in the human retinoblastoma gene: their application to genetic counseling. N Engl J Med 1989;321:1689–1695

Uveal Melanoma

M. Ronan Conlon, M.B., B.Ch.
Daniel M. Albert, M.D.

Uveal melanoma is the most common intraocular malignancy in adults. It is estimated that approximately 1,200 to 1,500 new cases are diagnosed each year in the United States [1]. Ocular melanoma comprises 79% of the noncutaneous melanomas, but its annual age-adjusted incidence of 0.6 per 100,000 population is only one-twentieth the rate of cutaneous melanoma [2, 3]. In contrast to skin melanomas, the incidence of which has doubled since 1980 in the United States (currently 12.5 per 100,000), the incidence of uveal melanoma has not increased significantly over the last 10 years [3]. It most commonly occurs in whites older than 50 years and rarely is seen in dark-skinned populations.

Despite an increased knowledge about the pathological, histochemical, and immunogenic properties of uveal melanoma, there has been no substantial increase in the survival rate. This has created a need to identify possible risk factors or markers that might be helpful in developing strategies to reduce the morbidity and mortality from this condition. To date, sunlight, environmental toxins, viruses, and preexisting nevi have been postulated as possible predisposing factors, but no one agent has emerged as the primary cause.

A resurgence of interest has developed in identifying recurring chromosomal abnormalities in tumors, as molecular examination of these abnormalities has led to the localization of growth-regulatory sequences (oncogenes) responsible for tumorigenesis. Recognition of specific chromosomal changes in cutaneous melanoma has heightened the interest in identifying such changes in uveal melanoma [4–9]. It is now known that genetic mutations are the initiating event in a variety of tumors, followed by a series of events leading to tumor growth, heterogeneity and, eventually, metastasis. The identification of these aberrant genes has allowed for the experimental manipulation of the genes through DNA recombinant technology in an effort to reverse the cancerous process [10].

The clearest evidence of a genetic component in the pathogenesis of uveal melanoma is its predominance in whites, its rare occurrence in dark-skinned individuals, and its virtual exclusion in blacks. A clearer understanding of the genetic factors involved will be important not only for identifying the cause of this tumor but also to gain further insight into its heterogeneity, progression, and spread.

■ Kindred Studies of Uveal Melanoma

The possibility of a heritable form of uveal melanoma was first proposed by Silcock in 1892 when he described the development of uveal melanoma in 3 successive generations [11]. Since then there have been numerous reports of familial uveal melanoma [11–23]. Although these reports represent a small fraction of the total number of melanoma patients, the clear line of transmission in these families strongly suggests a subset of uveal melanoma patients in which heredity plays an important role (Table).

The presence of uveal melanoma can be documented in the majority of affected families through 2 or more generations. In 7 families, 2 generations were affected, and in 2 families, 3 generations were affected. Parsons [12] and then Davenport [13] reported the development of uveal melanomas in additional members of the family initially reported by Silcock, increasing the total in that family to 7 members over 4 generations who had an eye enucleated; the eyes of 5 members had histologically proved uveal melanoma. Walker and co-workers [21] reported a family in which melanoma developed in 3 generations. In 4 families, melanoma was in a sibling [15, 18, 22, 23].

In the pedigrees described to date, there has been no clear consensus in the literature regarding the mode of transmission. The development of tumors in successive generations and the absence of a history of consanguinity have led some authors [11, 18] to speculate on an autosomal dominant mode of transmission. However, in a number of the families it has not been possible to confirm transmission through successive generations. Possible obscuring factors to the emergence of a clear mode of transmission include incomplete penetrance, delayed onset of symptoms, and incomplete family histories. Based on current knowledge, it would be reasonable to say an autosomal dominant transmission with incomplete penetrance is probable, but further cases are required before this can be confirmed.

The average age of patients in whom familial tumors were diagnosed was 42 years, compared to an average age of more than 50 years in larger series of nonfamilial tumors; the age difference is statistically significant [23]. The diagnosis of uveal melanoma in someone younger than 30 years is extremely uncommon, yet of 30 patients reported with familial melanoma, 5 were not yet 30 years old. Lynch and associates [18] noted that

Details from Case Reports of Familial Uveal Melanoma

Reference	Case/Relation	Gender	Year	Age (yr)	Eye	Outcome
Davenport [13]	Proband	F	1871	33	L	Died after 7 months
Silcock [11]	Daughter	F	1899	19	L	Died after 5 years
Parsons [12]	Daughter	F	1904	38	L	Died after 1 year
	Granddaughter	F	1918	29	L	Died after 4 years
	Granddaughter	F	1914	19	?	Alive after 10 years
Gutmann [14]	Proband	F	1891	32	R	Alive after 4 years
	Brother	M	?	?	R	Died 1899
Pfingst [15]	Proband	M	?	44	L	Alive at 3 years
	Brother	M	1921	47	L	Alive
Waardenberg [16]	Proband	F	1925	19	L	Died of metastases
	Uncle	M	1940	?	R	No follow-up
Bowen [17]	Proband	F	1953	45	L	Died at 1 year
	Daughter	F	1963	26	L	Alive at 6 months
Lynch [18]	Proband	M	1964	59	R	Died at 2 years
	Sister	F	1963	56	R	Alive at 3 years
	Proband	F	1962	33	L	Died at 1 year
	Uncle	M	?	?	R	Died at 57 years
Tasman [19]	Proband	F	?	58	R	No follow-up
	Daughter	F	1967	38	R	No follow-up
Green [20]	Proband	M	1976	50	L	No follow-up
	Father	M	1926	46	R	Died at 7 years
Walker [21]	Proband	M	1976	46	L	Alive at 3 years
	Father	M	1926	67	L	Died at 7 years
	Grandmother	F	?	44	?	No follow-up
Simons [22]	Proband	M	1974	?	?	Alive at 5 years
	Sister	F	1981	50	L	Alive at 2 years
Canning [23]	Proband	F	1986	63	L	Alive at 6 months
	Brother	M	1986	67	L	Alive at 4 months
	Proband	F	1962	33	L	Alive at 20 months
	Son	M	1976	20	L	Alive at 45 years

Source: Adapted from CR Canning and J Hungerford, Familial uveal melanoma. Br J Ophthalmol 1988;72:241.

this finding is consistent with the tendency for hereditary neoplasms to occur at a younger age than their histological somatic counterpart. The development of uveal melanoma at an earlier age in this group of patients is further evidence that they represent a distinctive subset of melanoma patients.

The higher-than-expected occurrence of other primary neoplasms in family members of patients with familial melanoma is noteworthy. In the family reported by Green and colleagues [20], 3 siblings died of other primary malignancies. One brother died of primary hepatic carcinoma, another brother of metastatic lung cancer from an undetermined primary, and a sister in her forties of a poorly differentiated carcinoma of undetermined origin. In cutaneous melanoma, in which a hereditable pattern is well established, investigators have found a higher-than-expected incidence of other primary malignancies in first-degree relatives [24]. The similar finding of a higher-than-expected incidence of other primary malignancies in relatives of patients with these two malignancies further supports the role of heredity in this group of ocular melanomas.

Those skeptical of the role of heredity in uveal melanoma would attribute the occurrence of cases in family members to chance alone. The statistical chance of this tumor arising independently in 2 family members is extremely low. The chance of the tumor arising in 3 successive generations is even lower: Walker and colleagues [21] estimate the probability to be 1 in 10^{16}. It would appear that some factor other than chance alone must account for the development of uveal melanoma within families. A possible resolving of this dispute would be a cytogenetic analysis of an involved family, but such an analysis has not been performed.

■ Dysplastic Nevus Syndrome

The dysplastic nevus syndrome is an autosomal dominant condition characterized by the presence of multiple atypical variegated nevi that are generally greater than 5 mm in size and distributed in the upper trunk region (Fig A, B). Individuals with this condition are at increased risk for developing cutaneous melanoma and other primary malignancies, often at a younger age than the general population. Dysplastic nevi are found in up to 90% of individuals with familial cutaneous melanoma and in 50% of individuals with nonfamilial forms. The significance of dysplastic nevi as a marker for melanoma is dependent mainly on the presence or absence of a family history of cutaneous melanoma. In melanoma kindreds, the presence of dysplastic nevi is associated with an almost 100% lifetime risk of malignant degeneration, whereas in the absence of a family history, the relative risk for developing melanoma is on the order of fourfold to tenfold [25]. The reported occurrence of ocular melanomas developing in patients with the dysplastic nevus syndrome has led to interest about a shared inheritance of cutaneous and uveal melanomas [26–28].

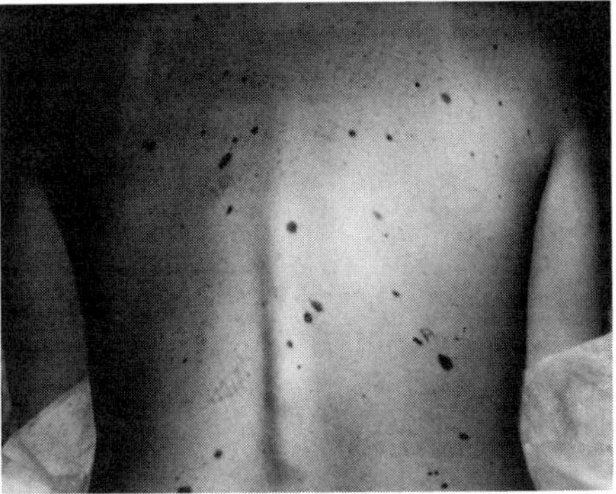

A

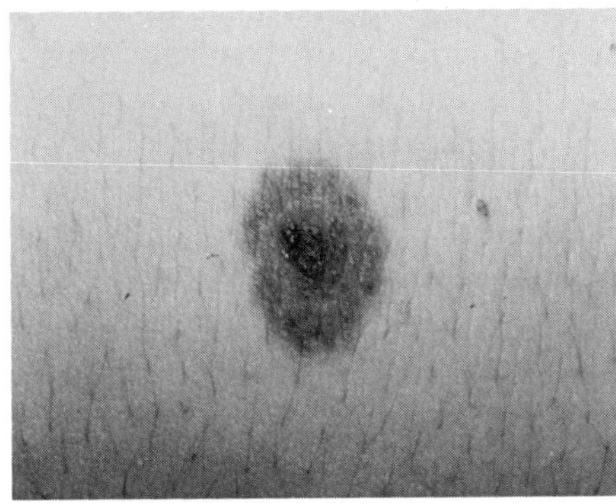

B

(A) Typical presentation of a patient with dysplastic nevi revealing prominence on the trunk and variability of mole size, outline, and color. (B) Magnified view of a dysplastic nevus in the same patient demonstrating the variegated appearance of the lesion. (Both photographs courtesy of Duane Whitaker, Iowa City.)

There have been 10 reported cases of combined cutaneous melanoma and uveal melanoma; in 7 there was a documented familial occurrence of pigmented lesions [29]. Features of the dysplastic nevus syndrome were noted in 4 of the families [29]. The occurrence of these cases challenges the belief that cutaneous and ocular melanomas are inherited separately, but there is considerable controversy about the association [28, 30–34].

Green and co-workers [32] studied the pedigrees of 26 patients with hereditary cutaneous melanoma or dysplastic nevus syndrome for evidence of uveal melanoma. They concluded there was no association between these two conditions [32]. However the methodology of their study has been criticized for "inadequate genetic investigations" [35]. A study by Taylor and colleagues [33] of 44 patients with uveal melanoma did not show a prevalence of dysplastic nevus syndrome higher than that found in the general population, and the authors concluded that the pathogenesis of intraocular and cutaneous melanomas is fundamentally different. This study also has been criticized, for inadequate documentation of pigmented lesions in the relatives of patients with uveal melanoma [36]. A study of 92 patients with the dysplastic nevus syndrome revealed a statistically significant increase in the occurrence of conjunctival, iris, and choroidal nevi over that found in the general population [36]. Given the common neural crest cell origin of cutaneous, iris, and choroidal melanocytes, it is not inconceivable that all these cells in genetically predisposed individuals have the potential to develop melanomas.

The practical significance of this debate has immediate implications for the appropriate management of a patient who presents with a uveal melanoma or cutaneous melanoma, or both. If one accepts the association between the two conditions, then all patients with the dysplastic nevus syndrome should have an ocular assessment to rule out uveal melanoma and, conversely, patients presenting with uveal melanoma should be asked about a family history of pigmented lesions and should be examined for evidence of the dysplastic nevus syndrome.

The question of association between the two conditions would be best answered through a large prospective study with matched controls, looking at the incidence of dysplastic nevi or cutaneous melanoma in newly diagnosed uveal melanoma patients. Because these conditions are relatively infrequent, the feasibility of conducting such a study is low. Until the proposed association can be definitively confirmed or denied, it would seem prudent to advise patients in whom dysplastic nevus syndrome is newly diagnosed to have an ocular examination for pigmented lesions and emphasize the importance of a dermatological examination in the systemic evaluation of patients with uveal melanoma.

■ Cytogenetics

Numerous cytogenetic studies of cutaneous malignant melanoma have identified chromosomal abnormalities specific to both the primary and the metastatic lesions. Abnormalities of chromosomes 1, 3, 5, 6, 7, 9, 10, 11, and 15 have been reported in primary cutaneous melanomas. Cytogenetic studies of uveal melanoma, although less extensive, have revealed chromosomal abnormalities that appear to be nonrandom [37–40]. Prescher and co-workers [37], reporting their findings on the cytogenetic features of tissue obtained from 14 patients with uveal melanoma, noted an increased prevalence of monosomy 3 in 6 patients (43%) and increased parts of chromosome 8 in 8 patients (57%). These findings have been supported by Horsman and colleagues [38], who also found monosomy 3 and trisomy 8 in a patient with uveal melanoma.

Both groups of investigators considered the increased amount of duplication of chromosome 8 and monosomy of chromosome 3 to be a specific aberration for uveal melanoma. The structural changes in chromosome 8 included reduplication of the 8q21 region. This is the same region to which the *myc* oncogene has been previously localized and suggests a possible role of this oncogene in the pathogenesis of uveal melanoma. Other oncogenes that map to the 8q region include *mos, lyn,* and *pvt-1* [41].

Monosomy 3 has been reported in renal carcinoma and breast and lung cancers as well [41].

Although cytogenetic studies yield useful insights into the structural changes of the genome, it is only through the use of the elegant techniques of molecular genetics that more specific information about the role of these chromosomes will be acquired. To date, there has been only one study of uveal melanoma at the molecular level. Mukai and Dryja [42], using DNA probes for which published evidence suggest that a locus important in cutaneous melanoma was present, searched the twenty-two autosomes and identified statistically significant loss of alleles on chromosome 2. However, cytogenetic analysis has not identified loss of the heterozygosity at this location.

■ Silver-Stained Nucleolar Organizing Regions

Ultrastructurally, nucleolar organizing regions (NORs) correspond to protrusions of the nucleolar DNA that directs ribosomal RNA transcription. The selective staining of these areas with modified silver stains (Ag-NORs) has proved a useful technique for determining the degree of malignancy in both cutaneous and uveal melanomas [43, 44]. Histopathological studies using the Ag-NORs have demonstrated an increased number of Ag-NORs per nucleus in malignant cutaneous melanomas compared with dysplastic nevi or benign nevi of the skin. However, a statistically significant difference in the number of NORs per cell between benign and dysplastic nevi was not found [45].

Applying the technique to the study of uveal melanoma, Marcus and co-workers [44] examined 130 specimens from the Collaborative Ocular Melanoma Study and found that malignant melanomas (spindle cell, mixed, and epithelioid) demonstrated a higher mean number of Ag-NORs than did benign nevi. They also noted that spindle cell, mixed cell, and epithelioid cell melanoma demonstrated a difference in the number of NORs counted, but the difference was not significant clinically. A correlation was seen between the number of Ag-NORs in uveal melanoma and tumor size and the number of mitoses. However, higher Ag-NOR counts were not found in epithelioid cell tumors or in tumors with scleral extension or ciliary body involvement, other known prognostic indicators. In the future, this technique may provide information useful in the management of patients with uveal melanoma.

■ HLA Typing of Uveal Melanoma

In an attempt to establish other genetic markers in uveal melanoma, two studies have been performed to look for an association between human leukocyte antigen (HLA) and this tumor. German investigators noted a prevalence of HLA-A32 in melanoma patients, but the difference from control was not statistically significant [46]. In a second study of HLA typing of 16 uveal melanoma patients, Martinetti and associates [47] attempted to correlate the immunogenetic polymorphic markers of the HLA region with the histological (phenotypical) expression of uveal melanoma. They found that the HLA class 1 antigens (A32, B27) were more prevalent in the less malignant spindle cell types and that HLA class 2 (DR3, DR7) and class 3 (Bf F) antigens strongly correlated with the more malignant histological types. In comparison with controls, an increase was noted in HLA-B4, -B27, -DR3, -DR7, and the heterozygous phenotype -DR3/DR7. The prevalence of the DR3/DR7 phenotype resulted in a relative risk of six compared with controls.

■ Comments

A better understanding of the genetic determinants of uveal melanoma will play an important role in our understanding of the development, progression, and spread of this tumor. Attention should be paid to the family history of a patient with uveal melanoma. Cytogenetic analysis of the tumor is beginning to provide useful information regarding karyotypic changes in this tumor. Chromosomes 3 and 8 appear to be most frequently altered, but further studies at the molecular level must be performed to gain further insight into the significance of these changes.

■ References

1. Scotto J, Fraumeni JF Jr, Lee JAH. Melanomas of the eye and other noncutaneous sites: epidemiological aspects. J Natl Cancer Inst 1976;56:489–491
2. Albert DM. Ocular melanoma. Presented at the 35th annual clinical conference and 24th annual special pathology program: advances in the biology and clinical management of melanoma, Houston, 1991
3. Rigel DS. The worldwide incidence of malignant melanoma. Presented at the 35th annual clinical conference and 24th annual special pathology program: advances in the biology and clinical management of melanoma, Houston, 1991
4. Kakati S, Song SY, Sandberg AA. Chromosomes and causation of human cancer and leukemia XXII. Karyotypic changes in malignant melanoma. Cancer 1977; 40:1173–1181
5. Balaban G, Herlyn M, Guerry D, et al. Cytogenetics of human malignant melanoma and premalignant lesions. Cancer Genet Cytogenet 1984;11:429–439
6. Pedersen MI, Bennett JW, Wang N. Nonrandom chromosome structural aberrations and oncogene loci in human malignant melanoma. Cancer Genet Cytogenet 1986;20:11–27
7. Cowan JM, Halaban R, Lane AT, et al. The involvement of 6p in melanoma. Cancer Genet Cytogenet 1986;20:255–261
8. Parmiter AH, Balaban G, Herlyn M, et al. A t(1;19) chromosome translocation in three cases of human malignant melanoma. Cancer Res 1986;46:1526–1529

9. Lynch HT, Fusaro RM, Danes BS, et al. A review of hereditary malignant melanoma including biomarkers in familial atypical multiple mole melanoma syndrome. Cancer Genet Cytogenet 1983;8:325–358

10. Rosenberg SA, Aebersold P, Cometta K. Gene transfer into humans: immunotherapy of patients with advanced melanoma using tumor infiltrating lymphocytes modified by retroviral gene transduction. Presented at the 35th annual clinical conference and 24th annual special pathology program: advances in the biology and clinical management of melanoma, Houston, 1991

11. Silcock A. Hereditary sarcoma of eyeball in three generations. Br Med J 1892; 1:1079

12. Parsons JH. Some anomalous sarcomata of the choroid. Trans Ophthalmol Soc UK 1905;25:193–242

13. Davenport RC. Family history of choroidal sarcoma. Br J Ophthalmol 1927; 11:443–445

14. Gutmann G. Casuisticher Beitrag zur Lehre von den Geschwülsten des Augapfels. Arch Augenheilkd 1895;31:158–180

15. Pfingst AO, Graves S. Melanosarcoma of the choroid occurring in brothers. Arch Ophthalmol 1921;50:431–439

16. Waardenburg PJ. Melanosarcoma van bet bij verschillende leden eener zelfde familie. Ned Tijdschr Geneeskd 1940;84:4718–4719

17. Bowen SF Jr, Brady H, Jones VL. Malignant melanoma of eye occurring in two successive generations. Arch Ophthalmol 1964;71:805–806

18. Lynch HT, Anderson DE, Krush AJ. Heredity and intraocular malignant melanoma: study of two families and review of forty-five cases. Cancer 1968;21:119–125

19. Tasman W. Familial intraocular melanoma. Trans Am Acad Ophthalmol Otolaryngol 1970;74:955–958

20. Green GJ, Hong WK, Everett JR, et al. Familial intraocular malignant melanoma: a case report. Cancer 1978;41:2481–2483

21. Walker JP, Weiter JJ, Albert DM, et al. Uveal malignant melanoma in three generations of the same family. Am J Ophthalmol 1979;88:723–726

22. Simons KB, Hale LM, Morrison HM Jr, et al. Choroidal malignant melanoma in siblings. Am J Ophthalmol 1983;96:675–680

23. Canning CR, Hungerford J. Familial uveal melanoma. Br J Ophthalmol 1988; 72:241–243

24. Wallace DC, Beardmore GL, Exton LA. Familial malignant melanoma. Ann Surg 1973;177:15–20

25. Elder DE. Dysplastic nevi as precursors and risk markers for melanoma (abstr). Presented at the 35th annual clinical conference and 24th annual special pathology program: advances in the biology and clinical management of melanoma. Houston, 1991

26. Bellet RE, Shields JA, Soll DB, et al. Primary choroidal and cutaneous melanomas occurring in a patient with the B-K mole syndrome phenotype. Am J Ophthalmol 1980;89:567–570

27. Abramson DH, Rodriguez-Sains RS, Rubman R. B-K mole syndrome: cutaneous and ocular malignant melanoma. Arch Ophthalmol 1980;98:1397–1399

28. Rodriguez-Sains RS. Are concurrent or subsequent malignant melanomas in the skin and eye related or coincidental? J Dermatol Surg Oncol 1980;6:915–918

29. Albert DM, Chang MA, Lamping K, et al. The dysplastic nevus syndrome. A pedigree with primary malignant melanomas of the choroid and skin. Ophthalmology 1985;92:1728–1734

30. Rodriguez-Sains RS. Uveal findings in patients with ocular and cutaneous melanoma. Am J Ophthalmol 1983;96:257–258

31. Albert DM, Searl SS, Forget B, et al. Uveal findings in patients with cutaneous melanoma. Am J Ophthalmol 1983;95:474–479

32. Greene MH, Sanders RJ, Chu FC, et al. The familial occurrence of cutaneous melanoma, intraocular melanoma and the dysplastic nevus syndrome. Am J Ophthalmol 1983;96:238–245

33. Taylor MR, Guerry DP IV, Bondi EE, et al. Lack of association between intraocular melanoma and cutaneous dysplastic nevi. Am J Ophthalmol 1984;98:478–482

34. Nordlund JJ, Kirkwood J, Forget BM, et al. Demographic study of clinically atypical (dysplastic) nevi in patients with melanoma and comparison subjects. Cancer Res 1985;45:1855–1861

35. Fusaro RM, Lynch HT. Dysplastic nevus syndrome (letter). Ophthalmology 1984;93:1371–1372

36. Rodriguez-Sains RS. Ocular findings in patients with dysplastic nevus syndrome. Ophthalmology 1986;93:661–665

37. Prescher G, Bornfeld N, Becher R. Nonrandom chromosomal abnormalities in primary uveal melanoma. J Natl Cancer Inst 1990;82:1765–1769

38. Horsman DE, Sroka H, Rootman J, et al. Monosomy 3 and isochromosome 8q in a uveal melanoma. Cancer Genet Cytogenet 1990;45:249–253

39. Griffin CA, Long PP, Schachat AP. Trisomy 6p in an ocular melanoma. Cancer Genet Cytogenet 1988;32:129–132

40. Rey JA, Bello MJ, de Campos JM, et al. Cytogenetic findings in a human malignant melanoma metastatic to the brain. Cancer Genet Cytogenet 1985;16:179–183

41. Trent JM, Kaneko Y, Mitelman F. Report of the committee on structural chromosome changes in neoplasia. Human gene mapping 9.5 (1988): update to the 9th international workshop on human gene mapping. Cytogenet Cell Genet 1988;49:236–253

42. Mukai S, Dryja TP. Loss of alleles at polymorphic loci on chromosome 2 in uveal melanoma. Cancer Genet Cytogenet 1986;22:45–53

43. Howat AJ, Giri DD, Wright AL, et al. Silver stained nucleoli and nucleolar organizer regions counts are of no prognostic value in thick cutaneous malignant melanoma. J Pathol 1988;156:227–232

44. Marcus DM, Minkovitz JB, Wardwell SD, et al. The value of nucleolar organizer regions in uveal melanoma. Am J Ophthalmol 1990;110:527–534

45. Howat AJ, Wright AL, Cotton DWK, et al. AgNORs in benign, dysplastic, and malignant melanocytic skin lesions. Am J Dermatopathol 1990;12:156–161

46. Bertrams J, Spitznas M, Rommelfanger M. Missing evidence for HLA antigen association with Eales' disease, chorioretinitis, central serous retinopathy, and malignant choroidal melanoma. Invest Ophthalmol Vis Sci 1978;17:918–920

47. Martinetti M, Tafi A, DePaoli F, et al. Immunogenetic heterogeneity of uveal melanoma. Cancer Detect Prev 1988;12:145–148

Genetics of Aniridia: The Aniridia–Wilms' Tumor Association

Mark A. Pavilack, M.D.
David S. Walton, M.D.

Aniridia is a group of closely related panocular disorders characterized primarily by iris hypoplasia [1]. The term *aniridia,* however, is actually a misnomer since it suggests total absence of the iris. Other ocular or systemic defects may be associated with aniridia.

A recent classification of aniridia illustrates the clinical and genetic diversity of this group of disorders (Table 1) [2, 3]. Most cases of aniridia are transmitted by autosomal dominant inheritance. Congenital aniridia in patients without family history of iris hypoplasia is referred to as *sporadic.* The majority of sporadic cases represent new autosomal dominant mutations, but a small percentage are caused by chromosomal deletions [1]. The total incidence of aniridia in the general population has been estimated at from 1 in 64,000 to 1 in 96,000 [4, 5]. No racial or sexual predilection is apparent.

■ Clinical Features of Aniridia

The clinical features of aniridia are summarized in Table 2. Variable expression of iris hypoplasia can range from minimal iris thinning with a round, normal-appearing pupil to near-total absence of the iris [6]. Associated ocular abnormalities typically may include cataracts, glaucoma, keratopathy, nystagmus, strabismus, ectopia lentis, and optic nerve and foveal hypoplasia. When aniridia occurs as a result of deletion of the 11p13 band of chromosome 11, concurrent systemic defects characteristically include mental retardation, genitourinary anomalies, and genetic predisposition to Wilms' tumor or nephroblastoma [7].

Although visual function can be relatively preserved [2, 7], many af-

Table 1 *Classification of Aniridia*

Type	Clinical Features	Inheritance
I	Iris hypoplasia, keratopathy, glaucoma, foveal hypoplasia, optic nerve hypoplasia, ectopia lentis, cataracts, nystagmus	AD
II	Iris hypoplasia, preserved visual function	AD[a]
III	Iris hypoplasia, cerebellar ataxia, mental retardation (Gillespie's syndrome)	AR
IV	Iris hypoplasia, Wilms' tumor, genitourinary anomalies, mental retardation (WAGR syndrome)	SP[b]
V	Iris hypoplasia with other malformative ocular syndromes, including Peter's anomaly, congenital aphakia, congenital anterior staphyloma, microcornea, and ectopia lentis	V
VI	Iris hypoplasia with other systemic syndromes or chromosomal abnormalities including Smith-Lemli-Opitz syndrome, absence of the patella, Beimond's syndrome, ring chromosome 6 (congenital glaucoma and hydrocephalus), and XXXXY chromosomal pattern	V

AD = autosomal dominant; AR = autosomal recessive; SP = sporadic; V = variable.
[a]Possible link to chromosome 2.
[b]Linked to deletion of chromosomal band 11p13.
Source: Modified from FJ Elsas et al, Familial aniridia with preserved ocular function. Am J Ophthalmol 1977;83:718–724; and EI Traboulsi et al, Hypoplasia of the iris: the aniridia spectrum. Int Pediatr 1990;5:275–278.

fected patients have visual acuity of 20/200 or worse [5]. Poor visual function in childhood is usually secondary to foveal hypoplasia. Further vision loss can occur from progressive cataracts, glaucoma, or keratopathy [8]. Congenital glaucoma is rare in aniridia, but glaucoma may occur in 6% to 75% of patients in later childhood [8–10].

Cataracts and ectopia lentis are common in aniridia. Small congenital

Table 2 *Ocular Anomalies Seen in Aniridia*

Iris hypoplasia
Keratopathy
Cataracts
Foveal hypoplasia
Nystagmus
Glaucoma
Ectopia lentis
Optic nerve hypoplasia
Strabismus
Congenital ptosis
Retinal lipoidal deposits
Microcornea
Optic nerve aplasia

anterior and posterior lens opacities may be present in early childhood. Prominent cortical, subcapsular, and lamellar cataracts begin in childhood and progress [2]. Ectopia lentis is present in up to 56% of patients [5, 6].

Corneal changes develop in the majority (up to 89%) of aniridia patients and have been observed at as early as 2 years of age [11]. The keratopathy begins in the corneal periphery as superficial opacification associated with fine vascularization [11]. The opacification is usually progressive, both circumferentially and centrally, and can result in further reductions in visual acuity when the visual axis is involved. Other associated anterior segment abnormalities, including microcornea and Peter's anomaly, have also been reported [1].

The high prevalence of pendular nystagmus in aniridia is believed to be a consequence of foveal hypoplasia and other secondary causes of poor visual acuity. Foveal hypoplasia is characterized by the lack of normal macular architecture, the presence of a poor foveal reflex, and the abnormal persistence of vessels within the foveal avascular zone. Variable degrees of optic nerve hypoplasia are also frequent. True aplasia of the optic nerve has been described in association with both complete and partial aniridia [12]. In a few patients, other abnormalities, including peripheral retinal lipoidal deposits, have been identified [6, 13]. Jesberg [13] proposed that these lipoidal deposits may represent a disorder of lipid metabolism, but no systemic metabolic defect has been identified.

Refractive errors and esotropia are common in patients with aniridia. Unrecognized anisometropia or strabismus can result in asymmetrical visual loss due to amblyopia. Varying degrees of congenital ptosis with decreased levator function have been observed in some families with autosomal dominant aniridia [14].

A number of disorders can be confused with congenital aniridia, including coloboma of the iris, corectopia, iridocorneal endothelial syndrome, anterior cleavage syndrome, colobomatous microphthalmos, and traumatic aniridia [1]. Thorough clinical histories and careful examination of both the patient, under anesthesia if necessary, and related family members usually will allow identification of patients with true aniridia.

■ Pathogenesis of Aniridia

The pathogenesis of aniridia is not known, but several theories have been proposed. Earlier reports have identified families with both ocular coloboma and aniridia, thus leading some to characterize aniridia as a colobomatous disorder. It has also been proposed that a defect in mesenchymal tissue (mesodermal theory) could result in abnormal development of the rim of the optic cup and secondarily cause hypoplasia of the iris [1, 15]. In contrast, others interpret the persistence of remnants of the tunica vasculosa lentis as evidence against a mesodermal defect [16]. Furthermore, the common association of retinal anomalies in aniridia and the absence of iris musculature, both derived from neuroectoderm, has given support to the concept of a developmental failure of neuroectoderm (ectodermal theory) [1]. Excessive remodeling and cell death have been offered as an alternative hypothesis for development of the iris hypoplasia [17].

Other factors such as environmental influences may also play a role in the pathogenesis of aniridia. For example, iris hypoplasia and genitourinary tract anomalies have been produced experimentally in mice following maternal vitamin A deficiency [18]. However, the role of vitamin A deficiency in the development of aniridia in humans has not been determined.

■ Genetic Research

Aniridia

Congenital aniridia is most often transmitted by autosomal dominant inheritance and is typically associated with other congenital or acquired abnormalities, including keratopathy, cataract, glaucoma, nystagmus, and foveal hypoplasia [5]. The penetrance of autosomal dominant aniridia is almost complete [1], though its expressivity may be highly variable [6]. Approximately two-thirds of all patients with aniridia have an affected parent [1]. Of the remaining sporadic cases, the majority are believed to result from new autosomal dominant mutations [1]. Only a small number of sporadic cases are caused by chromosomal deletions. Infrequently, aniridia is transmitted by autosomal recessive inheritance. Gillespie's syndrome is an autosomal recessive syndrome characterized by cerebellar ataxia, mental retardation, and partial aniridia [19].

Aniridia has been associated with several autosomal dominant syndromes, including one characterized by absence of the patella [20]. Rarely, other disorders with various inheritance patterns, such as Smith-Lemli-Opitz syndrome, Biemond's syndrome, and an XXXXY chromosomal pattern, involve associated iris hypoplasia [1]. Aniridia has also been described with bilateral gonadoblastoma and mental retardation [21].

Autosomal dominant aniridia has been mapped to chromosome 1 by linkage with Rh, Duffy, and PGM loci [22]. Ferrell and colleagues [23] have reported linkage with the chromosome 2p25 marker ACP1 for acid phosphatase-1 as evidence of a second aniridia locus on chromosome 2 (AN1). However, these studies did not investigate for possible linkage with 11p13 markers. In contrast, Mannens and co-workers [24] found close linkage of autosomal dominant aniridia to the chromosome 11p13 markers catalase and D11S151. As a result of these findings, it has been proposed that genes on several chromosomes contribute to the formation of the iris during embryogenesis [1].

The Aniridia–Wilms' Tumor Association

Nephroblastoma, commonly referred to as *Wilms' tumor,* is an embryonal malignancy of the kidney. Wilms' tumor is the most common solid tumor of childhood and accounts for approximately 20% of all childhood malignancies [25]. Its incidence has been estimated at between 1 in 10,000 and 1 in 50,000 live births [25]. This tumor usually occurs sporadically without other associated anomalies. However, Wilms' tumor can also be inherited by an autosomal dominant pattern, either in isolation or as part of a systemic syndrome. All bilateral cases and up to one-third of unilateral cases of Wilms' tumor are believed to be hereditary [26]. Bilateral and familial tumors constitute approximately 7% and 1%, respectively, of all Wilms' tumors and typically present at an earlier age than do unilateral or sporadic cases [27, 28].

Both Wilms' tumor and retinoblastoma are malignancies of embryonal origin. The two-hit hypothesis, as first described by Knudson for retinoblastoma, may also apply to Wilms' tumor [27]. Specifically, this hypothesis states that mutational events leading to genesis of these childhood neoplasms may occur in two distinct steps. In hereditary forms, the first predisposing mutation is postulated to be present at birth, inherited by germinal cells, and the second mutation in somatic cells, if it occurs, results in the development of the tumor. In sporadic cases, both mutations are believed to occur in somatic cells after birth, thus resulting in the later age (3 to 4 years) of tumor onset compared with patients with hereditary tumors (approximately 2 years) [27, 28]. Since most cases (95%) of Wilms' tumor are diagnosed within the first decade of life [28], it has been proposed that undifferentiated metanephric cells capable of Wilms' tumor formation are present only during gestation and are lost before birth [27].

In 1953, Brusa and Torricelli [29] first reported the association of Wilms' tumor with aniridia. Sporadic aniridia was later associated with Wilms' tumor, hemihypertrophy, and other congenital anomalies [30]. Miller and colleagues [30] found aniridia present with greatly increased frequency in patients with Wilms' tumor, up to 1 in 73; a later study found a prevalence of 1 in 69 [31]. Fraumeni and Glass [32] observed that one-third of all patients with sporadic aniridia developed Wilms' tumor compared with only a single known case of Wilms' tumor associated with autosomal dominantly inherited aniridia.

The rate of Wilms' tumor development is much greater when aniridia is accompanied by genitourinary anomalies and mental retardation (*AGR complex*) [7]. In fact, up to 50% of patients with the AGR complex will develop Wilms' tumor [31]. Other systemic defects, including tracheomalacia, craniofacial dysostosis, and dysmorphism, have also been described in patients with sporadic aniridia and Wilms' tumor [33].

The presence of Wilms' tumor, aniridia, genitourinary anomalies, and mental retardation, referred to as *WAGR syndrome,* has been attributed to partial deletion of the short arm of chromosome 11, specifically of the 11p13 band [7]. The risk of Wilms' tumor increases to more than 60% in cases of aniridia with cytogenetically detectable deletion of the distal region of the 11p13 band [34]. A few patients with aniridia and Wilms' tumor did not have detectable chromosomal abnormalities when evaluated by high-resolution chromosomal banding techniques; however, the presence of point mutations could not be excluded [31].

Recent studies have demonstrated close linkage of the aniridia locus (AN2) and the Wilms' tumor gene within the 11p13 band [35, 36]. A complete physical map of the WAGR region of 11p13 has localized the candidate Wilms' tumor gene (WT33) and limited the Wilms' tumor gene locus to a region of less than 345 kilobases [37]. Consistent with previous studies [35, 36], Rose and associates [37] have localized the gene for aniridia (AN2) to within the proximal portion of the WAGR region (Figure).

Transcripts from within the candidate Wilms' tumor locus (WT33) have been shown to encode for a zinc finger polypeptide that has features characteristic of a transcription regulator [38, 39]. These features include the presence of four zinc finger domains, suggesting potential for direct DNA binding, and a proline-glutamine-rich region, which has been found in several other transcription factors [38, 39]. This putative transcription factor is also believed to be involved in normal genitourinary development since it is expressed in the developing kidney [39, 40].

Markers used to narrow the localization of the WAGR region within the 11p13 band include genes encoding for follicle-stimulating hormone (β-FSH), erythrocyte catalase, and the cell surface antigen MIC1. The development of panels of restriction fragment length polymorphism (RFLP)

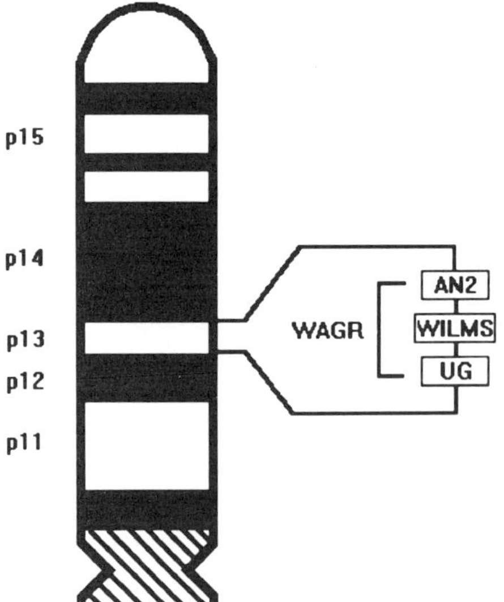

Schematic map of the WAGR gene complex (Wilms' tumor, aniridia, genitourinary anomalies, and mental retardation) on the short arm of chromosome 11. Loci for aniridia (AN2), Wilms' tumor (WILMS), and associated urogenital defects (UG) are shown. (Modified from EA Rose et al, Complete physical map of the WAGR region of 11p13 localizes a candidate Wilms' tumor gene. Cell 1990;60: 495–508.)

probes sublocalized within the chromosome band 11p13 will allow further investigation of the roles of individual genes in the development of aniridia, Wilms' tumor, and associated genitourinary anomalies [41]. New insights may also develop from a mouse model of a homologous genetic deletion that causes phenotypical ocular manifestations similar to aniridia in humans [42].

In addition to the WT33 gene within the 11p13 band, it appears that defects of alternative loci may also cause hereditary predisposition to Wilms' tumor [43, 44]. Still other studies have implicated mutations of the 11p15 region as contributory to sporadic Wilms' tumor [45, 46]. Further experimental investigation is needed to isolate and characterize these potential alternative loci of sporadic Wilms' tumor.

■ References

1. Nelson LB, Spaeth GL, Nowinski TS, et al. Aniridia: a review. Surv Ophthalmol 1984;28:621–642
2. Elsas FJ, Maumenee IH, Kenyon KR, Yoder F. Familial aniridia with preserved ocular function. Am J Ophthalmol 1977;83:718–724
3. Traboulsi EI, Jaafar MS, Wilson ME, Parks MM. Hypoplasia of the iris: the aniridia spectrum. Int Pediatr 1990;5:275–278
4. Mollenbach CJ. Congenital defects in the internal membrane of the eye. In: Nyt Nordiska Forlag, Opera ex Domo Biologiae Hereditariae Humanae Universitatis Hafniensis, vol 15. Copenhagen: Einer Munksgaard, 1947:164
5. Shaw MW, Falls HF, Neel JV. Congenital aniridia. Am J Hum Genet 1960;12:389–415
6. Hittner HM, Riccardi VM, Ferrell RE, et al. Variable expressivity in autosomal dominant aniridia by clinical, electrophysiologic, and angiographic criteria. Am J Ophthalmol 1980;89:531–539
7. Riccardi VM, Sujansky E, Smith AC, Francke V. Chromosomal imbalance in the aniridia–Wilms' tumor association: 11p interstitial deletion. Pediatrics 1978;61:604–610
8. Shaffer RN, Cohen JS. Visual reduction in aniridia. J Pediatr Ophthalmol 1975;12:220–222
9. Grant WM, Walton DS. Progressive changes in the angle in congenital aniridia with development of glaucoma. Am J Ophthalmol 1974;78:842–847
10. Walton DS. Aniridia with glaucoma. In: Chandler PA, Grant WM, eds. Glaucoma, ed 2. Philadelphia: Lea & Febiger, 1979:351–354
11. Mackman G, Brightbill FS, Opitz JM. Corneal changes in aniridia. Am J Ophthalmol 1979;87:497–502
12. Ginsberg J, Bove KE, Cuesta MG. Aplasia of the optic nerve with aniridia. Ann Ophthalmol 1980;12:433–439
13. Jesberg DO. Aniridia with retinal lipid deposits. Arch Ophthalmol 1962;68:331–336
14. Shields MB, Reed JW. Aniridia and congenital ptosis. Ann Ophthalmol 1975;7:203–205
15. Mann I. Persistence of capsulopupillary vessels as a factor in the production of abnormalities of the iris and lens. Arch Ophthalmol 1934;11:174–182
16. Hamming N, Wilensky J. Persistent pupillary membrane associated with aniridia. Am J Ophthalmol 1978;86:118–120

17. Beauchamp GR, Meisler DM. An alternative hypothesis for iris maldevelopment (aniridia). J Pediatr Ophthalmol Strabismus 1986;23:281–283

18. Warkany J, Schraffenberger E. Congenital malformations induced in rats by maternal vitamin A deficiency: I. Defects of the eye. Arch Ophthalmol 1946;35:150–169

19. Gillespie FD. Aniridia, cerebellar ataxia, and oligophrenia in siblings. Arch Ophthalmol 1965;73:338–341

20. Mirkinson AE, Mirkinson NK. A familial syndrome of aniridia and absence of the patella. Birth Defects 1975;11:129–131

21. Turleau C, de Grouchy J, Dufier JL, et al. Aniridia, male pseudohermaphroditism, gonadoblastoma, mental retardation, and del 11p13. Hum Genet 1981;57:300–306

22. Sloderbeck JD, Maumenee IH, Elsas FE, et al. Linkage assignment of aniridia to chromosome 1. Am J Hum Genet 1975;27:83A

23. Ferrell RE, Chakarvarti A, Hittner HM, Riccardi V. Autosomal dominant aniridia: probable linkage to acid phosphatase-1 locus on chromosome 2. Proc Natl Acad Sci 1980;77:1580–1583

24. Mannens M, Bleeker-Wagemakers EM, Bliek J, et al. Autosomal dominant aniridia linked to the chromosome 11p13 markers catalase and D11S151 in a large Dutch family. Cytogenet Cell Genet 1989;52:32–36

25. Glenn JF, Rhame RC. Wilms tumor: epidemiological experience. J Urol 1961;85:911–918

26. Diaz de Bustamante A, Delicado A, Garcia de Miguel P, et al. Balanced reciprocal translocation (X;20) limited to Wilms' tumor in a Wiedemann-Beckwith syndrome. Cancer Genet Cytogenet 1990;45:35–39

27. Knudson AG Jr, Strong LC. Mutation and cancer: a model for Wilms' tumor of the kidney. J Natl Cancer Inst 1972;48:313–324

28. Breslow N, Beckwith JB, Ciol M, Sharples K. Age distribution of Wilms' tumor: report from the National Wilms' Tumor Study. Cancer Res 1988;48:1653–1657

29. Brusa P, Torricelli C. Nefroblastoma di Wilms ed affezioni renali congenite nella casistica dell' I.P.P.A.I. di Milano. Minerva Pediatr 1953;5:457–463

30. Miller RW, Fraumeni JF Jr, Manning MD. Association of Wilms' tumor with aniridia, hemihypertrophy and other congenital malformations. N Engl J Med 1964;270:922–927

31. Narahara K, Kikkawa K, Kimira S, et al. Regional mapping of catalase and Wilms tumor—aniridia, genitourinary abnormalities, and mental retardation triad loci to the chromosome segment 11p1305—p1306. Hum Genet 1984;66:181–185

32. Fraumeni JF Jr, Glass AG. Wilms' tumor and congenital aniridia. JAMA 1968;206:825–828

33. Jotterand V, Boisjoly HM, Harnois C, et al. 11p13 deletion, Wilms' tumour, and aniridia: unusual genetic, non-ocular and ocular features of three cases. Br J Ophthalmol 1990;74:568–570

34. Turleau C, de Grouchy J, Tournade M-F, et al. Del 11p/aniridia complex: report of three patients and review of 37 observations from the literature. Clin Genet 1984;26:356–362

35. Compton DA, Weil MM, Jones C, et al. Long range physical map of the Wilms' tumor—aniridia region on human chromosome 11. Cell 1988;55:827–836

36. Davis LM, Stallard R, Thomas GH, et al. Two anonymous DNA segments distinguish the Wilms' tumor and aniridia loci. Science 1988;241:840–842

37. Rose EA, Glaser T, Jones C, et al. Complete physical map of the WAGR region of 11p13 localizes a candidate Wilms' tumor gene. Cell 1990;60:495–508

38. Call KM, Glaser T, Ito CY, et al. Isolation and characterization of a zinc finger polypeptide gene at the human chromosome 11 Wilms' tumor locus. Cell 1990;60:509–520

39. Gessler M, Poustka A, Cavenee W, et al. Homozygous deletion in Wilms tumours of a zinc-finger gene identified by chromosome jumping. Nature 1990;343:774–778

40. Pritchard-Jones K, Fleming S, Davidson D, et al. The candidate Wilms' tumour gene is involved in genitourinary development. Nature 1990;346:194–197
41. Huff V, Compton DA, Strong LC, Saunders GF. A panel of restriction fragment length polymorphisms for chromosomal band 11p13. Hum Genet 1990;84:253–257
42. Glaser T, Lane J, Housman D. A mouse model of the aniridia–Wilms tumor deletion syndrome. Science 1990;250:823–827
43. Grundy P, Koufos A, Morgan K, et al. Familial predisposition to Wilms' tumour does not map to the short arm of chromosome 11. Nature 1988;336:374–376
44. Huff V, Compton DA, Chao LV, et al. Lack of linkage of familial Wilms' tumour to chromosomal band 11p13. Nature 1988;336:377–378
45. Reeve AE, Sih SA, Raizis AM, et al. Loss of allelic heterozygosity at a second locus on chromosome 11 in sporadic Wilms' tumor cells. Mol Cell Biol 1989;9:1799–1803
46. Koufos A, Grundy P, Morgan K, et al. Familial Wiedemann-Beckwith syndrome and a second Wilms' tumor locus both map to 11p15.5. Am J Hum Genet 1989;44:711–719

IU/ml at birth, 20 IU/ml at age 1 year, and 40 IU/ml at 2 years. The levels peak at age 10 (140 IU/ml), then revert back to the levels seen in adults.

■ Control of IgE Production

Genetic studies of atopy have focused on the control of the production of IgE. Historically, the emphasis initially was on the variation in serum levels of IgE in atopic patients and in their family members [7]. Other researchers have demonstrated the significance of the presence of various immune response genes on the control of IgE production (see next section) [8]. Yodoi and Ishizaka [9] emphasized control of IgE production by suppressing and potentiating factors. Most recently, the control of IgE production has been linked to an interplay between interleukin 4 and gamma interferon [10].

IgE Levels in Families with Atopy

Increased serum and tear levels of IgE are found in patients with allergic conjunctivitis. No studies have been performed to examine exclusively the genetics of atopic ocular disease. In genetic studies of patients with nonocular atopy, including atopic dermatitis, hay fever, and asthma, the most consistent immune defect is elevated levels of IgE in the serum. Hence, an understanding of the genetic controls of IgE levels in patients with atopy would most closely approximate that of ocular atopic disease.

Historically, family studies have provided evidence for a gene regulation of IgE production. Early workers chose a level of 95 IU/ml IgE as separating low and high responders. They then found evidence for a recessive model of inheritance for high production of IgE [7]. Later work determined the production of IgE to fit a mixed model of recessive inheritance with polygenic influences [11]. Not all atopic patients have an elevated IgE level, and some nonatopic individuals do have elevated IgE levels. It is generally agreed that control of the serum IgE level involves a complex interaction of genetic and nongenetic factors, with a major gene involved in some but not most cases, and continued exposure of an allergic individual to a specific allergen playing a critical role in IgE level regulation.

Immune Response Genes and IgE Production

The immune response genes are found on the HLA-D regions of human chromosome 6. The HLA-D subregions—HLA-DR, -DQ, and -DP— each contain alpha and beta genes. These genes encode for the class II or immune response proteins, which are the cell surface markers responsible for immune recognition; they must be present, along with processed antigen, on the surface of antigen-presenting cells in order for antigen to be presented to T or B cells. There are striking associations between the HLA-DR/Dw2 gene and atopic responses to the ragweed antigen of the genus *Ambrosia*. Ninety-five percent of patients with serum IgE to *Ambrosia* were found to possess HLA-Dw2; only 22% of patients without *Ambrosia* IgE were HLA-Dw2-positive. Similar results were found for IgG to *Ambrosia* antigen [8].

IgE Binding Factors

Studies in rodents have shown that IgE levels are controlled by IgE binding factors (IgE-BF) that inhibit or potentiate IgE production [9]. These two factors are very similar molecules, differing only in their state of glycosylation [12]. Control over the state of glycosylation is directed by glycosylation-enhancing factor (GEF) or glycosylation-inhibiting factor (GIF). Thus, in the rodent the genetic control of GEF and GIF levels determines, to a very great extent, IgE production.

Cytokine Control of IgE Production

The study of cell-to-cell communication via cytokines has been a recent focus of research in the control of IgE synthesis. Interleukin 4 (IL-4) and gamma interferon have been shown reciprocally to regulate human IgE synthesis in vitro [10]. Recombinant human IL-4 along with a physical interaction of T and B cells induces IgE synthesis in vitro. This can be blocked by anti-IL-4 antibody; however, the B cells continue to make IgD and IgG [10].

■ Control of IgE Production in the Treatment of Atopic Disease

Knowledge of the various influences on the control of IgE production has helped to shape various approaches to treatment of atopic disorders. Hyposensitization or desensitization as immune therapy dates back to the 1800s. Today it consists of systemic injection of progressively increasing doses of allergens to which a patient has known sensitivities. Two possible changes are responsible for the effect of desensitizing patients to subsequent encounters with allergens [13, 14]. Usually, antigen-specific IgG appears in the serum of patients following hyposensitization therapy. This "blocking antibody" competes for antigen with cell-bound IgE and thereby reduces the available antigenic load that can interact with the IgE present on the cells. Second, reaginic antibody or IgE in the serum available to bind to tissue mast cells is reduced with hyposensitization, probably through the induction of antigen-specific suppressor T cells.

"Immunotoxin" therapy has been experimentally employed recently in rodents in an effort to regulate IgE production [15]. The type of immunotoxin employed was anti-IgE coupled with methotrexate. Experiments in rodents indicate extreme efficiency in inhibiting the generation of antigen-specific IgE [15]. The presumed mechanism is that of clearing IgE-bearing lymphocytes, through anti-IgE-methotrexate binding to IgE-bearing lymphocytes, with subsequent methotrexate-induced death of the cell. IgE is the immunoglobulin isotype generated late, and so clearing of B cells expressing IgE would not interfere with further production of the other immunoglobulins.

■ Summary

Atopy arises from a complex interplay between immunogenetic controls and complex environmental allergens. Family studies of atopic patients indicate a polygenic control of IgE production overlayed with exposure to certain ubiquitous environmental antigens. Ultrapurified antigen studies in families indicate that HLA-D immune response genes, notably HLA-DR/Dw2, are implicated in some atopic responses. IgE-binding factors and gene regulation of proteins controlling glycosylation of them also influence the serum levels of IgE, as do the levels of at least two cytokines, IL-4 and gamma interferon.

■ References

1. Cocoa AF, Cooke RA. On the classification of the phenomena of hypersensitiveness. J Immunol 1923;8:163–182
2. Prausnitz C, Kustner H. Studien Uber die Uberempfindlichkeit. Centralbl Bakt 1921;86:160
3. Ishizaka K, Ishizaka T. Identification of gamma E antibodies as carriers of reaginic activity. J Immunol 1967;99:1187–1198
4. Allansmith MR, Ross RN. Ocular allergy and mast cell stabilizers. Surv Ophthalmol 1968;30:229–244
5. Samra Z, Zavaro A, Barishak Y, Sompolinsky D. Vernal keratoconjunctivitis: the significance of immunoglobulin E levels in tears and serum. Int Arch Allergy Appl Immunol 1984;74:158–164
6. Ballow M, Donshik PC, Mendelson L, et al. IgG specific antibodies to rye grass and ragweed pollen antigens in the tear secretions of patients with vernal conjunctivitis. Am J Ophthalmol 1983;95:161–168
7. Marsh DG, Bias WB, Ishizaka K. Genetic control of basal serum immunoglobulin E level and its effect on specific reaginic sensitivity. Proc Natl Acad Sci USA 1974;71:3588–3592
8. Marsh DG, Hsu SH, Roebber M, et al. HLA-Dw2: a genetic marker for human

immune response to short ragweed pollen allergen Ra5: I. Response resulting primarily from natural antigenic exposure. J Exp Med 1982;155:1439–1451

9. Yodoi J, Ishizaka K. Lymphocytes bearing Fc receptors for IgE: IV. Formation of IgE-binding factor by rat T lymphocytes. J Immunol 1980;124:1322–1329

10. Del Prete G, Maggi E, Parronchi P, et al. IL-4 is an essential factor for the IgE synthesis induced in vitro by human T cell clones and supernatants. J Immunol 1988;140:4193–4198

11. Gerrard JW, Rao DC, Morton NE. A genetic study of immunoglobulin E. Am J Hum Genet 1978;30:46–58

12. Yodoi J, Hirashima M, Ishizaka K. Regulatory role of IgE-binding factors from rat T lymphocytes V. The carbohydrate moieties in IgE-potentiating factors and IgE-suppressive factors. J Immunol 1982;128:289–295

13. Sherman WB, Stull A, Cooke RA. Serologic changes in hayfever cases treated over a period of years. J Allergy 1940;11:225

14. Lichtenstein LM, Norman PS, Winkenwerder W. Clinical and in vitro studies of human ragweed allergies: changes in cellular and humoral activity associated with specific desensitization. J Clin Invest 1966;45:1126–1136

15. Whitaker RB, Galli SJ, Hannum LG. Immunotoxin suppression of IgE production. In: Streilein JW, ed. Proceedings of the 1990 Miami Bio/Technology Winter Symposium—the molecular biology of immune diseases and the immune response; advances in gene technology, 1990:195

HLA Antigens and the Development of Diabetic Retinopathy

Sashi K. Dharma, M.D.

Donald J. D'Amico, M.D.

Several histocompatibility cell surface antigens (human leukocyte antigens [HLA]) have been implicated as a risk factor in the development of diabetic retinopathy. This factor has especially been correlated with proliferative diabetic retinopathy in insulin-dependent diabetics. Diabetes mellitus is clinically and genetically a heterogeneous group of disorders characterized by glucose intolerance. Insulin-dependent diabetes mellitus (IDDM) has an abrupt onset and an increased incidence of ketosis with dependence on exogenous insulin to control the blood glucose level. In contradiction to the old definition of this disorder as juvenile-onset diabetes, IDDM can occur at any age [1]. Table 1 provides a classification of the various groups of disorders that constitute diabetes and glucose intolerance [2].

■ Role of Genetics in Diabetic Retinopathy

We sought to explore whether genetics play a role in the development of diabetic retinopathy. If so, what antigens are responsible for the development of retinopathy? The study by Tattersall and Pyke [3] of 96 pairs of identical twins, in which 65 pairs were concordant (both individuals had diabetes) and 31 pairs were discordant (one individual had diabetes but the other did not), was useful in answering the first question. A history of diabetes in the parents was strongly linked with concordant twin pairs having onset of diabetes after the age of 40 years (Table 2). The following conclusions can be drawn from this study: First, diabetes does not always occur in the identical twin of a diabetic. Second, if the identical twins are

Table 1 *Classification of Diabetes and Glucose Intolerance*

Class	Former Terminology
Insulin-dependent diabetes mellitus (IDDM); type I diabetes	Juvenile diabetes, juvenile-type diabetes, ketosis-prone or brittle diabetes
Non-insulin-dependent diabetes mellitus (NIDDM); type II diabetes Nonobese NIDDM Obese NIDDM NIDDM including diabetes mellitus	Adult-onset diabetes, maturity-onset-type diabetes, ketosis-resistant diabetes, stable diabetes
Secondary diabetes associated with certain conditions and syndromes Pancreatic disease Hormonally induced disease Drug- or chemical-induced disease Certain genetic syndromes	
Other types Gestational diabetes (GDM)	Gestational diabetes
Previous abnormality of glucose tolerance	Latent diabetes, prediabetes (prevAGT)
Potential abnormality of glucose tolerance	Prediabetes, potential diabetes (potAGT)
Impaired glucose tolerance (IGT) Nonobese (IGT)	Asymptomatic diabetes, chemical diabetes
Obese IGT	Subclinical or latent diabetes
IGT associated with certain conditions and syndromes Pancreatic disease Hormonally induced disease Drug- or chemical-induced disease Insulin receptor abnormalities Certain genetic syndromes	

Source: Adapted with permission from PH Morse, Practical management of diabetic retinopathy. Norwalk, CT: Appleton-Century-Crofts, 1985:1–51.

older than 50 years at diagnosis, the second twin is almost certain to be diabetic. Hence, heredity appears to be important in adult-onset diabetes.

Pyke and Tattersall [4] studied the occurrence of diabetic retinopathy in 13 pairs of concordant twins and 10 pairs of discordant twins. The mean duration of diabetes was 23.3 years and 21.9 years, respectively. Table 3

Table 2 *Number of Twin Pairs with a Diabetic Parent*

Group (by age)	Concordant	Discordant
All ages	21/65	1/31
Index twin in whom disease diagnosed at younger than 40 yr	6/30	1/28
Index twin in whom disease diagnosed at or after age 40 yr	15/35	0/3

Source: Data from RB Tattersall and DA Pyke, Diabetes in identical twins. Lancet 1972;2:1120–1125.

shows the severity of retinopathy in the two groups. The severity and progression of retinopathy were strikingly similar in the concordant pairs, with one exception. The greater frequency and severity of retinopathy in the concordant compared to the discordant twins suggests the importance of genetic factors in the etiology of diabetic retinopathy.

■ Correlation of HLA Antigens and Diabetic Retinopathy

Several studies have investigated the association of HLA antigens and the development of proliferative diabetic retinopathy. However, many of these studies may have been confounded by linkage disequilibrium [5, 6].

Definition of Linkage Disequilibrium

The HLA complex comprises at least seven closely linked loci on the short arm of chromosome 6. These loci are called *HLA-A, -B, -C, -D, -DR* (for *D-related*), *-DP*, and *-DQ*. One important characteristic of the HLA genes is that they are highly polymorphic—that is, several alleles exist at each locus. This makes HLA an ideal marker for genetic studies. Linkage disequilibrium is another important characteristic of HLA antigens. In a random mating population, the joint frequency of two alleles from two different loci will be the product of their individual gene frequencies. If the observed value of the joint frequency is significantly different from the expected frequency (the product of the individual allele frequencies), the two alleles are said to be in *linkage disequilibrium*. For example, the gene frequency of A1-B8 in North American whites is 0.138 and that of B8 is 0.090. The frequency of the A1-B8 haplotype should be 0.138 × 0.090 = 0.0124, but the observed frequency in this population is 0.0609. Thus, A1 and B8 antigens are said to be in linkage disequilibrium.

Table 3 *Severity of Retinopathy in Concordant and Discordant Twins*

Twin Types	No. of Pairs	No. of Pairs without Retinopathy	No. of Pairs with Microaneurysms Only	No. of Pairs with Hemorrhages or Exudates	No. of Pairs with Proliferative Retinopathy
Concordant	13	3	2	10	11 (5 blind, 2 partially sighted)
Discordant	10	5	2	2	1 (normal vision)

Source: Reprinted with permission from DA Pyke and RB Tattersall, Diabetic retinopathy in identical twins. Diabetes 1973;22:613–618.

Review of the Literature

A survey of studies of the correlation of HLA antigens and the development of diabetic retinopathy yields conflicting results. Rand and colleagues [7] found that the duration of diabetes, glycemic control, refractive error, and certain HLA-DR phenotypes were significantly linked to the appearance of proliferative retinopathy in diabetics. The association with myopia was especially interesting. The risk of retinopathy was not influenced by refractive error among patients with an HLA-DR phenotype of 3/4, 3/X, or 4/X. In patients with HLA-DR phenotypes, the susceptibility to proliferative diabetic retinopathy was ten to fifteen times higher in low myopia (less than 2 D) than in emmetropia and hyperopia.

Dornan and co-workers [8] studied 127 insulin-dependent diabetics at different stages of the disease. The incidence of retinopathy in insulin-dependent patients was higher in those with poor glycemic control. However, patients with the same mean blood glucose level who had retinopathy had a higher incidence of HLA-DR4 than those without retinopathy; the presence of HLA-DR4 and hyperglycemia also greatly increased the risk of retinopathy over that for individuals without HLA-DR4. The frequency of HLA-DR2 was highest (22%) in patients with poor glycemic control and no retinopathy and lowest in patients who developed retinopathy despite good control. HLA-DR4 was present in 61 of 87 patients (70%) with background or proliferative diabetic retinopathy and in 21 of 39 patients (54%) with no retinopathy.

Barbosa and associates [9] compared 100 insulin-dependent diabetic patients without proliferative diabetic retinopathy who were younger than 40 years with 200 insulin-dependent diabetic patients with proliferative diabetic retinopathy and a mean age of 35 to 38 years. Healthy blood donors (847) served as a control group. The comparison of proliferative and nonproliferative diabetic retinopathy showed a significant difference for HLA-B7 ($\chi^2 = 10.0$; $P_c < .03$). A diabetic who is HLA-B7-positive is approximately three times less likely to develop proliferative retinopathy than is a patient who is HLA-B7-negative.

Additionally, HLA-B15 is more common ($\chi^2 = 7.89$; $p^c < .03$) for the proliferative retinopathy group in the same subset of patients. When comparing these two groups, the relative risk for HLA-B7 is 0.19 and, for HLA-B15, 3.32. Hence, diabetics who are HLA-B7-positive are five times less likely, and diabetics who are HLA-B15-positive are three times more likely, to develop proliferative retinopathy than are diabetics with other antigens.

It is probable that the predictive value of HLA antigens is race- or region-specific. For example, in populations in which HLA-B7 is rare, such as Native Americans (2%) and Arabs (6%), the predictive value is limited.

In the study by Danielsen and colleagues [10] of 212 diabetic patients in Iceland, the relative risks of HLA-B8 and HLA-B15 were different from the results of Barbosa's group [9]. Insulin-dependent diabetics were divided into two groups—those with diabetes for 15 years or more and onset before age 30, and those with duration of diabetes of 10 years or more at any age. Each group was subdivided into those with and without retinopathy. HLA-B8 was similarly distributed in patients with and without retinopathy. HLA-B15 and HLA-DR4 showed a reduced frequency in the group with proliferative retinopathy. As in the study by Barbosa's group [9], HLA-B15 was more common in the proliferative retinopathy subset of patients. In Dornan's study [8], HLA-DR4 was found to have a higher incidence in insulin-dependent diabetics with retinopathy.

Gray and co-workers [11] found the incidence of HLA-B7 to be lower in insulin-dependent diabetics with retinopathy. They compared 112 type I diabetics with minimal or no retinopathy to 73 diabetics with severe background or proliferative diabetic retinopathy. The control group consisted of 100 normal nondiabetics. The patients were divided into four groups: Group A consisted of patients with no retinopathy; group B, pre-proliferative retinopathy; group C, proliferative retinopathy without nephropathy; and group D, proliferative retinopathy with nephropathy. HLA analysis showed HLA-A1 and HLA-B8 to be more common in all diabetics than in controls. HLA-A1 and HLA-B8 are in linkage disequilibrium. Additional studies showed a higher incidence of increased postprandial glucose levels, glycosylated HbA_{1c} concentration, and cigarette smoking among diabetics with retinopathy.

Becker and associates [12] found a significant increase in the prevalence of HLA-B8 and HLA-A1 in adult-onset diabetics without retinopathy. Again, HLA-B8 and HLA-A1 are in linkage disequilibrium. Among juvenile-onset diabetics, there was an increased incidence of HLA-B8 and a decreased incidence of HLA-B7; however, no differences were found between those with and without retinopathy.

Middleton and colleagues [13] studied two groups of insulin-dependent diabetics. One group consisted of 31 patients who had IDDM for 20 years without ophthalmoscopic evidence of background or proliferative diabetic retinopathy; all had been diabetic for 30 years or more. The second group consisted of 49 IDDM patients with severe bilateral proliferative retinopathy treated with panretinal photocoagulation; all had been diabetic for 15 years or more. No significant difference was found between the two groups in terms of HLA-DR antigen frequency.

Johnston and co-workers [14] studied two groups of patients who were matched for sex, age, and duration of diabetes. One group consisted of 57 patients who had had the disease for 15 years without ophthalmoscopic evidence of background or proliferative diabetic retinopathy. The age at onset of diabetes was less than 40 years in every patient. The second group consisted of 56 diabetic patients with severe bilateral proliferative retinopathy treated by panretinal laser photocoagulation. The diabetic patients and control population were typed for 22 HLA antigens: HLA types B14,

B15, and B17 were the major contributors. HLA-B15 was found more frequently in both diabetic groups, whereas HLA-B14 and -B17 were found less frequently than in the control group. No significant differences in HLA frequency were found between the two groups of diabetic patients.

■ Conclusions

Conflicting results were found concerning the incidence of HLA antigens, especially HLA-B antigens [15–18]. This may be secondary to linkage disequilibrium, or it may result from chance significant events, especially in relation to a highly polymorphic system such as the HLA antigens. The arbitrary division of data (for example, by age of onset) can produce chance significant results.

It is important to recognize gene pairs that are in linkage disequilibrium, such as HLA-B15 and HLA-DR4, and HLA-A1 and HLA-B8. Increased frequency of one antigen in the pair will necessarily show an increased incidence of the other. Variance from this rule is unusual but may be significant. Larkins and co-workers [18] found an increased incidence of HLA-B8 but not of HLA-A1 in 56% of IDDM patients with severe proliferative retinopathy.

The risk factors for the development of proliferative retinopathy in diabetics can be summarized as follows: duration of diabetes [7, 17], plasma blood glucose control [7, 11], presence or absence of certain HLA antigens [1, 18], cigarette smoking [11], hypertension with systolic blood pressure exceeding 170 without retinopathy [17], level of triglycerides [17], juvenile onset of disease [17], and refractive error [7].

■ References

1. Kohner EM. The evolution and natural history of diabetic retinopathy. Int Ophthalmol Clin 1978;18(4):1–16
2. Morse PH. Practical management of diabetic retinopathy. Norwalk, CT: Appleton-Century-Crofts, 1985:1–51
3. Tattersall RB, Pyke DA. Diabetes in identical twins. Lancet 1972;2:1120–1125
4. Pyke DA, Tattersall RB. Diabetic retinopathy in identical twins. Diabetes 1973;22: 613–618
5. Tiwari JL, Terasaki PI. HLA and disease associations. New York: Springer-Verlag, 1985
6. Frank RN. Etiologic mechanisms in diabetic retinopathy. In: Ryan SJ, ed. Retina, vol 2. St Louis: Mosby, 1989:301–325
7. Rand LI, Krolewski AS, Aiello LM, et al. Multiple factors in the prediction of risk of proliferative diabetic retinopathy. N Engl J Med 1985;313:1433–1438
8. Dornan TL, Ting A, McPherson CK, et al. Genetic susceptibility to the development of retinopathy in insulin-dependent diabetics. Diabetes 1982;31:226–231
9. Barbosa J, Ramsay RC, Knobloch WH, et al. Histocompatibility antigen frequencies in diabetic retinopathy. Am J Ophthalmol 1980;90:148–153

10. Danielsen R, Helgason T, Arnason A, Jonasson F. HLA and retinopathy in type 1 (insulin-dependent) diabetic patients in Iceland. Diabetologia 1982;22:297–298
11. Gray RS, Starkey IR, Rainbow S, et al. HLA antigens and other risk factors in the development of retinopathy in type 1 diabetes. Br J Ophthalmol 1982;66:280–285
12. Becker B, Shin DH, Burgess D, et al. Histocompatibility antigens and diabetic retinopathy. Diabetes 1977;26:997–999
13. Middleton D, Johnston PB, Gillespie EL. HLA-DR antigen association with proliferative diabetic retinopathy. Int Ophthalmol 1985;8:33–35
14. Johnston PB, Kidd M, Middleton D, et al. Analysis of HLA antigen association with proliferative diabetic retinopathy. Br J Ophthalmol 1982;66:277–279
15. Bodansky HJ, Wolf E. HLA association with diabetic retinopathy—fact or fancy? Diabetologia 1981;20:585
16. Barbosa J, Ramsay R. Of genes and proliferative retinopathy. Diabetologia 1981; 20:506
17. West KM, Erdreich LJ, Stober JA. A detailed study of risk factors for retinopathy and nephropathy in diabetes. Diabetes 1980;29:501–508
18. Larkins RG, Martin FI, Tait BD. HLA patterns and diabetic retinopathy. Br Med J 1978;1:1111

Inheritance of Glaucoma and Genetic Counseling of Glaucoma Patients

Peter A. Netland, M.D., Ph.D.

Janey L. Wiggs, M.D., Ph.D.

Evan B. Dreyer, M.D., Ph.D.

Varying patterns of inheritance may be present in different types of glaucoma. In some disorders associated with glaucoma, there is known mendelian inheritance or genetic defects, and genetic counseling can help families affected with these disorders. Primary open-angle glaucoma and certain other glaucomas are found in relatively low frequency within families but more commonly than in the general population, suggesting a polygenic or multifactorial inheritance. In primary open-angle glaucoma, family history information may aid in defining the relative risk in other family members and can provide information that is helpful in managing patients clinically. In contrast, certain types of glaucoma show no hereditary influence, and these patients may be informed that there is no increased risk in relatives.

■ Glaucomas with Mendelian Inheritance

Patients with aniridia may develop glaucoma, rarely early in life but usually in the preadolescent or adult years [1]. Developmental anomalies of the angle can occur or, more commonly, narrow-angle glaucoma can develop by progressive apposition of the rudimentary iris stump to the trabecular meshwork. The incidence of glaucoma in aniridia ranges from 6% to 75% in clinical studies [2]. There are several known patterns of inheritance of aniridia [3]. In the majority (approximately 85%) of patients, aniridia is inherited as an autosomal dominant trait, with complete penetrance and variable expressivity. Approximately 13% of patients have a sporadic form of aniridia that is associated with Wilms' tumor, genitourinary abnormalities, and mental retardation. This sporadic form of aniridia is frequently the result of a deletion on chromosome 11. Two percent of patients affected with aniridia have an autosomal recessive form that is associated with cerebellar ataxia and mental retardation. In the more common autosomal dominant form of aniridia, two-thirds of the patients have an affected parent (familial); the remaining one-third of cases are the result of new mutations.

Neurofibromatosis is inherited as an autosomal dominant trait with variable expressivity. Glaucoma can occur occasionally in patients with neurofibromatosis, usually in infancy or childhood. Typically, the glaucoma is unilateral and is associated with a plexiform neuroma of the upper eyelid. An association with congenital ectropion uveae has been reported [4, 5]. Various mechanisms of glaucoma can occur with neurofibromatosis, including anterior chamber angle developmental anomalies, infiltration of the angle by neurofibroma, or secondary angle closure, possibly due to neurofibromatous involvement of the choroid or ciliary body [6].

Angiomatosis retinae (von Hippel-Lindau syndrome) can be inherited as an autosomal dominant trait with incomplete penetrance. If untreated or unresponsive to treatment, the retinal angiomas may lead to exudative retinal detachment and secondary neovascular glaucoma.

In the Klippel-Trenaunay-Weber syndrome (irregular dominant inheritance), patients rarely develop glaucoma, and those who do usually have an associated facial nevus flammeus. Patients with Sturge-Weber syndrome often develop glaucoma, but this disorder does not appear to be hereditary. Other phakomatoses are rarely associated with glaucoma.

Approximately half of patients with the Axenfeld-Rieger syndrome may develop glaucoma, usually in childhood or young adulthood [7]. Although some cases are sporadic, most patients have a family history of the disorder, with an autosomal dominant pattern of inheritance. Axenfeld-Rieger syndrome should be distinguished from familial hypoplasia of the iris, which is an autosomal dominant congenital anomaly that may be associated with juvenile-onset glaucoma [8].

Oculodentodigital dysplasia (known also as *Meyer-Schwickerath and Weyers syndrome* and as *microphthalmos syndrome*) is a rare autosomal dominant condition that includes hypoplastic dental enamel, syndactyly, microphthalmos, microcornea, and glaucoma [9]. Various etiologies of glaucoma have been described in this disorder, including congenital angle anomalies [9], narrow-angle glaucoma [10], and adult-onset open-angle glaucoma [11].

Congenital microcoria is a rare autosomal dominant disorder in which there is maldevelopment of the iris dilator. In this disorder, the glaucoma is usually associated with goniodysgenesis [12, 13], although narrow-angle glaucoma has been reported [14]. Autosomal dominant microcoria associated with megalocornea and congenital glaucoma has also been described [15].

Glaucoma occurs in approximately 13% of patients with posterior polymorphous dystrophy, which is inherited in an autosomal dominant pattern with variable expression [16]. The glaucoma in posterior polymorphous dystrophy can be adult open-angle, adult narrow-angle, or juvenile [17–20].

Autosomal dominant open-angle glaucoma has also been reported in association with microcornea and absence of frontal sinuses [21]. Familial histiocytic dermatoarthritis is a rare autosomal dominant disorder manifesting histiocytic skin nodules, arthritis (hands and wrists especially), cataracts, uveitis, and glaucoma [22]. In this disorder, it is unclear whether the glaucoma is primary or secondary to the uveitis. Osteogenesis imperfecta is usually autosomal dominantly inherited and may be associated with open-angle glaucoma, generally developing in the first or second decade of life [23, 24].

Stickler's syndrome is an autosomal dominant connective tissue disorder characterized by ocular and generalized skeletal abnormalities and by orofacial anomalies that overlap with the Pierre Robin syndrome [25]. Patients with Stickler's syndrome may have high myopia, cataracts, vitreoretinal degeneration, retinal detachment, and glaucoma [25, 26]. Stickler's syndrome may be associated with open-angle glaucoma or neovascular glaucoma, related to chronic retinal detachment [27, 28].

A large pedigree of autosomal dominant neovascular inflammatory vitreoretinopathy has been described [29]. In this disorder, patients develop vitreous cells and selective loss of the B-wave on the electroretinogram early in adulthood. Later, pigmentary retinopathy, neovascularization of the retina or optic disc, cystoid macular edema, vitreous hemorrhage, tractional retinal detachment, and neovascular glaucoma (in half of the patients older than 60 years) can cause profound visual loss. This disorder can be classified with other autosomal dominantly inherited vitreoretinal dystrophies [29] that may be associated with secondary glaucoma.

Autosomal dominant pedigrees of primary juvenile open-angle glaucoma have been described (Fig 1). This type of glaucoma affects individuals in the first and second decades of life. Affected patients develop a severe high-pressure glaucoma that is rapidly progressive [30]. Gonioscopy of affected individuals demonstrates normal angle structures without excessive pigmentation or an increased number of iris processes [31]. Although an asymptomatic carrier state has not been identified, this disease is inherited as an autosomal dominant trait with high penetrance [32–36; also JL Wiggs and colleagues, unpublished report, 1992].

Ectopia lentis is frequently associated with glaucoma and may occur with or without systemic predisposing factors. Simple ectopia lentis is usually autosomal dominantly inherited and is characterized by spontaneous onset, normal pupils, frequent association with secondary glaucoma, and absence of systemic or ocular factors predisposing to lens dislocation [37, 38]. Although the age of onset may be during childhood, several pedigrees

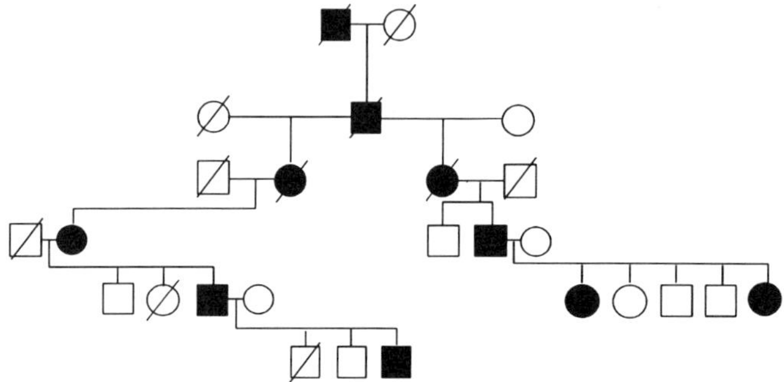

Figure 1 *Pedigree of a six-generation family affected with autosomal dominant juvenile open-angle glaucoma. Affected individuals are represented by the solid circles (female) or squares (male). Circles or squares crossed with a line represent deceased individuals.*

have been reported in which lens dislocation occurs between 20 and 70 years of age, known as genetic spontaneous late subluxation of the lens [39, 40].

Marfan's syndrome is an autosomal dominant disorder with high penetrance that is associated with lens dislocation in up to 80% of patients [41]. In Marfan's syndrome, glaucoma occurs in approximately 8% of eyes with ectopic lenses. Approximately one-third of these cases are caused by pupillary block and the remaining two-thirds are the result of other phacogenic mechanisms [42].

Weill-Marchesani syndrome is characterized by brachymorphia, brachydactyly, and microspherophakia, and may be associated with secondary glaucoma. Inheritance of Weill-Marchesani syndrome is usually autosomal recessive, but dominant inheritance has been described [43, 44].

Homocystinuria is an autosomal recessive disorder that is characterized by increased concentrations of homocystine in the blood and urine. Lens dislocation occurs in up to 90% of cases, and up to one-fourth of the patients with ectopia lentis develop secondary glaucoma [42].

Ectopia lentis et pupillae is an autosomal recessive, bilateral disorder in which the lenses and pupils are displaced in opposite directions, and it may be associated with secondary glaucoma [45, 46].

Zellweger's (cerebrohepatorenal) syndrome is a rare autosomal recessive disorder in which patients have cerebral dysgenesis, hepatic dysfunction, and polycystic kidneys, with death often occurring in the first year of life. Ocular findings in Zellweger's syndrome include cataracts with a prominent Y suture, corneal clouding, pigmentary retinopathy, optic atrophy, microphthalmos, and glaucoma; iridocorneal adhesions and angle closure were also documented in 1 case [47, 48].

Although glaucoma is uncommon in the mucopolysaccharidoses, it has been reported in several cases of autosomal recessively inherited Morquio's syndrome [49]. Glaucoma has also been reported in association with Hurler's syndrome [50] and Hunter's syndrome [51], which are autosomal recessive and X-linked recessive, respectively. Nanophthalmos may be sporadic, dominant, or recessive, and may be associated with narrow-angle glaucoma. Nanophthalmos with progressive retinal pigmentary degeneration and narrow-angle glaucoma has been reported in autosomal recessive and autosomal dominant pedigrees [52, 53]. The Walker-Warburg syndrome is a lethal, autosomal recessive disorder characterized by lissencephaly (agenesis of cerebral gyrations), cerebellar malformations, and ocular abnormalities, which include microphthalmos, retinal detachment, and glaucoma [54, 55]. Although cystinosis has been reported in association with pupillary block glaucoma [56], this is an uncommon manifestation of this rare autosomal recessive disorder.

The oculocerebrorenal syndrome of Lowe is an X-chromosome-linked recessive disorder characterized by congenital cataracts, renal tubular dysfunction, and mental retardation [57]. The majority of patients develop glaucoma, which may be due to angle abnormalities or secondary to microphakia [58–60]. Although patients may live to young adulthood, the prognosis is poor; there is reduced life expectancy and severe mental retardation. Female carriers can be identified by characteristic punctate, white to gray cortical lens opacities [61]. The gene for Lowe's syndrome has been localized to the distal long arm of the X chromosome at Xq24-q26 [62–64]. Linkage analysis has shown that some probes are tightly linked to the disease gene, which is promising for carrier assessment and prenatal diagnosis [65, 66].

Disorders that are associated with glaucoma and have a mendelian inheritance pattern are listed in Table 1. As in the mendelian disorders, a strong genetic influence is apparent in congenital syndromes with known chromosomal abnormalities. Glaucoma may be associated with certain chromosomal abnormalities, including partial trisomy 3q, trisomy 18 syndrome (Edward's syndrome), and partial deletion syndromes of chromosome 18 [67, 68]. Although usually fatal in the first few months of life, trisomy 13 may involve congenital glaucoma. Glaucoma has also been reported in trisomy 21 (Down's syndrome), Turner's syndrome, and ring chromosome 6 syndrome [68]. When glaucoma occurs in association with chromosomal abnormalities, it is usually (but not always) due to anterior chamber angle dysgenesis.

■ Glaucomas with Polygenic or Multifactorial Inheritance

Polygenic inheritance results from the influence of multiple genes with small, additive, but individually indeterminate effects. The term *multifactorial inheritance* implies that a combination of genetic and environmental

Table 1 *Disorders Associated with Glaucoma and Having a Mendelian Inheritance Pattern*

Disorder	Inheritance Pattern
Aniridia	Autosomal dominant[a]
Neurofibromatosis	Autosomal dominant
von Hippel-Lindau syndrome	Autosomal dominant
Axenfeld-Rieger syndrome	Autosomal dominant[b]
Familial hypoplasia of the iris	Autosomal dominant
Oculodentodigital dysplasia	Autosomal dominant
Familial microcoria	Autosomal dominant
Posterior polymorphous dystrophy	Autosomal dominant
Microcornea and absence of frontal sinuses	Autosomal dominant
Familial histiocytic dermatoarthritis	Autosomal dominant
Osteogenesis imperfecta	Autosomal dominant[b]
Stickler's syndrome	Autosomal dominant
Neovascular inflammatory vitreoretinopathy	Autosomal dominant
Juvenile glaucoma	Autosomal dominant[b]
Ectopia lentis	
Simple ectopia lentis	Autosomal dominant
Marfan's syndrome	Autosomal dominant
Weill-Marchesani syndrome	Autosomal recessive[c]
Homocystinuria	Autosomal recessive
Ectopia lentis et pupillae	Autosomal recessive
Zellweger's syndrome	Autosomal recessive
Morquio's syndrome	Autosomal recessive
Hurler's syndrome	Autosomal recessive
Nanophthalmos with retinal degeneration	Autosomal recessive[c]
Walker-Warburg syndrome	Autosomal recessive
Cystinosis	Autosomal recessive
Hunter's syndrome	X-linked recessive
Lowe's syndrome	X-linked recessive

[a]Aniridia may also be associated with a deletion on chromosome 11 or an autosomal recessive inheritance pattern.
[b]Some cases are sporadic.
[c]Autosomal dominant inheritance has also been described.

factors are responsible for a disease but does not specify the nature of the genetic influence. Some common polygenic or multifactorial traits include cleft lip and palate, schizophrenia, rheumatoid arthritis, ischemic heart disease, pyloric stenosis, and refractive errors [69].

In polygenic and multifactorial inheritance, there is a higher risk of the disorder among relatives of the affected person compared with the general population. Usually, the risk is approximately 3% to 5% for first-degree relatives and approximately half that much for second-degree relatives. The risk increases with increasing numbers of affected relatives and with increased severity of the trait. If individuals of the affected person's gender are less usually affected, there is increased risk in relatives.

Hereditary Patterns in Primary Open-Angle Glaucoma

Primary open-angle glaucoma is not inherited according to simple mendelian predictions. However, most studies suggest that relatives of patients affected with glaucoma have a higher risk of developing the disease than does the general population [70]. Because there is no definite role of environmental influences in the etiology of glaucoma, a multifactorial or polygenic mechanism is probable.

Twin studies have demonstrated some genetic influences in primary open-angle glaucoma. Teikari [71] reported the results of the Finnish twin cohort study, which is the largest population-based study of twins and chronic open-angle glaucoma. In this study population, there were 29 monozygotic and 79 dizygotic twin pairs, of which 3 monozygotic and 3 dizygotic pairs were concordant for chronic open-angle glaucoma, whereas 26 monozygotic and 76 dizygotic pairs were discordant. This degree of concordance is consistent with polygenic or multifactorial inheritance. For comparison, the degree of concordance was less than that for schizophrenia, cleft lip and palate, essential hypertension, and peptic ulcer. Individual case reports and similar studies of twins affected with open-angle glaucoma have also demonstrated a similar percentage of concordance for primary open-angle glaucoma [71, 72].

Family studies have provided further information about the genetic influences in primary open-angle glaucoma. An increased prevalence of glaucoma was seen in close relatives of patients affected with open-angle glaucoma, ranging from 2.8% to 13.5% [73–81], with a median prevalence of approximately 6%. Because the prevalence of glaucoma in the white adult population is nearly 1% to 2% [82], the prevalence of glaucoma in close relatives of affected patients was approximately three to six times that of the general population. The incidence of new cases of glaucoma in first-degree relatives has been reported as 2.7% over 10 years, which is two and a half times that found in the general population [78]. Others have reported a three to five times higher incidence of primary open-angle glaucoma among first-degree relatives of patients with primary open-angle glaucoma compared with the general population [73, 74]. The higher prevalence of primary open-angle glaucoma among black Americans compared with white Americans may reflect an underlying genetic difference in susceptibility to this disease [82]. Although pedigrees of autosomal dominant primary open-angle glaucoma have been reported [83], these are rare and usually represent juvenile glaucoma. In nearly all cases, the familial pattern of primary open-angle glaucoma is consistent with a polygenic or multifactorial inheritance.

The ocular characteristics associated with glaucoma have been found in moderate familial patterns. In case-control studies, elevated intraocular pressure is markedly more likely in individuals with a family history of primary open-angle glaucoma compared with the general population [84, 85]. Intraocular pressure has been significantly correlated among close relatives [76, 77, 86, 87], the correlation coefficient in parent-offspring pairs being 0.3 to 0.49 and in sibling-sibling pairs 0.25 to 0.47 [88]. Although similarities in intraocular pressure in husband-wife pairs may suggest a role for environmental factors [89], Armaly [90] found that the intraocular pressure of spouses of patients with primary open-angle glaucoma does not differ markedly from the general population. Facility of outflow has a correlation coefficient of 0.30 to 0.36 in sibling pairs, suggesting a genetic influence [87], and other studies have found a higher prevalence of decreased outflow facility among close relatives [76–78].

Similarities in cup-to-disc ratio among first-degree relatives have been demonstrated in several studies [70, 91], as have similarities in other ocular dimensions [92]. Clinically, it can be helpful to compare optic nerve contour between patients and their relatives, such as when distinguishing low-tension glaucoma from a familial tendency toward large optic nerve cups. We examined stereophotographs of the optic nerve head of 25 pairs of primary relatives followed on the Glaucoma Consultation Service at the Massachusetts Eye and Ear Infirmary. In masked comparisons, we found that 8 pairs (32%) showed marked similarities in cup-to-disc ratio and optic nerve contour (Fig 2).

Although potentially helpful in detecting patients at risk and in facilitating gene studies, the search for traits genetically linked to primary open-angle glaucoma has not been rewarding. A relationship of glaucoma to increased intraocular pressure in response to steroids has been suggested, but this hypothesis has not been supported by twin and other studies [93, 94]. An association of diabetes mellitus and glaucoma has been proposed [95], but this relationship is likely to be multifactorial and does not necessarily represent genetically linked traits. There is no known association of histocompatibility antigens or blood markers [70, 96, 97]. An interesting observation has been reported regarding the inability of glaucoma patients to taste phenylthiocarbamide (PTC). In the normal population, approximately 30% of subjects do not taste PTC (black populations have a lower prevalence of nontasters). In one study, 53% of primary open-angle glaucoma patients were nontasters, whereas 17% of narrow-angle glaucoma patients were nontasters [98]. However, this association has not been consistently reproducible in other populations [99].

Figure 2 *Similarities of optic nerve appearance in primary relatives. The optic nerve pairs shown are from (A) a mother and (B) son, (C) a father and (D) daughter, (E) a father and (F) son, and (G,H) a pair of brothers. The black spot that appears on the disc in A and B are artifacts.*

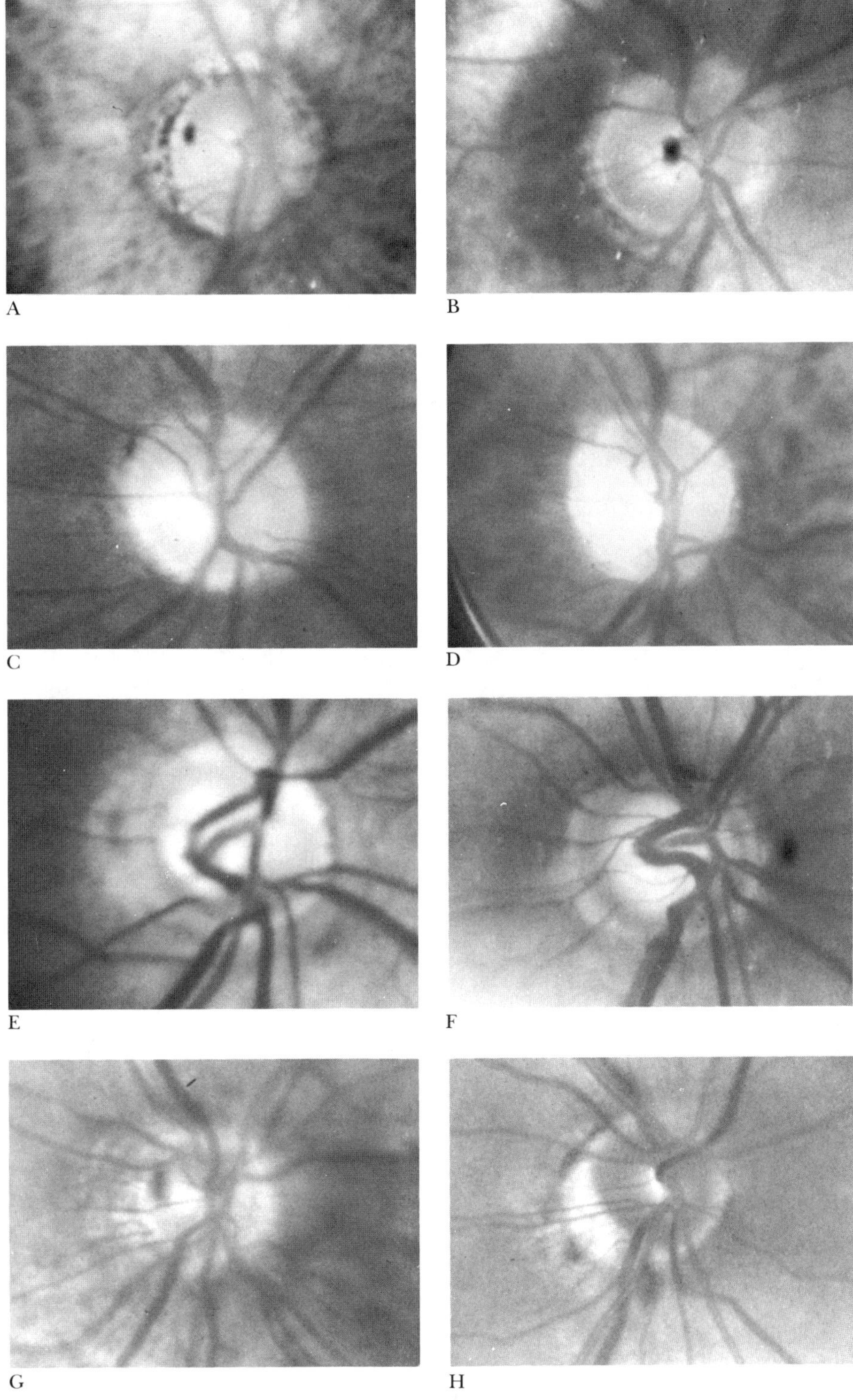

A
B
C
D
E
F
G
H

Current research is directed toward the isolation of genetic markers from the gene(s) responsible for hereditary types of glaucomas. Many of these hereditary glaucomas affect the pediatric age group, and often the diagnosis of glaucoma is not made until after the patient has sustained permanent damage to the optic nerve. A DNA-based diagnostic test that would identify individuals at risk for hereditary glaucoma at premorbid stages of the disease before any damage to the eye has occurred would be extremely valuable. Finding a genetic marker that is linked to the disease trait in affected patients would lead to the prompt development of such a DNA test.

Hereditary Patterns in Narrow-Angle Glaucoma

Inheritance of narrow-angle glaucoma is probably polygenic or multifactorial. Ocular characteristics related to narrow-angle glaucoma are more common in close relatives of affected patients than in the general population; these characteristics include anterior position of the lens, increased lens thickness, and a shallow anterior chamber [100–105]. Estimates of the prevalence of primary narrow-angle glaucoma among first-degree relatives in the white population have ranged from 1% to 12%, which is higher than the 0.1% prevalence in the general population [76, 100, 101, 106–109]. There are also racial differences, with a higher prevalence among Eskimos (2% to 8%) and Asians (0.3% to 1.4%) compared to whites (0.1%), suggesting a genetic predisposition to this disorder [110]. First-degree relatives of Eskimos with primary narrow-angle glaucoma have a three and a half times greater risk of developing the disorder compared with the general Eskimo population [111]. In the white population, François [105] identified a 2% to 5% risk in first-degree relatives and a 1% to 2.5% risk in second-degree relatives, which is consistent with polygenic or multifactorial inheritance. Monogenetically inherited diseases show 100% concordance in monozygotic twins. In the Finnish twin cohort study, 2 monozygotic pairs were concordant for angle-closure glaucoma, 5 monozygotic pairs were discordant, and 13 dizygotic pairs were discordant, which supports polygenic or multifactorial inheritance of angle-closure glaucoma [112].

Other Glaucomas with Polygenic or Multifactorial Inheritance

In primary congenital glaucoma, there is a 3% to 5% risk of congenital glaucoma in siblings, suggesting a polygenic or multifactorial inheritance [113, 114]. However, approximately 10% of the cases are found in a hereditary pattern, usually autosomal recessive with variable penetrance [115–117]. François found a high rate of concordance among monozygotic twin pairs, suggesting monogenetic inheritance in these families [118].

In low-tension glaucoma, there is a low risk of the disorder among

Table 2 *Glaucomas with Polygenic or Multifactorial Inheritance*

Primary open-angle glaucoma
Narrow-angle glaucoma
Primary congenital glaucoma[a]
Low-tension glaucoma[b]

[a]Hereditary patterns have been described, usually autosomal recessive.
[b]Autosomal dominant pedigrees have been reported.

close relatives, although the risk is higher than that of the general population, suggesting a polygenic or multifactorial mode of inheritance [119]. A rare autosomal dominant form of low-tension glaucoma has been reported in two pedigrees [120, 121].

Most primary glaucomas appear to follow a polygenic or multifactorial inheritance pattern (Table 2), with the exception of autosomal dominant juvenile glaucoma. It is likely that genetic factors will play an important role in many of these glaucomas but that environmental factors are also important. More research directed toward the genetic origin of these conditions is indicated in an effort to define better their genetic basis.

Glaucomas with Reported Clusters of Cases in Families

Although they are probably sporadic, polygenic, or multifactorial, certain types of glaucoma have been reported to occur in several family members in some affected pedigrees (Table 3). Fuchs' heterochromic iridocyclitis has been observed in families and twins [122]. Pigmentary glaucoma has been reported in families [115, 123, 124] and has appeared in pedigrees with a possible autosomal recessive [125] or dominant [126, 127] inheritance. Pseudoexfoliation syndrome may occur in high prevalence in Scandinavian, Greek, and other populations, suggesting a genetic predis-

Table 3 *Glaucomas with Reported Clusters of Cases in Families*

Fuchs' heterochromic iridocyclitis
Pigment dispersion syndrome
Pseudoexfoliation syndrome
Peters' anomaly
Idiopathic elevated episcleral venous pressure
Keratoderma
Sclerocornea

position to this disorder [128–130]. Pseudoexfoliation has been reported in first-degree relatives of affected patients [131, 132], and an autosomal dominant mode of inheritance with varying penetrance has been suggested [133]. Although there may be a higher prevalence of pseudoexfoliation in close relatives of affected patients [134, 135], there is usually no clear pattern of inheritance. In Peters' anomaly, infantile or juvenile glaucoma may occur in approximately half of patients, or glaucoma may occur as a late complication after penetrating keratoplasty [136, 137]. Peters' anomaly is usually sporadic; however, clusters of cases in some affected pedigrees have suggested autosomal recessive inheritance [138–140] or autosomal dominant inheritance with reduced penetrance [141–143]. Idiopathic elevated episcleral venous pressure with glaucoma is usually sporadic, but a familial pattern has been reported [144]. Familial keratoderma associated with congenital glaucoma also has been described [145]. Although most cases are sporadic, autosomal dominant and recessive inheritance of sclerocornea has been reported [146–148].

■ Glaucomas with No Apparent Genetic Influence

There is no apparent genetic influence in certain glaucomas (Table 4). Knowledge of family history is not helpful in posttraumatic glaucomas. Similarly, there is no genetic pattern in postsurgical glaucomas, such as malignant glaucoma, epithelial ingrowth, or glaucoma associated with aphakia, penetrating keratoplasty, or scleral buckling. Also, uveitic glaucoma, lens-induced glaucoma, Schwartz's syndrome, and neovascular glaucoma have no known hereditary influence. Certain congenital ocular disor-

Table 4 *Glaucomas with No Genetic Influence*

Posttraumatic glaucomas
Postsurgical glaucomas
Uveitic glaucoma
Lens-induced glaucoma
Schwartz's syndrome
Neovascular glaucoma
Sturge-Weber syndrome
Cutis marmorata telangiectasia congenita
Rubinstein-Taybi syndrome
Krause's syndrome
Congenital rubella with glaucoma
Congenital ectropion uveae
Persistent hyperplastic primary vitreous
Congenital microcornea

ders with glaucoma have no hereditary pattern, including congenital ectropion uveae [5, 149], congenital corneal staphyloma, cornea plana, iridoschisis, persistent hyperplastic primary vitreous, microphthalmos, and microcornea. Congenital ectropion uveae, which is nearly always associated with glaucoma, may occur as an isolated defect or may be associated with neurofibromatosis, Prader-Willi syndrome, or other abnormalities [4, 5, 149]. Rubinstein-Taybi syndrome [150–152], Sturge-Weber syndrome, cutis marmorata telangiectasia congenita [153–155], nevus of Ota, and Krause's syndrome (mental retardation with cerebral dysplasia or hydrocephaly) may be associated with glaucoma and are nonhereditary. Likewise, congenital rubella with cataract and glaucoma is not hereditary.

■ Genetic Counseling for Glaucoma Patients

Genetic counseling for glaucoma patients usually includes providing information about the risks of glaucoma in children and other close relatives. It is the physician's responsibility to inform patients and their relatives of the risk of developing the disease and the implications of the disease for their health. Also, patients must be informed of the need for early, regular monitoring in potentially affected offspring. Rarely, glaucoma patients in their reproductive years may make reproductive decisions based on information from the physician. Some disorders associated with glaucoma in which genetic counseling may have an important role are listed in Table 1. In particular, there have been promising developments in understanding the genetics of Lowe's syndrome, which may have applications in carrier identification and prenatal diagnosis [62–66]. As the genes for other forms of glaucoma are identified, additional DNA-based diagnostic tests that can identify individuals at risk for developing these glaucomas will become available.

In the glaucomas associated with polygenic or multifactorial inheritance, the role for genetic counseling is less obvious than in glaucomas associated with disorders exhibiting mendelian inheritance. In many of these glaucomas, patients are past their reproductive years. However, affected patients should be informed of the low overall but higher-than-normal risk in relatives. Also, the family history may help identify relatives at risk and may help in managing individual clinical cases. In certain cases such as congenital glaucoma, patients may be reassured to know of the low risk of glaucoma in siblings or offspring.

Although patients with primary open-angle glaucoma are frequently in non-child-bearing age groups, a family history of primary open-angle glaucoma can help identify patients at risk for glaucoma and can help tailor individual therapy. For example, the clinician may observe a glaucoma suspect more closely if several of that patient's siblings are affected with severe primary open-angle glaucoma. Also, patients with primary open-angle glaucoma can be reassured of the small risk to first-degree relatives compared with the higher risk in, for example, autosomal dominant disorders.

■ References

1. Grant WM, Walton DS. Progressive changes in the angle in congenital aniridia, with development of glaucoma. Am J Ophthalmol 1974;78:842–847
2. Nelson LB, Spaeth GL, Norvinski TS, et al. Aniridia: a review. Surv Ophthalmol 1984;28:621–642
3. Hittner HM. Aniridia. In: Ritch R, Shields MB, Krupin T, eds. The glaucomas. St Louis: Mosby, 1989:869–884
4. Wolter JR, Butler RG. Pigment spots of the iris and ectropion uveae with glaucoma in neurofibromatosis. Am J Ophthalmol 1963;56:964–973
5. Ritch R, Forbes M, Hetherington J Jr, et al. Congenital ectropion uveae with glaucoma. Ophthalmology 1984;91:326–331
6. Grant WM, Walton DS. Distinctive gonioscopic findings in glaucoma due to neurofibromatosis. Arch Ophthalmol 1968;79:127–134
7. Shields MB. Axenfeld-Rieger syndrome: a theory of mechanism and distinctions from the iridocorneal endothelial syndrome. Trans Am Ophthalmol Soc 1983;81:736–784
8. Jerndal T. Goniodysgenesis and hereditary juvenile glaucoma. Acta Ophthalmol (Copenh) 1970;suppl 107:1–100
9. Judisch GF, Martin-Casals A, Hanson JW, Olin WH. Oculodentodigital dysplasia: four new reports and a literature review. Arch Ophthalmol 1979;97:878–884
10. Sugar HS. Oculodentodigital dysplasia syndrome with angle-closure glaucoma. Am J Ophthalmol 1978;86:36–38
11. Dudgeon J, Chisolm IA. Oculo-dento-digital dysplasia. Trans Ophthalmol Soc UK 1974;94:203–210
12. Tawara A, Inomata H. Familial cases of congenital microcoria associated with late onset congenital glaucoma and goniodysgenesis. Jpn J Ophthalmol 1983;27:63–72
13. Mazzeo V, Gaiba G, Rossi A. Hereditary cases of congenital microcoria and goniodysgenesis. Ophthalmic Paediatr Genet 1986;7:121–125
14. Hyams SW, Neumann E. Congenital microcoria and combined mechanism glaucoma. Am J Ophthalmol 1969;68:326–327
15. Pearce WG. Autosomal dominant megalocornea with congenital glaucoma: evidence for germ-line mosaicism. Can J Ophthalmol 1991;26:21–26
16. Rodrigues MM, Phelps CD, Krachmer JH, et al. Glaucoma due to endothelialization of the anterior chamber angle: a comparison of posterior polymorphous dystrophy of the cornea and Chandler's syndrome. Arch Ophthalmol 1980;98:688–696
17. Cibis GW, Krachmer JH, Phelps CD, Weingeist TA. The clinical spectrum of posterior polymorphous dystrophy. Arch Ophthalmol 1977;95:1529–1537
18. Pratt AW, Saheb NE, Leblanc R. Posterior polymorphous corneal dystrophy and juvenile glaucoma: a case report and brief review of the literature. Can J Ophthalmol 1976;11:180–185
19. Krachmer JH. Posterior polymorphous corneal dystrophy: a disease characterized by epithelial-like endothelial cells which influence management and prognosis. Trans Am Ophthalmol Soc 1985;83:413–475
20. Bourgeois J, Shields MB, Thresher R. Open-angle glaucoma associated with posterior polymorphous dystrophy: a clinicopathologic study. Ophthalmology 1984;91:420–423

21. Holmes LB, Walton DS. Hereditary microcornea, glaucoma, and absent frontal sinuses: a family study. J Pediatr 1969;74:968–972
22. Zayid I, Farraj S. Familial histiocytic dermatoarthritis: a new syndrome. Am J Med 1973;54:793–800
23. Buyse M, Bull MJ. A syndrome of osteogenesis imperfecta, microcephaly, and cataracts. Birth Defects 1978;14:95–98
24. Ruedemann AD Jr. Osteogenesis imperfecta congenita and blue sclerotics: a clinicopathologic study. Arch Ophthalmol 1953;49:6–16
25. Blair NP, Albert DM, Liberfarb RM, Hirose T. Hereditary progressive arthro-ophthalmopathy of Stickler. Am J Ophthalmol 1979;88:876–888
26. Stickler GB, Belau PG, Farrell FJ, et al. Hereditary progressive arthro-ophthalmopathy. Mayo Clin Proc 1965;40:433–455
27. Phelps CD. Glaucoma associated with retinal disorders. In: Ritch R, Shields MB, eds. The secondary glaucomas. St Louis: Mosby, 1982:150–161
28. Young NJA, Hitchings RA, Sehmi K, Bird AC. Stickler's syndrome and neovascular glaucoma. Br J Ophthalmol 1979;63:826–831
29. Bennett SR, Folk JC, Kimura AE, et al. Autosomal dominant neovascular inflammatory vitreoretinopathy. Ophthalmology 1990;97:1125–1136
30. Walton DS. Juvenile open-angle glaucoma. In: Epstein DL, ed. Chandler and Grant's glaucoma, ed 3. Philadelphia: Lea & Febiger, 1986:528–529
31. Courtney RH, Hill E. Hereditary juvenile glaucoma simplex. JAMA 1931;97:1602–1609
32. Johnson AT, Stone EM, Cannon RL, Alward WLM. Autosomal dominant juvenile glaucoma in a six-generation family. Invest Ophthalmol Vis Sci 1991;32:813
33. Dorozynski A. Privacy rules blindside French glaucoma effort. Science 1991;252:369–370
34. Crombie AL, Cullen JF. Hereditary glaucoma occurrence in five generations of an Edinburgh family. Br J Ophthalmol 1964;48:143–147
35. Martin JP, Zorab EC. Familial glaucoma in nine generations of a South Hampshire family. Br J Ophthalmol 1974;58:536–542
36. Lee DA, Brubaker RF, Hruska L. Hereditary glaucoma: a report of two pedigrees. Ann Ophthalmol 1985;17:739–741
37. Casper DS, Simon JW, Nelson LB, et al. Familial simple ectopia lentis: a case study. J Pediatr Ophthalmol Strabismus 1985;22:227–228
38. Falls HF, Cotterman CW. Genetic studies on ectopia lentis: a pedigree of simple ectopia of the lens. Arch Ophthalmol 1943;30:610–620
39. McCulloch C. Hereditary lens dislocation with angle closure glaucoma. Can J Ophthalmol 1979;14:230–234
40. Malbran ES, Croxatto JO, D'Alessandro C, Charles DE. Genetic spontaneous late subluxation of the lens. Ophthalmology 1989;96:223–229
41. Cross HE. Ectopia lentis in systemic heritable disorders. Birth Defects 1974;10:113–119
42. Cross HE, Jensen AD. Ocular manifestations in the Marfan syndrome and homocystinuria. Am J Ophthalmol 1973;75:405–420
43. Rosenthal JW, Kloepfer HW. The spherophakia-brachymorphia syndrome. Arch Ophthalmol 1956;55:28–35
44. Young ID, Fielder AR, Casey TA. Weill-Marchesani syndrome in mother and son. Clin Genet 1986;30:475–480
45. Cross HE. Ectopia lentis et pupillae. Am J Ophthalmol 1979;88:381–384
46. Townes PL. Ectopia lentis et pupillae. Arch Ophthalmol 1976;94:1126–1128
47. Haddad R, Font RL, Friendly DS. Cerebro-hepato-renal syndrome of Zellweger: ocular histopathologic findings. Arch Ophthalmol 1976;94:1927–1930
48. Stanescu B, Dralands L. Cerebro-hepato-renal (Zellweger's) syndrome: ocular involvement. Arch Ophthalmol 1972;87:590–592

49. Cahane M, Treister G, Abraham FA, Melamed S. Glaucoma in siblings with Morquio syndrome. Br J Ophthalmol 1990;74:382–383
50. Spellacy E, Bankes JLK, Crow J, et al. Glaucoma in a case of Hurler disease. Br J Ophthalmol 1980;64:773–778
51. Kaiden JS, Schechter R, Bader BF, Podos SM. Angle-closure glaucoma in a patient with Hunter's syndrome. J Ocul Ther Surg 1982;1:250–252
52. MacKay CJ, Shek MS, Carr RE, et al. Retinal degeneration with nanophthalmos, cystic macular degeneration, and angle closure glaucoma: a new recessive syndrome. Arch Ophthalmol 1987;105:366–371
53. Hermann P. Le syndrome microphtalmie-rétinite pigmentaire-glaucome. Arch Ophthalmol 1958;18:17–24
54. Gershoni-Baruch R, Mandel H, Miller B, et al. Walker-Warburg syndrome with microtia and absent auditory canals. Am J Med Genet 1990;37:87–91
55. Murphy KJ, PeBenito R, Storm RL, et al. Walker-Warburg syndrome: case report and literature review. Ophthalmic Paediatr Genet 1990;11:103–108
56. Wan WL, Minckler DS, Rao NA. Pupillary-block glaucoma associated with childhood cystinosis. Am J Ophthalmol 1986;101:700–705
57. Charnas LR, Bernardini I, Rader D, et al. Clinical and laboratory findings in the oculocerebrorenal syndrome of Lowe, with special reference to growth and renal function. N Engl J Med 1991;324:1318–1325
58. Walton DS. Congenital glaucoma associated with congenital cataract. In: Epstein DL, ed. Chandler and Grant's glaucoma, ed 3. Philadelphia: Lea & Febiger, 1986:515–517
59. Curtin VT, Joyce EE, Ballin N. Ocular pathology in the oculo-cerebro-renal syndrome of Lowe. Am J Ophthalmol 1967;64:533–543
60. Johnson BL, Hiles DA. Ocular pathology of Lowe's syndrome in a female infant. J Pediatr Ophthalmol 1976;13:204–210
61. Cibis GW, Waeltermann JM, Whitcraft CT, et al. Lenticular opacities in carriers of Lowe's syndrome. Ophthalmology 1986;93:1041–1045
62. Silver DN, Lewis RA, Nussbaum RL. Mapping the Lowe oculocerebrorenal syndrome to Xq24-q26 by use of restriction fragment length polymorphisms. J Clin Invest 1987;79:282–285
63. Wadelius C, Fagerholm P, Pettersson U, Annerén G. Lowe oculocerebrorenal syndrome: DNA-based linkage of the gene to Xq24-q26 using tightly linked flanking markers and the correlation to lens examination in carrier diagnosis. Am J Hum Genet 1989;44:241–247
64. Mueller OT, Hartsfield JK Jr, Gallardo LA, et al. Lowe oculocerebrorenal syndrome in a female with a balanced X;20 translocation: mapping of the X chromosome breakpoint. Am J Hum Genet 1991;49:804–810
65. Reilly DS, Lewis RA, Ledbetter DH, Nussbaum RL. Tightly linked flanking markers for the Lowe oculocerebrorenal syndrome, with application to carrier assessment. Am J Hum Genet 1988;42:748–755
66. Gazit E, Brand N, Harel Y, et al. Prenatal diagnosis of Lowe's syndrome: a case report with evidence of de novo mutation. Prenat Diagn 1990;10:257–260
67. Chrousos GA, O'Neill JF, Traboulsi EI, et al. Ocular findings in partial trisomy 3q: a case report and review of the literature. Ophthalmic Paediatr Genet 1988;9:127–130
68. Cantor LB. Glaucoma associated with congenital disorders. In: Ritch R, Shields MB, Krupin T, eds. The glaucomas. St Louis: Mosby, 1989:931–960
69. Carter CO. Multifactorial genetic disease. In: McCusick VA, Claiborne R, eds. Medical genetics. New York: HP Publishing, 1973:199–208
70. Teikari JM. Genetic influences in open-angle glaucoma. Int Ophthalmol Clin 1990;30:161–168

71. Teikari JM. Genetic factors in open-angle (simple and capsular) glaucoma: a population-based twin study. Acta Ophthalmol (Copenh) 1987;65:715–720

72. Goldschmidt E. The heredity of glaucoma. Acta Ophthalmol (Copenh) 1973; suppl 120:27–31

73. Miller SJH. Genetics of glaucoma and family studies. Trans Ophthalmol Soc UK 1978;98:290–292

74. Rosenthal AR, Perkins ES. Family studies in glaucoma. Br J Ophthalmol 1985; 69:664–667

75. Perkins ES. Family studies in glaucoma. Br J Ophthalmol 1974;58:529–535

76. Becker B, Kolker AE, Roth FD. Glaucoma family study. Am J Ophthalmol 1960;50:557–567

77. Davies TG. Tonographic survey of the close relatives of patients with chronic simple glaucoma. Br J Ophthalmol 1968;52:32–39

78. Paterson G. A nine-year follow-up of studies on first-degree relatives of patients with glaucoma simplex. Trans Ophthalmol Soc UK 1970;90:515–525

79. Jay B, Paterson G. The genetics of simple glaucoma. Trans Ophthalmol Soc UK 1970;90:161–171

80. François J, Heintz-De Bree C. Personal research on the heredity of chronic simple (open-angle) glaucoma. Am J Ophthalmol 1966;62:1067–1071

81. Kellerman L, Posner A. The value of heredity in the detection and study of glaucoma. Am J Ophthalmol 1955;40:681–685

82. Tielsch JM, Sommer A, Katz J, et al. Racial variations in the prevalence of primary open-angle glaucoma: the Baltimore eye survey. JAMA 1991;266:369–374

83. Kitsos G, Cote G, Psilas K. Un exemple d'hérédité dominante pour la transmission du glaucome primitif à angle ouvert dans une région du nord-ouest de la Grèce. J Fr Ophtalmol 1988;11:859–864

84. Wilson MR, Hertzmark E, Walker AM, et al. A case-control study of risk factors in open angle glaucoma. Arch Ophthalmol 1987;105:1066–1071

85. Seddon JM, Schwartz B, Flowerdew G. Case-control study of ocular hypertension. Arch Ophthalmol 1983;101:891–894

86. Levene RZ, Workman PL, Broder SW, et al. Heritability of ocular pressure in normal and suspect ranges. Arch Ophthalmol 1970;84:730–734

87. Armaly MF, Monstavicius BF, Sayegh RE. Ocular pressure and outflow facility in siblings. Arch Ophthalmol 1968;80:354–360

88. Armaly MF. The genetic determination of ocular pressure in the normal eye. Arch Ophthalmol 1967;78:187–192

89. Bengtsson B. Resemblance between tonometer readings on relatives and spouses. Acta Ophthalmol (Copenh) 1976;54:27–40

90. Armaly MF. Applanation pressure in husband-wife pairs. Am J Ophthalmol 1966;62:635–639

91. Armaly MF. Genetic determination of cup/disc ratio of the optic nerve. Arch Ophthalmol 1967;78:35–43

92. Tomlinson A, Leighton DA. Ocular dimensions and the heredity of open-angle glaucoma. Br J Ophthalmol 1974;58:68–74

93. Schwartz JT, Reuling FH, Feinleib M, et al. Twin study on ocular pressure following topically applied dexamethasone. Arch Ophthalmol 1973;90:281–286

94. Lewis JM, Priddy T, Judd J, et al. Intraocular pressure response to topical dexamethasone as a predictor for the development of primary open-angle glaucoma. Am J Ophthalmol 1988;106:607–612

95. Becker B. Diabetes mellitus and primary open-angle glaucoma. The XXVII Edward Jackson Memorial Lecture. Am J Ophthalmol 1971;71:1–16

96. Kass MA, Palmberg P, Becker B, Miller JP. Histocompatibility antigens and primary open-angle glaucoma. Arch Ophthalmol 1978;96:2207–2208

97. Ritch R, Podos SM, Henley W, et al. Lack of association of histocompatibility antigens with primary open-angle glaucoma. Arch Ophthalmol 1978;96:2204–2206

98. Becker B, Morton WR. Phenylthiourea taste testing and glaucoma. Arch Ophthalmol 1964;72:323–327

99. Kubickova Z, Kloucek F, Kraus H, Dvorakova M. ABO blood groups, secretory behavior and PTC testing of glaucoma patients. Klin Monatsbl Augenheilkd 1972;161:32–35

100. Lowe RF. Primary angle-closure glaucoma: family histories and anterior chamber depths. Br J Ophthalmol 1964;48:191–195

101. Lowe RF. Primary angle-closure glaucoma: inheritance and environment. Br J Ophthalmol 1972;56:13–20

102. Tornquist R. Chamber depth in primary acute glaucoma. Br J Ophthalmol 1956;40:421–429

103. Alsbirk PH. Anterior chamber depth, genes, and environment: a population study among long-term Greenland Eskimo immigrants in Copenhagen. Acta Ophthalmol (Copenh) 1982;60:223–234

104. Spaeth GL. Gonioscopy: uses old and new—the inheritance of occludable angles. Ophthalmology 1978;85:222–232

105. François J. Multifactorial or polygenic inheritance in ophthalmology. In: Henkind P, ed. Acta: 24th international congress of ophthalmology, 1982, vol 1. Philadelphia: Lippincott, 1983:1–24

106. Alsbirk PH. Anterior chamber depth and primary angle-closure glaucoma: II. A genetic study. Acta Ophthalmol (Copenh) 1975;53:436–449

107. Leighton DA. Survey of the first-degree relatives of glaucoma patients. Trans Ophthalmol Soc UK 1976;96:28–32

108. Lowe RF. Clinical types of primary angle closure glaucoma. Aust NZ J Ophthalmol 1988;16:245–250

109. Paterson G. Studies on siblings of patients with both angle-closure and chronic simple glaucoma. Trans Ophthalmol Soc UK 1961;81:561–576

110. Congdon N, Wang F, Tielsch JM. Issues in the epidemiology and population-based screening of primary angle-closure glaucoma. Surv Ophthalmol 1992;36:411–423

111. Alsbirk PH. Primary angle-closure glaucoma: oculometry, epidemiology and genetics in a high risk population. Acta Ophthalmol (Copenh) 1976;suppl 127:5–31

112. Teikari JM. Closed-angle glaucoma in 20 pairs of twins. Can J Ophthalmol 1988;23:14–16

113. Demenais F, Bonaiti C, Briard ML, et al. Congenital glaucoma genetic models. Hum Genet 1979;46:305–317

114. Jay MR, Rice NSC. Genetic implications of congenital glaucoma. Metab Ophthalmol 1978;2:257–258

115. Shaffer RN. Genetics and the congenital glaucomas. Trans Am Acad Ophthalmol Otolaryngol 1965;69:253–268

116. Westerlund E. On the heredity of congenital hydrophthalmus. Acta Ophthalmol (Copenh) 1944;21:330–348

117. Gencik A. Epidemiology and genetics of primary congenital glaucoma in Slovakia: description of a form of primary congenital glaucoma in gypsies with autosomal-recessive inheritance and complete penetrance. Dev Ophthalmol 1989;16:76–115

118. François J. Congenital glaucoma and its inheritance. Ophthalmologica 1980;181:61–73

119. Levene RZ. Low tension glaucoma: a critical review and new material. Surv Ophthalmol 1980;24:621–664

120. Sandvig K. Pseudoglaucoma of autosomal dominant inheritance: a report on three families. Acta Ophthalmol (Copenh) 1961;39:33–43

121. Bennett SR, Alward WLM, Folberg R. An autosomal dominant form of low-tension glaucoma. Am J Ophthalmol 1989;108:238–244

122. Makley TA Jr. Heterochromic cyclitis in identical twins. Am J Ophthalmol 1956;41:768–772

123. Kaiser-Kupfer MI, Kupfer C, McCain L. Asymmetric pigment dispersion syndrome. Trans Am Ophthalmol Soc 1983;81:310–324

124. Epstein DL. Chandler and Grant's glaucoma, ed 3. Philadelphia: Lea & Febiger, 1986:201–210

125. Stankovic I. Ein Beitrag zur Kenntnis der Vererbung des Pigmentglaukoms. Klin Monatsbl Augenheilkd 1961;139:165–174

126. Mandelkorn RM, Hoffman ME, Olander KW, et al. Inheritance and the pigmentary dispersion syndrome. Ophthalmic Paediatr Genet 1985;6:325–331

127. Roth A, Royer J, Jouary-Letoublon G, Noir A. L'hérédité du syndrome de dispersion pigmentaire. Bull Mem Soc Fr Ophtalmol 1977;89:211–218

128. Dell WM. The epidemiology of the pseudo-exfoliation syndrome. J Am Optom Assoc 1985;56:113–119

129. Forsius H. Prevalence of pseudoexfoliation of the lens in Finns, Lapps, Icelanders, Eskimos, and Russians. Trans Ophthalmol Soc UK 1979;99:296–298

130. Sugar HS, Harding C, Barsky D. The exfoliation syndrome. Ann Ophthalmol 1976;8:1165–1181

131. Gifford H Jr. A clinical and pathologic study of exfoliation of the lens capsule. Am J Ophthalmol 1958;46:508–524

132. Tarkkanen A, Voipio H, Koivusalo P. Family study of pseudoexfoliation and glaucoma. Acta Ophthalmol (Copenh) 1965;43:679–683

133. Tarkkanen HA. Exfoliation syndrome. Trans Ophthalmol Soc UK 1986;105:233–236

134. Aasved H. Study of relatives of persons with fibrillopathia epitheliocapsularis (pseudoexfoliation of the lens capsule). Acta Ophthalmol (Copenh) 1975;53:879–886

135. Pohjanpelta P, Hurskainen L. Studies on relatives of patients with glaucoma simplex and patients with pseudoexfoliation of the lens capsule. Acta Ophthalmol (Copenh) 1972;50:255–261

136. Waring GO III, Rodrigues MM, Laibson PR. Anterior chamber cleavage syndrome: a stepladder classification. Surv Ophthalmol 1975;20:3–27

137. Schanzlin DJ, Goldberg DB, Brown SI. Transplantation of congenitally opaque corneas. Ophthalmology 1980;87:1253–1264

138. Boel M, Timmermans J, Emmery L, et al. Primary mesodermal dysgenesis of the cornea (Peters' anomaly) in two brothers. Hum Genet 1979;51:237–240

139. Eggink CA, Mooy CM, Pinckers A. Peters' anomaly: an unusual case. Ophthalmic Paediatr Genet 1991;12:19–22

140. Tabuchi A, Matsuura M, Hirokawa M. Three siblings with Peters' anomaly. Ophthalmic Paediatr Genet 1985;5:233–240

141. Kresca LJ, Goldberg MF. Peters' anomaly: dominant inheritance in one pedigree and dextrocardia in another. J Pediatr Ophthalmol Strabismus 1978;15:141–146

142. Ferrell RE, Hittner HM, Kretzer FL, Antoszyk JH. Anterior segment mesenchymal dysgenesis: probable linkage to the MNS blood group on chromosome 4. Am J Hum Genet 1982;34:245–249

143. Hittner HM, Kretzer FL, Antoszyk JH, et al. Variable expressivity of autosomal dominant anterior segment mesenchymal dysgenesis in six generations. Am J Ophthalmol 1982;93:57–70

144. Minas TF, Podos SM. Familial glaucoma associated with elevated episcleral venous pressure. Arch Ophthalmol 1968;80:202–208

145. Slade MP, Brooks AMV, Gillies WE. Two cases of hereditary keratoderma with congenital glaucoma. Aust NZ J Ophthalmol 1989;17:445–450
146. Elliott JH, Feman SS, O'Day DM, Garber M. Hereditary sclerocornea. Arch Ophthalmol 1985;103:676–679
147. Howard RO, Abrahams IW. Sclerocornea. Am J Ophthalmol 1971;71:1254–1260
148. Goldstein JE, Cogan DG. Sclerocornea and associated congenital anomalies. Arch Ophthalmol 1962;67:761–768
149. Dowling JL Jr, Albert DM, Nelson LB, Walton DS. Primary glaucoma associated with iridotrabecular dysgenesis and ectropion uveae. Ophthalmology 1985;92:912–921
150. Shihab ZM. Pediatric glaucoma in Rubinstein-Taybi syndrome. Glaucoma 1984;6:288–290
151. Levy NS. Juvenile glaucoma in the Rubinstein-Taybi syndrome. J Pediatr Ophthalmol 1976;13:141–143
152. Ziring PR, Weiss DI, Cooper LZ. The association of congenital glaucoma with the Rubinstein-Taybi syndrome. J Pediatr Ophthalmol 1974;11:203–206
153. Sato SE, Herschler J, Lynch PJ, et al. Congenital glaucoma associated with cutis marmorata telangiectatica congenita: two case reports. J Pediatr Ophthalmol Strabismus 1988;25:13–17
154. Miranda I, Alonso MJ, Jiminez M, et al. Cutis marmorata telangiectatica congenita and glaucoma. Ophthalmic Paediatr Genet 1990;11:129–132
155. Mayatepek E, Krastel H, Völcker HE, et al. Congenital glaucoma in cutis marmorata telangiectatica congenita. Ophthalmologica 1991;202:191–193

Hereditary Primary Childhood Glaucomas

Cynthia Mattox, M.D.
David S. Walton, M.D.

■ Primary Forms of Childhood Glaucoma

Childhood glaucomas are associated with a variety of systemic and ocular conditions. To provide appropriate counseling and timely referrals and examinations for glaucoma and other ocular diseases, the ophthalmologist must know which conditions are and which are not associated with known patterns of inheritance. Tables 1 through 3 group the various conditions associated with glaucoma according to these inheritance patterns. In the primary childhood glaucomas, the conditions adequate for the development of glaucoma are present congenitally in association with the systemic syndrome or the ocular abnormality. Secondary childhood glaucomas usually arise from such things as trauma, lens dislocation, ocular tumor, uveitis, or neovascularization.

Primary Congenital Open-Angle Glaucoma

The occurrence of primary congenital open-angle glaucoma [1, 2] is sporadic, but evidence for autosomal recessive inheritance with variable penetrance does exist [1, 2]. Congenital glaucoma is usually recognized in the first 6 months of life. In 65% to 80% of patients, it is bilateral. It presents with an enlarged corneal diameter, increased intraocular pressure (IOP), and often a cloudy, edematous cornea from a break in Descemet's membrane. Buphthalmos, an enlarged globe, may result. The child may exhibit tearing and photophobia. The cause of the increased pressure is a decreased outflow facility from improper angle development. In the more distensible infantile eye, corneal enlargement and buphthalmos occur. With early lowering of the IOP, the corneal edema and optic nerve cupping may resolve, but the corneal enlargement is permanent. Treatment consists of surgical goniotomy or trabeculotomy, which relieves the outflow

Table 1 *Primary Childhood Glaucomas with Autosomal Dominant Inheritance*

Neurofibromatosis type 1
Juvenile glaucoma
Stickler syndrome
Oculodentodigital dysplasia
Open-angle glaucoma associated with microcornea and absent frontal sinuses
Osteogenesis imperfecta
Congenital microcoria
Aniridia
Sclerocornea
Familial hypoplasia of the iris
Axenfeld-Rieger syndrome
Posterior polymorphous dystrophy
Marfan's syndrome

obstruction. With early recognition and prompt surgical intervention, cure rates are 80% to 100%. If the condition is first recognized after age 2, the prognosis is worse.

Juvenile Glaucoma

The occurrence of juvenile glaucoma is sporadic, but autosomal dominant pedigrees exist [2]. The presentation resembles that of adult-onset open-angle glaucoma, only it presents in the first to third decade. Examination often reveals a normal-appearing open angle. Axial myopia may be more common among patients with juvenile-onset glaucoma than in age-matched controls. The high incidence of juvenile glaucoma in myopic black boys has been reported [3].

Table 2 *Primary Childhood Glaucomas with Autosomal Recessive or X-linked Inheritance*

Autosomal recessive
   Zellweger's (hepatocerebrorenal) syndrome
   Mucopolysaccharidosis (except MPS II)
   Cystinosis
   Warburg's syndrome
X-linked
   Lowe's (oculocerebrorenal) syndrome
   MPS II (Hunter's syndrome)

Table 3 *Primary Childhood Glaucomas Occurring Sporadically*

Primary congenital glaucoma

Juvenile glaucoma

Sturge-Weber syndrome

Rubinstein-Taybi syndrome

Chromosomal trisomies and deletions

Cutis marmorata telangiectasia congenita

Microcornea

Aniridia

Congenital ocular melanosis

Sclerocornea

Peter's anomaly

Iridogoniodysgenesis with ectropion uveae

Elevated episcleral venous pressure

Anterior corneal staphyloma

Congenital lens-iris-angle membrane

■ Childhood Glaucomas Associated with Systemic Abnormalities

Sturge-Weber Syndrome

The occurrence of Sturge-Weber syndrome is sporadic, and there is no sex predilection. Encephalotrigeminal angiomatosis consists of (1) a vascular nevus of the face, which is bilateral in 25% of cases; (2) seizures from leptomeningeal angiomas found ipsilateral to the skin lesion (calcium deposition is seen in the middle and outer cortical zones); (3) varying degrees of mental retardation; and (4) possible contralateral hemiparesis in one-third of cases. Thirty percent of Sturge-Weber patients develop glaucoma, 60% of these before age 2 and 40% at older ages. Upper eyelid involvement correlates with the incidence of glaucoma [4]. Abnormal angle structure or increased episcleral venous pressure may be responsible for the increased IOP [5].

Neurofibromatosis Type 1

The inheritance pattern of neurofibromatosis type 1 is autosomal dominant. Recently, the gene was located near the centromere on chromosome 17 [6]. A significant proportion of cases are due to mutations at a single locus. Neurofibromatosis type 2, the hallmark of which is bilateral acoustic neuromas, is more rare and has been linked to chromosome 22 [7].

The glaucoma mechanisms are related to the abnormal angle, which involves a high insertion of the iris stromal tissue over the trabecular meshwork. When plexiform neuromas of the eyelid are present, they are accompanied by ipsilateral glaucoma in approximately 50% of cases [8]. Iris nodules, also known as *Lisch nodules,* may suggest the diagnosis [9]. However, the nodules may not be present in younger children, although by the age of 5 years 92% of patients will have them [10]. Younger children with neurofibromatosis and congenital glaucoma often have ectropion uveae and no iris nodules.

Stickler's Syndrome

The inheritance pattern of Stickler's syndrome is autosomal dominant. The COL2A1 gene on chromosome 12, which codes for type II collagen, is believed to be involved [11–13]. There is a progressive arthroophthalmopathy characterized by vitreoretinal degeneration, high myopia, cataracts, glaucoma in 15%, and musculoskeletal abnormalities. The onset of glaucoma usually occurs by age 30 to 50 years [14, 15].

Marfan's Syndrome

The inheritance pattern of Marfan's syndrome is autosomal dominant. Rarely, primary open-angle glaucoma develops in these patients. The angle is maldeveloped. More commonly, secondary glaucoma develops after lens dislocation or retinal detachment.

Lowe's (Oculocerebrorenal) Syndrome

The oculocerebrorenal syndrome is X-linked, on the long arm in the 24-26 region (Xq24-q26) [16]. This syndrome consists of renal tubular dysfunction with acidosis, congenital cataracts and glaucoma, hypotonia, bone disease, mental retardation, and death in the second decade [17]. Female carriers may be identified by the number of cortical lens opacities; more than 100 opacities indicates the mutated gene [18].

Zellweger (Hepatocerebrorenal) Syndrome

The inheritance pattern of the hepatocerebrorenal syndrome is autosomal recessive. Alteration of any of three different genes can cause the syndrome [19]. The underlying error is defective biogenesis of the peroxisome (the cellular organelle responsible for very long chain fatty acid and phytanic acid degradation, as well as others). The clinical syndrome presents with infantile hypotonia, seizures, craniofacial dysmorphism with high forehead and hypertelorism, hepatomegaly, and jaundice. Death occurs within the first year of life. Ocular findings are corneal opacification, cataract, glaucoma, a typical pigmentary retinopathy at the equator, and optic atrophy [19].

Rubinstein-Taybi Syndrome

The inheritance pattern of the Rubinstein-Taybi syndrome is unknown. A reciprocal translocation of the short arm of chromosomes 2 and 16 has been reported [20]. The syndrome consists of broad-based fingers and toes, mental retardation, low-set ears, microcephaly, hypertelorism, strabismus, antimongoloid slant, a high arched palate, short stature, and glaucoma [21–24]. It can be confused clinically with trisomy 13.

Oculodentodigital Dysplasia

Oculodentodigital dysplasia usually follows an autosomal dominant inheritance pattern, but a recessive variety probably exists [25]. These patients are similar to Hallermann-Streiff patients in appearance, with a long face, narrow nose with hypoplastic alae, and narrow and short palpebral fissures with scanty eyebrows. The patients also exhibit dysplastic dental enamel with microdontia and skeletal abnormalities of digits and toes. Glaucoma can develop in infancy or later, usually as a result of abnormal angle development.

Open-Angle Glaucoma Associated with Microcornea and Absence of Frontal Sinuses

In one family, open-angle glaucoma associated with microcornea and absence of the frontal sinuses has been reported [26]. The inheritance pattern is autosomal dominant.

Mucopolysaccharidosis

All forms of mucopolysaccharidosis (MPS) are autosomal recessive, except for MPS type II (Hunter's syndrome) which is X-linked recessive [2]. A small number of case reports document glaucoma in these patients. Chronic angle closure, which was treated successfully with laser iridectomies, was reported in a patient with Hunter's syndrome [27]. The authors proposed two possible mechanisms: (1) narrowing of the angle due to the thickened anterior segment tissues and (2) decreased outflow facility because of deposition of mucopolysaccharide in the trabecular meshwork. Other reports in Hurler, Scheie, and Morquio patients do not describe the angle appearance because of corneal clouding [28].

Chromosomal Trisomies and Deletions

The most common ocular abnormality in *trisomy 13* is microphthalmos. Congenital glaucoma with an immature-appearing angle structure has been reported [29]. Other ocular abnormalities such as persistent hyperplastic primary vitreous may cause secondary glaucoma.

Trisomy 18 appears mostly in female individuals. Most patients die in infancy. Congenital glaucoma may be due to immature angle structures, with anomalies of the iris and ciliary body, or to the presence of sclerocornea.

Congenital glaucoma has only rarely been associated with *trisomy 21* [30].

Turner's syndrome is associated with the XO genotype. Congenital open-angle glaucoma has been reported [2]. Secondary angle closure from other ocular abnormalities, such as microcornea and microphthalmos, may occur.

The most frequent ocular anomaly associated with *ring chromosome 6* is microphthalmos. Aniridia, congenital ectropion uveae, and Rieger's anomaly have also been reported [2] and may be associated with glaucoma. Primary congenital glaucoma has occurred as well [2].

Cutis Marmorata Telangiectasia Congenita

There is no known genetic pattern for cutis marmorata telangiectasia congenita (CMTC). The skin of affected patients has a characteristic marblelike appearance from telangiectasias, which often resolves in the first two decades of life [31]. In 3 of the 65 reported cases, there was congenital glaucoma and buphthalmos and a nevus flammeus in the trigeminal distribution [32]. The glaucoma seemed to be related to an abnormal angle and not to increased episcleral venous pressure. However, a recent case report describes an intraoperative choroidal hemorrhage in a patient with CMTC, a complication usually seen in patients with increased episcleral venous pressure [33].

Cystinosis

The inheritance pattern of cystinosis is autosomal recessive. The childhood nephropathic form is the most common presentation of this disorder of amino acid metabolism. Renal rickets and growth retardation occur. Cystine crystals deposit in the kidney, liver, spleen, lymph nodes, and bone marrow. In the eye, cystine crystals are found in the cornea, iris, ciliary body, choroid, retinal pigment epithelium, and optic nerve [34]. A case of angle closure due to pupillary block from an iris thickened with cystine crystals was reported. Systemic and topical cysteamine eye drops are now available to treat this disease [35].

Krause's Syndrome

Krause's syndrome, characterized by mental retardation with cerebral dysplasia or hydrocephalus, probably results from a chromosomal anomaly [2]. Glaucoma may result from various causes and has been reported [2] with a shallow or flat anterior chamber, peripheral anterior synechiae, neovascularization, posterior synechiae, and immature angle structures.

Osteogenesis Imperfecta

The inheritance pattern of osteogenesis imperfecta is usually autosomal dominant, although autosomal recessive and sporadic cases have been reported [2]. The classic triad of findings consists of brittle bones, blue sclera, and deafness. Open-angle glaucoma may present in the first or second decade of life.

Prader-Willi Syndrome

An interstitial deletion of the proximal long arm of chromosome 15, 15-del (15q)(q11-q13), has been found in approximately 50% of patients with the Prader-Willi syndrome [2]. Other anomalies of chromosome 15 have been found in other patients.

The systemic findings include muscular hypotony, mental retardation, and hypogonadism. Strabismus and oculocutaneous albinism are frequent eye findings. Iridogoniodysgenesis is frequently seen, with variable amounts of iris stromal hypoplasia. Large iris processes and broad peripheral anterior synechiae have been noted in the angle. Congenital ectropion uveae with the late development of open-angle glaucoma is also found in this syndrome.

Warburg's Syndrome

The inheritance pattern of Warburg's syndrome is autosomal recessive. Ocular abnormalities are severe, with bilateral microphthalmos and congenital nonattachment of the retina. Lissencephaly, or agenesis of cerebral gyrations, is the central nervous system anomaly. Death occurs in infancy [36]. In 11 of 12 patients, the pathological examination revealed closed angles with uninterrupted endothelial tissue extending over an undeveloped trabecular meshwork [37, 38].

■ Childhood Glaucomas Associated with Congenital Ocular Abnormalities

Congenital Microcoria

Congenital microcoria exhibits an autosomal dominant inheritance pattern. The iris dilator muscle is maldeveloped, resulting in a pupil size of less than 2 mm. The angle reveals goniodysgenesis, and late-onset congenital glaucoma often develops. Rarely, acute angle closure with pupillary block occurs and requires iridectomy.

Microcornea

The occurrence of microcornea is sporadic. Corneal diameter is 10 mm or less. Often it is associated with other ocular anomalies, but the eye may be normal. The glaucoma may be the result of goniodysgenesis or of a crowded anterior segment causing angle closure [2].

Microphthalmos

The inheritance of microphthalmos is sporadic, autosomal dominant or recessive or, rarely, X-linked, depending on the associated systemic or ocular anomalies [2]. Many systemic and ocular conditions have associated microphthalmos. Nanophthalmos is characterized by short axial lengths, hyperopia, small corneas, and narrow angles with acute or chronic angle closure glaucoma.

Aniridia

Aniridia usually presents sporadically. Rarely in these patients, a chromosomal deletion (11p13 deletion) may be found, which increases the risk of Wilms' tumor. More commonly, a gene mutation is present that is expressed in an autosomal dominant fashion. Recently, the mutation responsible for autosomal dominant aniridia has been located on the short arm of chromosome 11 [39].

The amount of iris tissue present varies tremendously, from tiny stubs of iris visible in the periphery to normal-appearing irides with mild stromal atrophy [40, 41]. The peripheral cornea manifests a pathognomonic haze with an irregular border that exhibits a characteristic stippling pattern with fluorescein stain. Cataract develops in 50% to 85% of patients, usually during the first two decades of life. Zonular dehiscence and ectopia lentis may occur. Poor visual acuity is common. Refractive error, foveal hypoplasia, amblyopia, cataract, and glaucoma may contribute to the visual loss. Rarely, glaucoma may be present at birth, with the angle findings indistinguishable from primary congenital glaucoma [42]. More commonly, glaucoma develops late as the iris tissue progressively becomes apposed to the trabecular meshwork with fine sawtoothlike attachments [43]. This can be prevented with frequent gonioscopy and prophylactic goniosurgery when apposition becomes evident [44].

Only one report exists of a familial aniridia patient who developed Wilms' tumor. The overall risk of developing Wilms' tumor in sporadic cases of aniridia is 33%. However, in the presence of the 11p13 deletion, the risk increases to more than 60%. Periodic ultrasound examinations can detect early tumor masses prior to extension outside the kidney [45].

Congenital Ocular Melanosis (Nevus of Ota)

Congenital ocular melanosis, or nevus of Ota, occurs sporadically. Two case reports found associated ipsilateral glaucoma with heavy slate-gray coloration to the trabecular meshwork [46, 47].

Sclerocornea

An autosomal dominant inheritance pattern of sclerocornea has been reported in four pedigrees. Its occurrence is usually sporadic. A severe form of total sclerocornea may be inherited as an autosomal recessive trait [48].

Scleralization of the peripheral or total cornea is present at birth and is nonprogressive. The affected areas are opaque and vascularized with superficial or deep arcades. Sclerocornea may occur as a primary anomaly but usually is associated with cornea plana [49]. All the reported autosomal dominant cases are accompanied by cornea plana. Ninety percent of cases are bilateral. Other anterior segment developmental abnormalities, including glaucoma, may be found [50].

Familial Hypoplasia of the Iris

The inheritance pattern of familial hypoplasia of the iris is autosomal dominant. There is hypoplasia of the iris stroma, allowing pigment epithelium and sphincter muscle to be viewed through fine strands of remaining stroma. Abnormal trabecular structure is observed, but Schwalbe's line is in a normal location and there is no bridging iris tissue as in Axenfeld-Rieger syndrome [51–54].

Axenfeld-Rieger Syndrome

The Axenfeld-Rieger syndrome often demonstrates an autosomal dominant inheritance pattern, but it may also be sporadic. Typically bilateral, there is a spectrum of findings. A prominent, anteriorly displaced Schwalbe's line is seen in conjunction with peripheral iris strands that bridge the angle and adhere to the line. Often the iris insertion is just posterior to the trabecular meshwork. The central iris may be normal or may exhibit mild thinning to extensive atrophy, with hole formation, corectopia, and ectropion uveae. Slightly more than 50% of patients develop glaucoma, which may present any time from infancy to young adulthood. Systemic findings associated with this syndrome include abnormal teeth, maxillary hypoplasia, umbilical defects, hypospadias, and oculocutaneous albinism. Pituitary gland abnormalities also may be seen. The syndrome is believed to represent a developmental arrest of neural crest cell migration [55, 56].

Peter's Anomaly

Most cases of Peter's anomaly are sporadic. Reports of autosomal recessive inheritance exist. Chromosome 4, 18, and 11 deletions, ring 21, and 13-15 trisomy have been associated with this condition [2].

A central corneal leukoma with loss of Descemet's membrane and the posterior stroma is present at birth. Iridocorneal adhesions are seen at the edge of the corneal defect. The anterior chamber is often shallow. A central keratolenticular adhesion may sometimes occur, and an anterior polar cataract is common. Glaucoma occurs in 50% to 70% of cases. The mechanism of the decreased outflow facility is not fully understood. Peter's anomaly is bilateral in 80% of cases [55, 57].

Iridogoniodysgenesis with Congenital Ectropion Uveae

The occurrence of iridogoniodysgenesis with congenital ectropion uveae is sporadic, but it may occur in neurofibromatosis, which is autosomal dominant [58]. This condition results from the proliferation of pigment epithelium on the anterior surface of the iris ruff and is not a true ectropion. It is usually unilateral. Ectropion is present at birth, but glaucoma may not develop until later. The eye generally shows angle dysgenesis and abnormal iris stroma. Ptosis is common [59].

Posterior Polymorphous Dystrophy

The inheritance pattern of posterior polymorphous dystrophy is autosomal dominant. Bilateral, usually nonprogressive, vesicular, grayish patches are seen at the level of the endothelium. Epitheliallike cells are found histologically. A recessive inheritance pattern has also been described [60]. Recently, a study of Thai patients with Alport's syndrome (usually an X-linked disorder) showed a high incidence of posterior polymorphous dystrophy [61].

Idiopathic or Familial Elevated Episcleral Venous Pressure

One report of a mother and daughter with glaucoma, tortuous episcleral vessels, and increased episcleral venous pressure appears in the literature [62]. Other cases are sporadic [63].

Anterior Corneal Staphyloma

Anterior corneal staphyloma occurs sporadically [64]. At birth, the cornea is totally opacified and ectatic, often protruding through the palpebral fissure. The condition may be unilateral or bilateral. If unilateral, the eye often has associated anomalies such as microphthalmos, keratoglobus, cornea plana, and keratoconus. The epithelium and Bowman's layer are normal, but the stroma is disorganized and hypercellular, and Descemet's membrane and the endothelium are completely absent. Iris pigment epithelium is often found adherent to the posterior cornea, and the IOP is usually elevated. This anomaly is believed to be due to a failure of the migration of neural crest cells.

Congenital Lens-Iris-Angle Membrane

The occurrence of a congenital lens-iris-angle membrane is sporadic. The condition is usually unilateral and microcoria exists, with an abnormal fibrous membrane that attaches to the lens and pupillary border and inserts in the angle [65]. Pupillary block can occur. Excision of the membrane may require lensectomy.

■ **References**

1. DeLuise VP, Anderson DR. Primary infantile glaucoma. Surv Ophthalmol 1983; 28:1–19
2. Ritch R, Shields MB, Krupin T. The glaucomas, vols 1, 2. St Louis: Mosby, 1989
3. Lotufo D, Ritch R, Szmyd L Jr, Burris JE. Juvenile glaucoma, race, and refraction. JAMA 1989;261:249–252
4. Cibis GW, Tripathi RC, Tripathi BJ. Glaucoma in Sturge-Weber syndrome. Ophthalmology 1984;91:1061–1071
5. Iwach AG, Hoskins HD Jr, Hetherington J Jr, Shaffer RN. Analysis of surgical and medical management of glaucoma in Sturge-Weber syndrome. Ophthalmology 1990;97:904–909
6. Barker D, Wright E, Nguyen K, et al. Gene for von Recklinghausen neurofibromatosis is in the pericentromeric region of chromosome 17. Science 1987;236: 1100–1102
7. Richards S, Bachynski BN. Ophthalmic manifestations of neurofibromatosis type 2. Int Pediatr 1990;5:270–274
8. Kobrin JL, Blodi FC, Weingeist TA. Ocular and orbital manifestations of neurofibromatosis. Surv Ophthalmol 1979;24:45–51
9. Lubs ME, Bauer M, Formas ME, et al. Iris hamartomas in the diagnosis of neurofibromatosis-1. Int Pediatr 1990;5:261–265
10. Lewis RA, Riccardi V. von Recklinghausen neurofibromatosis. Ophthalmology 1981;88:348–354
11. Ahmad NN, Ala KL, Knowlton RG, et al. Stop codon in the procollagen II gene (*COL2A1*) in a family with the Stickler syndrome (arthro-ophthalmopathy). Proc Natl Acad Sci USA 1991;88:6624–6627

12. Knowlton RG, Weaver EJ, Struyk AF, et al. Genetic linkage analysis of hereditary arthro-ophthalmopathy (Stickler syndrome) and the type II procollagen gene. Am J Hum Genet 1989;45:681–688

13. Priestley L, Kumar D, Sykes B. Amplification of the COL2A1 3' variable region used for segregation analysis in a family with the Stickler syndrome. Hum Genet 1990;85:525–526

14. Spallone A. Stickler's syndrome: a study of 12 families. Br J Ophthalmol 1987;71:504–509

15. Liberfarb RM, Hirose T, Holmes L. The Wagner-Stickler syndrome: a study of 22 families. J Pediatr 1981;99:394–399

16. Wadelius C, Fagerholm P, Pettersson U, Anneren G. Lowe oculocerebrorenal syndrome: DNA-based linkage of the gene to Xq24-q26. Am J Hum Genet 1989;44:241–247

17. Abbassi V, Lowe CU, Calcagno PL. Oculo-cerebro-renal syndrome: a review. Am J Dis Child 1986;135:145–168

18. Cibis GW, Waeltermann JM, Whitcraft CT, et al. Lenticular opacities in carriers of Lowe's syndrome. Ophthalmology 1986;93:1041–1045

19. Folz SJ, Trobe JD. The peroxisome and the eye. Surv Ophthalmol 1991;35:353–368

20. Rubinstein JH. Broad thumb–hallux (Rubinstein-Taybi) syndrome 1957–1988. Am J Med Genet Suppl 1990;6:3–16

21. Shihab ZM. Pediatric glaucoma in Rubinstein-Taybi syndrome. Glaucoma 1984;6:288–290

22. Ziring PR, Weiss DI, Cooper LZ. The association of congenital glaucoma with the Rubinstein-Taybi syndrome. J Pediatr Ophthalmol 1974;11:203–206

23. Levy NS. Juvenile glaucoma in the Rubinstein-Taybi syndrome. J Pediatr Ophthalmol 1976;13:141–143

24. Gellis SS, Feingold M. Rubinstein-Taybi syndrome. Am J Dis Child 1971;121:327–328

25. Traboulsi EI, Parks MM. Glaucoma in oculo-dento-osseous dysplasia. Am J Ophthalmol 1990;109:310–313

26. Holmes LB, Walton DS. Hereditary microcornea, glaucoma, and absent frontal sinuses: a family study. J Pediatr 1969;74:968–972

27. Kaiden JS, Schechter R, Bader BF, Podos SM. Angle closure glaucoma in a patient with Hunter's syndrome. J Ocul Ther Surg 1982;250–252

28. Spellacy E, Bankes JLK, Crow J, et al. Glaucoma in a case of Hurler disease. Br J Ophthalmol 1980;64:773–778

29. Lichter PR, Schmickel RD. Posterior vortex vein and congenital glaucoma in a patient with trisomy 13 syndrome. Am J Ophthalmol 1975;80:939–942

30. Catalano RA. Down syndrome. Surv Ophthalmol 1990;34:385–398

31. Gellis S, Feingold M, Merritt TA, Slaughter R. Cutis marmorata telangiectasia congenita. Am J Dis Child 1977;131:1027–1028

32. Sato SE, Herschler J, Lynch PJ, et al. Congenital glaucoma associated with congenital generalized phlebectasia: two case reports. J Pediatr Ophthalmol Strabismus 1988;25:13–17

33. Kremer I, Metzker A, Yassur Y. Intraoperative suprachoroidal hemorrhage in congenital glaucoma associated with cutis marmorata telangiectatica congenita. Arch Ophthalmol 1991;109:1199–1200

34. Kaiser-Kupfer MI, Caruso RC, Minkler DS, Gahl WA. Long-term ocular manifestations in nephropathic cystinosis. Arch Ophthalmol 1986;104:706–711

35. Kaiser-Kupfer MI, Gazzo MA, Datiles MB, et al. A randomized placebo-controlled trial of cysteamine eye drops in nephropathic cystinosis. Arch Ophthalmol 1990;108:689–693

36. Levine RA, Gray DL, Gould N, et al. Warburg syndrome. Ophthalmology 1983;90: 1600–1603
37. Murphy KJ, PeBenito R, Storm RL, et al. Walker-Warburg syndrome: case report and literature review. Ophthalmic Paediatr Genet 1990;11:103–108
38. Pagon RA, Clarren SK, Milam DF Jr, Hendrickson AE. Autosomal recessive eye and brain anomalies: Warburg syndrome. J Pediatr 1983;102:542–546
39. Glaser T, Walton DS, Maas RL. Genomic structure, evolutionary conservation and aniridia mutations in the human PAX6 gene. Nat Genet 1992;2:232–238
40. Nelson LB, Spaeth GL, Nowinski TS, et al. Aniridia: a review. Surv Ophthalmol 1984;28:621–642
41. Traboulsi EI, Jaafar MS, Wilson ME, et al. Hypoplasia of the iris: the aniridia spectrum. Int Pediatr 1990;5:275–278
42. Margo CE. Congenital aniridia: a histopathologic study of the anterior segment in children. J Pediatr Ophthalmol Strabismus 1983;20:192–198
43. Grant WM, Walton DS. Progressive changes in the angle in congenital aniridia, with development of glaucoma. Am J Ophthalmol 1974;78:842–847
44. Walton DS. Aniridic glaucoma: the results of gonio-surgery to prevent and treat this problem. Trans Am Ophthalmol Soc 1986;84:59–70
45. Friedman AL. Wilms' tumor detection in patients with sporadic aniridia: successful use of ultrasound. Am J Dis Child 1986;140:173–174
46. Weiss DI, Krohn DL. Benign melanocytic glaucoma complicating oculodermal melanocytosis. Ann Ophthalmol 1971;3:958–963
47. Foulks GN, Shields MB. Glaucoma in oculodermal melanocytosis. Ann Ophthalmol 1977;9:1299–1304
48. Elliott JH, Feman SS, O'Day DM, Garber M. Hereditary sclerocornea. Arch Ophthalmol 1985;103:676–679
49. Goldstein JE, Cogan DG. Sclerocornea and associated congenital anomalies. Arch Ophthalmol 1962;67:761–768
50. Howard RO, Abrahams IW. Sclerocornea. Am J Ophthalmol 1971;71:1254–1260
51. Weatherill JR, Hart CT. Familial hypoplasia of the iris stroma associated with glaucoma. Br J Ophthalmol 1969;53:433–438
52. Jerndal T. Dominant goniodysgenesis with late congenital glaucoma: a reexamination of Berg's pedigree. Am J Ophthalmol 1972;74:28–33
53. Pearce WG, Wyatt HT, Boyd TAS, et al. Autosomal dominant iridogoniodysgenesis: genetic features. Can J Ophthalmol 1983;18:7–10
54. Wyatt HT, Pearce WG, Boyd TAS, et al. Autosomal dominant iridogoniodysgenesis: glaucoma management. Can J Ophthalmol 1983;18:11–14
55. Waring GO III, Rodrigues MM, Laibson PR. Anterior chamber cleavage syndrome. Surv Ophthalmol 1975;20:3–27
56. Shields MB, Buckley E, Klintworth GK, Thresher R. Axenfeld-Rieger syndrome. A spectrum of developmental disorders. Surv Ophthalmol 1985;29:387–409
57. DeRespinis PA, Wagner RS. Peters' anomaly in a father and son. Am J Ophthalmol 1987;104:545–546
58. Ritch R, Forbes M, Hetherington J Jr, et al. Congenital ectropion uveae with glaucoma. Ophthalmology 1984;91:326–331
59. Dowling J, Walton DS, Richardson TM, et al. Glaucoma with congenital ectropion uveae. Ophthalmology 1985;92:912–921
60. Cibis GW, Krachmer JA, Phelps CD, et al. The clinical spectrum of posterior polymorphous dystrophy. Arch Ophthalmol 1977;95:1529–1537
61. Teekhasaenee C, Nimmanit S, Wutthiphan S, et al. Posterior polymorphous dystrophy and Alport syndrome. Ophthalmology 1991;98:1207–1215
62. Minas TF, Podos SM. Familial glaucoma associated with elevated episcleral venous pressure. Arch Ophthalmol 1968;80:202–208

63. Talusan ED, Fishbein SL, Schwartz B. Increased pressure of dilated episcleral veins with open-angle glaucoma without exophthalmos. Ophthalmology 1983;90:257–265
64. Schanzlin DJ, Robin JB, Erikson G, et al. Histopathologic and ultrastructural analysis of congenital corneal staphyloma. Am J Ophthalmol 1983;95:506–514
65. Cibis GW, Waeltermann JM, Hurst E, et al. Congenital pupillary-iris-lens membrane with goniodysgenesis (a new entity). Ophthalmology 1986;93:847–852

Corticosteroid-induced Glaucoma

Robert C. Urban, Jr., M.D.

Evan B. Dreyer, M.D., Ph.D.

In the early 1950s, ophthalmologists first became aware that corticosteroids could cause an elevation of intraocular pressure (IOP).

Topical and Systemic Administration

In 1963, Becker and Mills [1] demonstrated that a proportion of normal individuals showed a rise in IOP after the topical administration of corticosteroids. These investigators also found that this response was more common in close relatives of patients with open-angle glaucoma than in those without such a history. Also in 1963, Armaly [2] studied the effect on IOP and fluid dynamics in the normal eye of topical application of 0.1% dexamethasone three times daily for 4 weeks. He found an increase in IOP and a reduction in both outflow facility and the rate of aqueous formation. The magnitude of the effect was significantly greater in older subjects than in younger ones, and the response was more pronounced in glaucomatous than in nonglaucomatous eyes [3].

It is now well documented that topical corticosteroids may cause a rise in IOP. The rise is variable in onset but almost invariably disappears some weeks after steroid withdrawal. However, some patients sustain protracted elevation of IOP, necessitating surgical intervention, even after corticosteroid use is stopped [4].

Kalina [5] described 4 patients with moderate increases in IOP after subconjunctival injection of methylprednisolone acetate. The increased pressures were medically controlled, and IOP returned to normal within 3 months with no further treatment. Herschler [4] described a single patient with medically intractable increased IOP that developed after a sub-tenon's injection of triamcinolone acetonide. Numerous other reports in the ophthalmic and dermatological literature support the notion that periocular corticosteroids may cause IOP to rise.

Systemic corticosteroids are also implicated in producing a rise in IOP, although generally not as frequently as with local therapy. Typically, the patients that show a marked increase in IOP are on a long-term, high-dose therapeutic regimen. Long [6], however, reported a case of ocular hypertension in a 20-year-old woman after only 12 days of systemic prednisone therapy for poison ivy dermatitis.

■ Individual Susceptibility

The susceptibility of patients to develop a rise in IOP secondary to corticosteroid use has been an area of much study and debate. The steroid response is typically greater in patients with primary open-angle glaucoma and their relatives and in glaucoma suspects than in normal subjects [1, 3, 7]. When a normal population was subjected to short-term topical corticosteroid testing, 58% showed a minimal increase in IOP, 36% a moderate rise, and 6% a marked increase [1].

■ Genetic Studies

On the basis of studies of glaucoma patients, glaucoma suspects, and normal subjects, Becker [1] and Armaly [2, 3] independently proposed the concept that corticosteroid responsiveness is determined by a single gene pair. Both investigators classified corticosteroid response as high, intermediate, or low, but each used different criteria.

Evidence against the concept of a single gene was found in a study of corticosteroid responses in twins. Schwartz and co-workers [8] tested 37 monozygotic and 26 dizygotic twin pairs using topical dexamethasone and found that the frequency of similar responses was not significantly different in the two types of twins. They concluded that environmental, not genetic, factors are the dominant determinants of the corticosteroid response.

A partial explanation for the discrepancy between the results of the twin study and the earlier studies is found in the analysis by Palmberg and colleagues [7] of the reproducibility of the corticosteroid provocative test. When a group of normal subjects was tested, the proportion of low, intermediate, and high responders was the same on each of several testing occasions, but the subjects in each response group differed from test to test. Considerable crossover occurred between the low and intermediate response groups, but high responders the first time tended to be high responders on subsequent testing. This suggested that only the high responders emerged consistently owing to spontaneous variation of IOP. Because few of the twins were high responders, this study could not conclusively prove or disprove the genetic nature of the response.

In a study of bilateral response, Kitazawa and associates [9] found that the eyes of 6 of 40 glucocorticoid responders showed unequal responsiveness toward the development of a rise in IOP, suggesting that a single genetic influence is not likely to be the sole determinant of the steroid response.

Subsequent work by Kitazawa [10] and others suggested that the steroid response is, at least in part, dose-related. Significant correlations were found between elevation in IOP and potency, concentration, frequency of instillation, and duration of use of the steroid.

In addition, there are differences in the ability of the various corticosteroid preparations to elicit this response. Cantrill and co-workers [11] compared the IOP response to various topically applied corticosteroids in each of 10 corticosteroid-sensitive patients. The rises in IOP (in mm Hg) were as follows: dexamethasone 0.1%, 22.0 ± 2.9; prednisone 1.0%, 10.0 ± 1.7; dexamethasone 0.005%, 8.2 ± 1.7; fluorometholone 0.1%, 6.1 ± 1.4; hydrocortisone 0.5%, 3.2 ± 1.0; tetrahydrotriamcinolone 0.25%, 1.8 ± 1.3; and medrysone 1.0%, 1.0 ± 1.3.

Herschler [4] studied 12 patients with IOP elevation induced by repository corticosteroids. He found the duration and severity of the pressure elevation to be directly related to the decreasing solubility of the agent employed. Injectable corticosteroid preparations include water-soluble, short-acting compounds, such as dexamethasone sodium phosphate (Decadron) and hydrocortisone sodium succinate (Solu-Cortef); suspensions of moderately soluble compounds in polyethylene glycol, such as triamcinolone diacetate (Aristocort) and methylprednisolone acetate (Depo-Medrol); suspensions of minimally soluble compounds, such as triamcinolone acetonide (Kenalog) and triamcinolone hexacetonide (Aristospan); and mixtures of soluble and moderately soluble compounds, such as betamethasone sodium phosphate and betamethasone acetate (Celestone). Herschler's work is also important because, of the 12 patients who had IOP elevations induced by repository corticosteroids, 10 had received intensive topical corticosteroids before injection, resulting in no IOP elevation during that period. Two of the patients who developed marked IOP elevation after repository corticosteroid injection did not manifest a positive response on subsequent topical corticosteroid testing.

■ Proposed Response Mechanisms

The mechanism by which corticosteroids bring about an elevation of IOP has not been fully elucidated. However, studies on both animal and human eyes suggest that the primary mechanism relates to impaired outflow facility through the trabecular meshwork. Most of the attention has focused on the role of glycosaminoglycans.

François [12] has put forward the hypothesis that glucocorticoid-induced IOP elevation is due in part to the accumulation in the angle of a mucopolysaccharide sensitive to hyaluronidase (hyaluronic acid) and that this mucopolysaccharide, in concert with the corticoid, inhibits aqueous outflow. Corticosteroids do not liberate mucopolysaccharides but rather act on their catabolism. François's theory is based on the following premises: (1) The lysosomal membrane of one or several clones of fibroblasts in the anterior chamber angle is genetically more sensitive to the action of the corticosteroids. (2) The lysosomal membrane, reinforced by the action of glucocorticoids, prevents the liberation of the catabolic enzymes of mucopolysaccharides. (3) As a consequence, the mucopolysaccharides accumulate in the anterior chamber angle. (4) The retention of water by the mucopolysaccharides obstructs the trabeculae. (5) The process continues as long as the action of the corticosteroids continues. (6) When the corticosteroid action ceases, the IOP tends to normalize.

Glucocorticoid receptors have been identified in trabeculectomy specimens from both normal and glaucomatous eyes. Johnson and co-workers [13] have shown that dexamethasone caused a 92% increase in glycosaminoglycans in the trabecular meshwork after 14 to 21 days, lending further credence to the association of glycosaminoglycans with corticosteroid therapy.

Southren and colleagues [14] have shown that 5β-dihydrocortisol, a substance that accumulates abnormally in cells derived from the outflow region of the eye from patients with primary open-angle glaucoma, potentiates the action of topical dexamethasone to raise IOP. This is likely one of the reasons that glaucoma patients typically show a higher incidence of IOP rise on corticosteroid testing.

Much work remains to be done to elucidate fully the genetic basis of corticosteroid-induced glaucoma and the mechanism of the response.

■ References

1. Becker B, Mills DW. Corticosteroids and intraocular pressure. Arch Ophthalmol 1963;70:500–507
2. Armaly MF. Effect of corticosteroids on intraocular pressure and fluid dynamics: I. The effect of dexamethasone in the normal eye. Arch Ophthalmol 1963;70:482–491
3. Armaly MF. Effect of corticosteroids on intraocular pressure and fluid dynamics: II. The effect of dexamethasone in the glaucomatous eye. Arch Ophthalmol 1963;70:492–499
4. Herschler J. Increased intraocular pressure induced by repository corticosteroids. Am J Ophthalmol 1976;82:90–93
5. Kalina RE. Increased intraocular pressure following subconjunctival corticosteroid administration. Arch Ophthalmol 1969;81:788–790
6. Long WF. A case of elevated intraocular pressure associated with systemic steroid therapy. Am J Optom Physiol Optics 1977;54:248–250
7. Palmberg PF, Mandell A, Wilensky JT, et al. The reproducibility of the intraocular pressure response to dexamethasone. Am J Ophthalmol 1975;80:844–856

8. Schwartz JT, Reuling FH, Feinleib M, et al. Twin study on ocular pressure following topically applied dexamethasone: II. Inheritance of variation in pressure response. Arch Ophthalmol 1973;90:281–286
9. Kitazawa Y, Nosé H, Saitoh S. On the bilaterality of the corticosteroid responsiveness of intraocular pressure in man. Acta Soc Ophthalmol Jpn 1972;76:1277–1285
10. Kitazawa Y. Increased intraocular pressure induced by corticosteroids. Am J Ophthalmol 1976;82:492–495
11. Cantrill HL, Palmberg PF, Zink HA, et al. Comparison of in vitro potency of corticosteroids with ability to raise intraocular pressure. Am J Ophthalmol 1975;79:1012–1017
12. François J. Corticosteroid glaucoma. Ophthalmologica 1984;188:76–81
13. Johnson DH, Bradley JMB, Acott TS. The effect of dexamethasone on glycosaminoglycans of human trabecular meshwork in perfusion organ culture. Invest Ophthalmol Vis Sci 1990;31:2568–2571
14. Southren AL, Gordon GG, l'Hommedieu D, et al. 5β-Dihydrocortisol: possible mediator of the ocular hypertension in glaucoma. Invest Ophthalmol Vis Sci 1985;26:393–395

Genetic Basis of Color Vision

Gary D. Haynie, M.D.
Shizuo Mukai, M.D.

We have witnessed remarkable advances in our understanding of color vision in recent years. The structure of rhodopsin has been elucidated and, from this, the means by which light is transduced into a neural signal has been clarified. Now, each of the human genes that encodes a photoreceptor pigment has been identified. The mode of inheritance and phenotypic character of color vision defects are largely explained by the physical organization of these genes, and this genetic structure has implications regarding the evolution of color vision.

Such advances have been accomplished chiefly through the efforts of Jeremy Nathans and co-workers. Their novel approach employed the known structure of an animal photoreceptor pigment, bovine rhodopsin, to create a nucleotide probe that would identify the photopigment genes in the human genome [1–4]. With the knowledge of the precise location and sequence of these genes, Nathans and others have been able to characterize the genetic alterations that underly the phenotypic variations seen in so-called color blindness and to provide insights on how the pigments are "tuned" to their respective wavelengths [5–10].

Color Vision Defects

Color vision in humans is based on three distinct photosensitive proteins (pigments), each of which absorbs light over a range of wavelengths, with peak absorbance in the middle of the range. In humans, the peak sensitivities of these pigments are 552 or 557 (red), 530 (green), and 426 nm (blue), respectively [11]. (Two alternative peaks are given for the red pigment owing to a phenotypic variation in subjects with normal color vision, as is described later.) These pigments, found in cone photoreceptors, are functional in bright light. Rod photoreceptors, which subserve vision in dim light, contain rhodopsin, which absorbs maximally at approximately 500 nm. The absorbance spectra of the pigments, though maximal at the wavelengths just cited, are sufficiently broad to cover the entire visible spectrum of light.

Persons with normal color vision have all three pigments and are known as *trichromats*. Those in whom one pigment is absent are known as *dichromats*—*protanopic* dichromats if the red-cone pigment is missing and *deuteranopic* if the green-cone pigment is missing. If all pigments are present but one has an altered absorption spectrum, the term *anomalous trichromat* is applied. Defects of the red and green pigments are vastly more common than those involving the blue pigment. Approximately 8% of white men and 0.5% of white women have some form of red-green color vision defect, of which three-fourths are anomalous trichromats. *Deuteranomalous* trichromats have abnormal green-cone pigment and outnumber *protanomalous* trichromats, who have abnormal red-cone pigment, by approximately 5 to 1. *Tritanopes* (with blue pigment defects) are very rare. Subjects who lack both the red and green pigments are also rare and are said to have *achromacy* or *blue-cone monochromacy;* since rhodopsin and the blue pigment are active in distinct spectral environments, these patients live in a monochrome world.

In 1802, Thomas Young [12] proposed that human vision is trichromatic, utilizing the following reasoning:

> Now, as it is almost impossible to conceive each sensitive point of the retina to contain an infinite number of particles, each capable of vibrating in perfect unison with every possible undulation, it becomes necessary to suppose the number limited, for instance, to the three principal colors.

Later in the same century, neuropsychological evidence for trichromacy was supplied by Rayleigh's anomaloscope [13]. In its present form (little different from the original), the anomaloscope projects three monochromatic lights onto a screen in view of the subject. On the left, red and green lights are projected so that they overlap and mix; on the right is a single yellow light. The subject adjusts the ratio of red and green lights on the left side as well as the intensity of the yellow light on the right, until the two halves of the screen are indistinguishable. Normal subjects always match the yellow light with a reproducible ratio of red to green light. Dichromats can match the yellow light using either the red or green light alone, because in them the yellow light excites only one of the two typical pigments. This reasoning can be extended to explain the behavior of anomalous trichromats. Protanomalous trichromats create ratios containing more red than normal, whereas deuteranomalous trichromats require more green [13].

■ Photoreceptor Structure

Photoreceptors are highly specialized cells. Each has an outer segment comprised of a stack of discs, each of which is a flattened membrane sac derived from the plasma membrane. The outer segment discs are metabolized and regenerated continuously. In rhesus monkeys, the average life span of a disc is 10 days; approximately ninety discs are generated daily at the base of the outer segment [14].

The visual pigment is a membrane protein, comprising 95% of the membrane protein of the outer segment. All visual pigments are proteins (opsins) coupled to a photosensitive moiety, 11-*cis*-retinal, via a covalent bond between the ϵ-amino group of a lysine residue and the aldehyde group of retinal. On activation by a photon, the retinal is isomerized to all-*trans*-retinal, triggering a conformational change in the attached apoprotein. All-*trans*-retinal is then released from the apoprotein and enzymatically restored to the 11-*cis* configuration before being reattached to the photopigment [14].

Until recently, bovine rhodopsin was the most extensively studied photopigment. Its amino acid sequence has been completely determined and found to contain 348 amino acids. The carboxy-terminus is in the cytosol, and the amino-terminus faces the lumen (intradiscal space). Approximately half of the protein molecule lies within the plasma membrane as a series of membrane-spanning alpha helices [14]. Unlike bovine rhodopsin, human rhodopsin and all cone pigments have not been available in sufficient quantities to be characterized.

Nathans and co-workers [1, 14] assumed that the cone pigments are structurally similar to rhodopsin and that the cone pigments may have evolved from rhodopsin in the following steps: (1) The primordial photopigment gene is duplicated. (2) One of the duplicated genes is altered in such a way as to change the spectral absorbance of the pigment. (3) Regulation of gene expression is altered so that the novel pigment is expressed in a separate set of cells from the original pigment. (4) The neural connections from the photoreceptors are modified in such a way as to recognize independently the new set of cells [14]. Based on these assumptions, a three-part plan was proposed by Nathans and Hogness [1]: First, isolate and characterize the bovine rhodopsin gene. Second, use this gene to identify at least one of the human opsin (pigment) genes. Third, use this human DNA to identify the remaining opsin genes in the human genome. The first step was accomplished in 1983 when the bovine rhodopsin gene was isolated [1].

Isolation of the Bovine Rhodopsin Gene

A synthetic oligonucleotide was prepared which, when conceptually translated, corresponded to a small part (five residues) of the known amino acid sequence for bovine rhodopsin. Of the multiple deoxynucleotide sequences that would code for this amino acid sequence, one was selected that was similar in sequence to those previously observed to prime bovine opsin messenger RNA (mRNA). Using this primer, complementary DNA (cDNA) was prepared from bovine retinal mRNA. The cDNA was then hybridized to fragments of bovine genomic DNA that had been amplified by recombinant technology. In this way, two genomic fragments were isolated that hybridized to the cDNA probe and whose sequence revealed a gene structure and a derived amino acid sequence that were fully consistent with the known structure of rhodopsin [1].

The bovine rhodopsin gene contains a coding region of 348 codons. The coding region consists of five expressed regions (exons), interrupted at four sites by introns. Conceptual translation of the 348 codons reveals an amino acid sequence identical to the known sequence for bovine rhodopsin. Rhodopsin, therefore, is the primary translation product of this gene, and there appears to be no posttranslation modification of the product protein [1].

The three-dimensional structure of rhodopsin could now be considered based on the amino acid sequence determined from the nucleotide sequence of the gene. A model for this was found in bacteriorhodopsin, a membrane protein in *Halobacterium haobium*. In this organism, bacteriorhodopsin is found in the "purple membrane," where it functions as a light-driven hydrogen ion pump. By electron microscopy and crystallography, this protein has been found to contain seven helical segments, each perpendicular to, and embedded in, the lipid membrane [15]. An analogous structure was postulated for bovine rhodopsin. Indeed, analysis of the amino acid sequence of bovine rhodopsin reveals seven relatively hydrophobic regions, each of sufficient length to span the lipid bilayer (Fig 1). Further, rhodopsin's carboxy-terminus is known to reside in the cytoplasm and the amino-terminus in the disc lumen; this requires that the protein span the membrane an odd number of times. As expected, cleavage sites for limited proteolysis of the embedded membrane protein all lie outside the membrane-spanning segments [1].

Isolation of the Human Rhodopsin Gene

The second step in the plan outlined by Nathans and Hogness [1] was the identification of the human rhodopsin gene using bovine DNA. To accomplish this, a library of restriction fragments from human genomic DNA was prepared from a male individual with normal color vision. These restriction fragments were hybridized to the radiolabeled bovine cDNA representing the bovine rhodopsin gene. In this manner, several overlapping human genomic DNA fragments were identified that hybridized the bovine cDNA probe. Sequencing of these fragments revealed homology between the bovine and human genes at 89.7% of the nucleotides. For

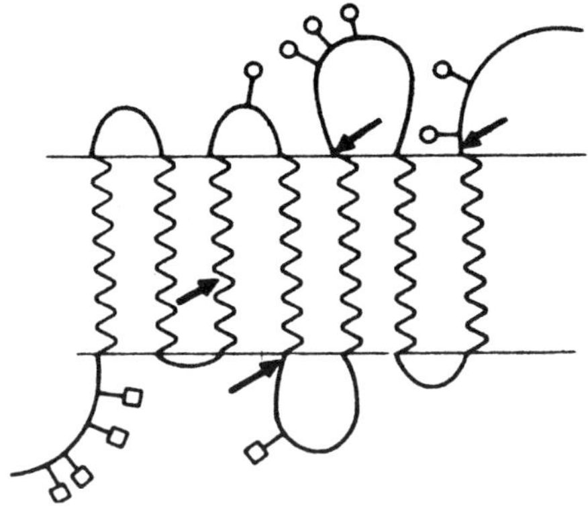

Figure 1 *Topographical structure of rhodopsin. Wavy lines represent transmembrane segments. Arrows indicate positions of introns. Protease cleavage sites on the cytoplasmic surface are indicated by open circles, whereas cleavage sites on the intradiscal surface are indicated by open squares. (Reprinted with permission from J Nathans and DS Hogness, Isolation, sequence analysis, and intron-exon arrangement of the gene encoding bovine rhodopsin. Cell 1983;34:807–814.)*

the amino acid sequences deduced by conceptual translation of the DNA sequences, there was 93.4% homology. This high degree of homology was expected since this approach was based on the assumption that the bovine and human rhodopsin genes were very similar. Like the bovine gene, the human gene is divided into five exons. In the intervening introns, there is a high degree of sequence homology in the regions immediately adjacent to the exons; the degree of homology declines progressively as one proceeds toward the interior of the intron [2]. Using a panel of hybrid mouse-human cell lines, the human rhodopsin gene was mapped to the long arm of chromosome 3, since only DNA from those cell lines retaining the human 3q21-3qter region hybridized the gene [3].

Additional observations supported the assertion that the human DNA clone just described (roJHN) is the human rhodopsin gene. Hybridization of the roJHN DNA to mRNA isolated from human retinas protected the DNA from digestion by S1 nuclease. It was shown that approximately 0.5% of the total retinal mRNA was protective. This corresponds well with the fact that rhodopsin mRNA constitutes approximately 0.5% of the total human retinal mRNA [2].

The functional importance of certain regions of the rhodopsin molecule is implied by the conservation of certain amino acid residues between human and bovine rhodopsin. The conserved residues include Lys(296), to which the retinal chromophore is attached, as well as six of seven targets of phosphorylation (serine and threonine residues) and both of two sites for glycosylation. In addition, the three cytoplasmic loops are entirely conserved, suggesting their functional importance [2].

Isolation of the Human Cone Pigment Genes

The stage was now set for the identification of the human cone pigment genes using bovine rhodopsin cDNA. Modifications were made in the hybridization technique to promote the identification of weakly hybridizing

DNA fragments. Under these less stringent conditions, bovine rhodopsin cDNA hybridized to two classes of DNA fragments from a human genomic library. When sequenced, the first of these classes was found to contain five exons exhibiting moderate homology to those of bovine rhodopsin. After conceptual translation, the amino acid sequence was identical to human rhodopsin at 42% of the residues. An additional 33% of the residues were similar with regard to chemical features such as size and charge [4].

Two pieces of evidence suggested that this first class of DNA fragments contained the blue-cone pigment. First, when human retinal mRNA was screened for homology to the putative blue pigment gene, significant homology was found for only 1/30,000 of the total retinal mRNA; the abundance of this mRNA population was only 1/150 of that noted for rhodopsin. This corresponded adequately to the observed ratio of blue cones to rods of approximately 1/200 [4]. Second, again using a panel of mouse-human hybrid cell lines, the putative blue-cone pigment gene mapped to human chromosome 7, an unlikely position for the red or green pigment, whose defects are X-linked [3].

The second class of weakly hybridizing fragments was found to contain two subsets, distinguished by restriction fragment length polymorphisms. Subsequent mapping in color-blind men would show this group of DNA fragments to represent the red and green pigment genes. Sequencing of the exons showed that one subset consisted of two pigment genes (green) that differed from each other by a single, "silent" nucleotide substitution. The other subset was a single pigment gene (red) that differed from the green pigment gene by 19 or 20 nucleotides (12 amino acids). The red and green pigment genes were nearly equally divergent from both the blue-cone pigment gene and the rhodopsin gene, with approximately 40% amino acid sequence identity for either (Fig 2). The red and green pigment genes contained five exons which, based on their homology, corresponded to those in bovine rhodopsin; an additional sixth exon was found in the 5′ end of the nucleotide sequence of both the red and green pigment genes. The abundance of human retinal mRNA homologous to these genes was found to be approximately one-fifteenth of that for rhodopsin mRNA, corresponding adequately to the known ratio of red and green cones to rods (1:30) [4]. The gene was preserved only in mouse-human hybrid cell lines that retain the human X chromosome, and it co-segregated with glucose-6-phosphate dehydrogenase (G6PD) activity. (The G6PD gene is on the X chromosome [3].)

It was proposed that the red pigment and green pigment genes are aligned in a tandem array on the X chromosome, with the red pigment gene in the 5′ (upstream) end of the array [5]. This was supported by many observations. Genomic DNA from 18 color-normal men was studied using probes for the red pigment and green pigment genes. The intensities of the bands on the separating gel varied in such a way as to suggest variability among the subjects in the proportion of red and green pigment

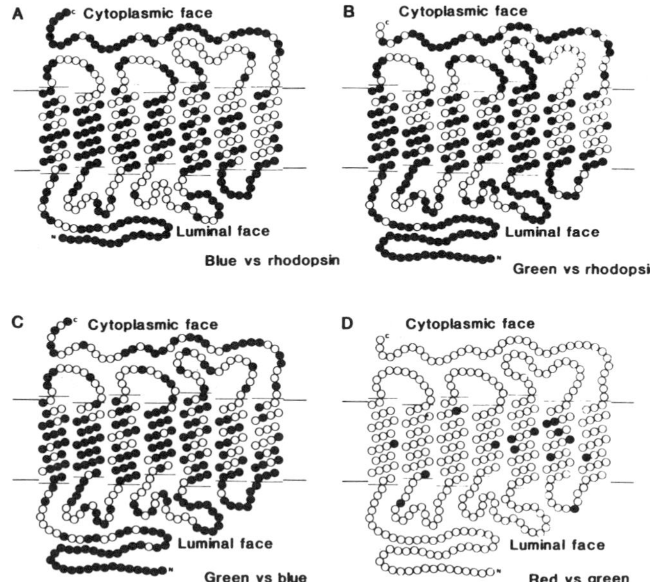

Figure 2 *Pairwise comparisons of human visual pigments showing positions where amino acids are identical* (white) *and different* (black). *(A) Blue versus rhodopsin. (B) Green versus rhodopsin. (C) Green versus blue. (D) Red versus green. (Reprinted with permission from J Nathans et al, Molecular genetics of human color vision: the genes encoding blue, green, and red pigments. Science 1986;232:193–202. Copyright © 1986 by the AAAS.)*

genes. Each subject had one red pigment gene and one, two, or three green pigment genes [4]. Presumably, the multiplication of green pigment genes had resulted from unequal crossing over, resulting in gene duplication (Fig 3). Since the red pigment gene was always present as a single copy, it was logical to place it upstream, where adjacent nonhomologous DNA inhibits crossing over. Indeed, divergent DNA was found just 195 base pairs upstream from the red pigment gene, corroborating its upstream position. The repeat length in the red-green pigment gene array has been found to be 39 kilobases [5].

Unlike humans and Old World monkeys, New World monkeys have only one long-wavelength cone pigment. Therefore, the duplication event that resulted in the generation of separated red pigment and green pigment genes must have occurred since the divergence of Old World and New World monkeys 30 to 40 million years ago [16]. Similarly, comparison of the homology among rhodopsin genes from humans, cows, and *Drosophila,* relative to the homology noted among all the human pigment genes, permits one to posit that the three main pigment genes (rhodopsin, blue pigment, and the long-wavelength pigments) all diverged between 500 million and 1 billion years ago [4].

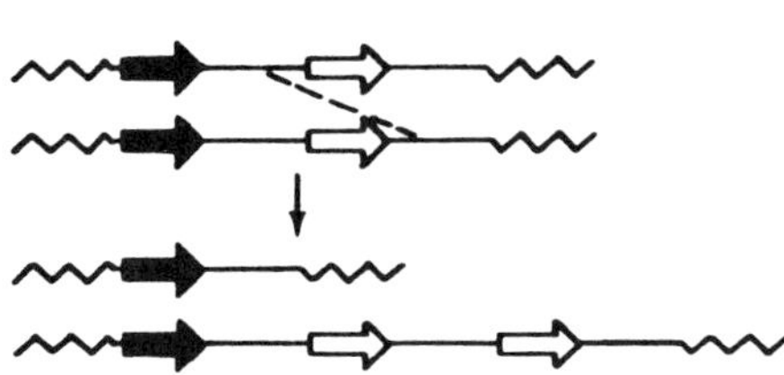

Figure 3 *The copy number of green pigment genes may be altered by unequal crossing over in the region between genes. This produces one chromosome with fewer and one chromosome with more green pigment genes. (Reprinted with permission from J Nathans et al, Molecular genetics of human color vision: the genes encoding blue, green, and red pigments. Science 1986;232:193–202. Copyright © 1986 by the AAAS.)*

■ Correlating the Phenotypic and Genotypic Variations

In the same way that unequal crossing over can delete or duplicate whole genes, red-green fusion genes may also be created. Analysis of the phenotypes associated with these genes has provided insights regarding the impact of such recombination events on the character (red or green) of the expressed pigment. The visual defects of 25 color-variant men were characterized using the Rayleigh anomaloscope previously described. The DNA of each was then characterized using well-defined restriction fragments from the red and green pigment genes. Replacement of the 3′ (downstream) end of the red pigment gene by green pigment DNA correlated with protanopic dichromacy (absence of red-wavelength detection) or protanomalous trichromacy (alteration of the wavelength detected by red pigment cones). Likewise, replacement of the 3′ end of all copies of the green pigment gene by red pigment DNA resulted in deuteranopic dichromacy or deuteranomalous trichromacy. Thus, minor and major changes in the absorption spectra of the pigments can be explained by changes in the 3′ end of the genes [3].

A similar analysis has been applied to subjects with blue-cone monochromacy (X-linked absence of red and green pigment activity). Detailed restriction fragment analysis revealed two genetic explanations for this phenotype, represented by two subsets of patients. In the first, the patients were found to have a single long-wavelength gene (red or red-green fusion); in addition, sequence analysis revealed a critical point mutation in each gene that eliminated the activity of the product of this single gene. In the second subset, a deletion of DNA upstream from the red pigment gene was present in each. These data suggest that a region of 579 or fewer base pairs located approximately 4 kilobases upstream of the red pigment gene is necessary for the expression of both red and green pigment genes [6].

■ Spectral Tuning

As noted earlier, in most color-blind individuals—namely, the anomalous trichromats—all three cone types are present. However, one of the pigments—most often the green pigment—is "tuned" to an abnormal wavelength. Even among subjects with normal color vision, sensitive psychophysical testing reveals minute differences in the wavelengths at which the red and green pigments absorb maximally [17–20]. These differences in spectral tuning are undoubtedly explained by variations in the amino acid sequences of the pigment opsins.

The retinal chromophore bound to the opsins in the photoreceptor pigments is an aromatic compound. Electrons are distributed in π orbitals along the length of the molecule. It has been shown for this and similar molecules that delocalization of these electrons along the molecule stabilizes the bonds, including the C11-C12 bond, resisting rotation between the *cis* and *trans* positions. Any alteration of the electronic milieu that reduces the electron delocalization promotes the appearance of alternating single and double bonds, enabling the *cis-trans* isomerization. Presumably, amino acid substitutions that result in changes in the net charge or molecular dipole moment in the vicinity of the chromophore would induce changes in the spectral absorption of the affected pigment [14]. With this in mind, it has been noted that the net charge for all amino acid residues believed to lie within the plasma membrane (potentially adjacent to the chromophore) is +1 for the blue pigment, 0 for rhodopsin, and −1 for both the red and green pigments [4]. To test the prediction that changes in the charges adjacent to the chromophore result in alteration of the absorption spectra, site-directed mutations were induced in six of the charged amino acids in the membrane-spanning segments of bovine rhodopsin. No change in the absorption spectrum of the pigment was noted [21]. However, a striking change in the absorbed wavelength—from 500 nm to 380 nm—was observed when glutamine was substituted for glutamate at position 113, just outside the putative intramembrane portion of the molecule [22, 23]. This example does not clarify fully the specific tuning of each of the human pigments. (The amino acid at position 113 in human rhodopsin and at the corresponding positions in all three human cone pigments is glutamate.) However, the example does prove that substitution of the charged residues by nonpolar ones may alter the spectral tuning of the pigment.

In other studies, there is evidence that may indicate which parts of the opsin molecule—perhaps even which specific residues—account for the precise tuning of each opsin. For example, an examination of the amino acid sequences from eight primate photoreceptor pigments has been undertaken. Two of the pigments were from humans, one a deuteranope and the other a protanope. Between them there were nonhomologous

Amino Acid Substitutions that Determine the Difference in Absorbance Peaks Between the Red- and Green-Cone Pigments

	Amino Acid Substitution Between		Change in Absorbance Peak (nm)
Position	Red Pigment	Green Pigment	
180	Ser	Ala	6
277	Tyr	Phe	9
285	Thr	Ala	15
Total			30

amino acid substitutions at seven positions; these were therefore candidates to be the critical substitutions in the spectral difference between the two pigments. The absorbance peaks of the two human pigments were separated by 31 nm. Six additional pigments, with absorbance peaks intermediate between the human pigments, were found in monkeys. Pairwise comparisons among the pigments revealed that substitutions at just three amino acid positions (180, 277, 285) accounted for the differences in the absorbance peaks (Table) [7].

Recently, systems have been devised for producing visual pigments in transfected cells [8–10]. Using cells expressing synthetic genes for the cone pigments, the impact of specific mutations on spectral tuning has been explored. By inducing mutations at all the sites where the amino acid sequence of the red pigment differed from that of the green, it has been found that substitutions at three positions accounted for all or nearly all of the spectral difference between the red- and green-cone pigments; not surprisingly, these were the same positions identified to be different in the comparison of primate photoreceptor pigments just described (DD Oprian, personal communication).

Other investigators have found that the small differences in color matching noted among subjects with normal color vision may also be explained by alterations in the amino acid sequences of the photopigments. The alteration accounting for the most commonly noted polymorphism among normal subjects is at position 180 of the red pigment, although in some, a contribution by substitutions at position 230 or 233 cannot be excluded [24].

■ Comments

The first description of color blindness was offered in 1798 by John Dalton, the English chemist well known for the atomic theory. In addition to lucidly describing his own abnormal visual sensations, Dalton [25] offered these comments:

It is remarkable that, out of twenty-five pupils I once had, to whom I explained this subject, two were found to agree with me; and, on another similar occasion, one . . . Our family consisted of three sons and one daughter . . . of whom two sons are circumstanced as I have described . . . I do not find that the parents or children in any of the instances have been so . . . It is remarkable that I have not heard of one female subject to this peculiarity.

Although he was totally unfamiliar with the modes of Mendelian inheritance, Dalton accurately described the inheritance of red-green color vision defects. Later, the X-linked nature of these defects would be established, and the linkage between the loci for color-blindness and hemophilia would be demonstrated in another classic publication [26]. The biochemistry of vision was explored by Wald [27] and others, but detailed analysis of the chemical differences among the pigments was impossible. Now, through a novel application of the techniques of molecular genetics—exploiting the anticipated homology among mammalian visual pigments—the genes for the pigments have been isolated and sequenced. This has yielded insight into the physical arrangement of the genes and the genetic defects that underlie the known phenotypes. Furthermore, knowledge of the nucleotide sequences has made possible a more detailed evaluation of the chemistry of the opsin proteins, which previously had not been isolated. Through molecular genetics we have an understanding of the chemistry of visual pigments that was otherwise inaccessible.

■ References

1. Nathans J, Hogness DS. Isolation, sequence analysis, and intron-exon arrangement of the gene encoding bovine rhodopsin. Cell 1983;34:807–814
2. Nathans J, Hogness DS. Isolation and nucleotide sequence of the gene encoding human rhodopsin. Proc Natl Acad Sci USA 1984;81:4851–4855
3. Nathans J, Piantanida TP, Eddy RL, et al. Molecular genetics of inherited variation in human color vision. Science 1986;232:203–210
4. Nathans J, Thomas D, Hogness DS. Molecular genetics of human color vision: the genes encoding blue, green, and red pigments. Science 1986;232:193–202
5. Vollrath D, Nathans J, Davis RW. Tandem array of human visual pigment genes at Xq28. Science 1988;240:1669–1672
6. Nathans J, Davenport CM, Maumenee IH, et al. Molecular genetics of human blue cone monochromacy. Science 1989;245:831–838
7. Neitz M, Neitz J, Jacobs GH. Spectral tuning of pigments underlying red-green color vision. Science 1991;252:971–974
8. Oprian DD, Molday RS, Kaufman RJ, Khorana HG. Expression of a synthetic bovine rhodopsin gene in monkey kidney cells. Proc Natl Acad Sci USA 1987; 84:8874–8878
9. Oprian DD, Asenjo AB, Lee N, Pelletier SL. Design, chemical synthesis, and expression of genes for the three human color vision pigments. Biochemistry 1991;30: 11367–11372

10. Nathans J, Weitz CJ, Agarwal N, et al. Production of bovine rhodopsin by mammalian cell lines expressing cloned cDNA: spectrophotometry and subcellular localization. Vision Res 1989;29:907–914

11. Merbs SL, Nathans J. Absorption spectra of human cone pigments. Nature 1992;356:433–435

12. Young T. The Bakerian lecture. On the theory of light and colours. Philos Trans R Soc Lond 1802(part 1):12–48

13. Nathans J. The genes for color vision. Sci Am 1989;260:42–49

14. Nathans J. Molecular biology of visual pigments. Annu Rev Neurosci 1987;10:163–194

15. Henderson R, Unwin PNT. Three-dimensional model of purple membrane obtained by electron microscopy. Nature 1975;257:28–32

16. Jacobs GH, Neitz J. Inheritance of color vision in a New World monkey (*Saimiri sciureus*). Proc Natl Acad Sci USA 1987;84:2545–2549

17. Neitz J, Jacobs GH. Polymorphism of the long-wavelength cone in normal human colour vision. Nature 1986;323:623–625

18. Mollon JD. Perception: questions of sex and colour. Nature 1986;323:578–579

19. Piantanida T. The molecular genetics of color vision and color blindness. Trends Genet 1988;4:319–323

20. Neitz J, Jacobs GH. Polymorphism in normal human color vision and its mechanism. Vision Res 1990;30:621–636

21. Nathans J. Determinants of visual pigment absorbance: role of charged amino acids in the putative transmembrane segments. Biochemistry 1990;29:937–942

22. Zhukovsky EA, Oprian DD. Effect of carboxylic acid side chains on the absorption maximum of visual pigments. Science 1989;246:928–930

23. Nathans J. Determinants of visual pigment absorbance: identification of the retinylidene Schiff's base counterion in bovine rhodopsin. Biochemistry 1990;29:9746–9752

24. Winderickx J, Lindsey DT, Sanocki E, et al. Polymorphism in red photopigment underlies variation in colour matching. Nature 1992;356:431–433

25. Dalton J. Extraordinary facts relating to the vision of colours: with observations. Mem Lit Philos Soc Manchester 1798;5:28–45

26. Bell J, Haldane JBS. The linkage between the genes of colour-blindness and haemophilia in man. Proc R Soc Lond [Biol] 1937;123:119–150

27. Wald G. The molecular basis of visual excitation. Nature 1968;219:800–807

Leber's Hereditary Optic Neuropathy

Nicholas J. Volpe, M.D.
Simmons Lessell, M.D.

Leber's hereditary optic neuropathy (LHON) is a devastating disorder that typically causes a subacute, sequential optic neuropathy with profound visual loss in young, otherwise healthy individuals. Since Leber described the disorder in 1871 [1], the clinical profile of Leber's disease has been well established, although it can be highly variable in members of the same pedigree. Men are affected more often than women, and the disease usually presents in the second or third decade of life.

Characteristic funduscopic changes, including circumpapillary telangiectatic microangiopathy, pseudoedema of the nerve fiber layer, and absence of fluorescein angiographic staining of the disc, are recognized in many cases [2]. Rarely, spontaneous visual acuity does occur. With knowledge of these characteristics alone, clinicians have been able to diagnose LHON with considerable accuracy. It became clear from numerous pedigrees that the disease was maternally inherited, which prompted Wallace and associates [3, 4] to search for a cytoplasmic determinant of inheritance, and attention was focused on the mitochondrial DNA (mtDNA). An mtDNA mutation in which a nucleotide substitution occurred at position 11778 was identified in 9 of 11 families. The substitution converts a highly conserved guanine to adenine and results in a substitution of histidine for arginine as the three hundred fortieth amino acid of reduced nicotinamide adenine-dinucleotide (NADH) dehydrogenase subunit 4. This mutation has been identified in approximately half of the available LHON pedigrees. Other mtDNA mutations have also been found. Although these discoveries have provided increased diagnostic reliability, the mutation alone cannot explain the variability in clinical expression of the disease. In the future, the hope is that we will understand better the biochemical failure in oxidative phosphorylation and mitochondrial energy production and the peculiar susceptibility of the optic nerve fibers. Ultimately, this understanding could lead to rational therapy.

■ Historical Perspective

The first descriptions of LHON, which appeared in the middle of the nineteenth century, were by Von Graefe [5] and Leber [1]. Leber reported that the disease occurred primarily in men between the ages of 18 and 23. However, he initially concluded that the condition was inflammatory. Numerous pedigrees with LHON have since been identified throughout the world. Studies of families in the 1960s and 1970s [6–10] failed to explain satisfactorily the mode of transmission. X-linked recessive transmission was initially suspected based on the preponderance of affected men and transmission in the maternal lineage, but this explanation proved inadequate. In 1963, van Senus [6] recognized that the disease was never transmitted by male individuals. No man who did not marry a carrier had a female offspring that was affected or was a carrier. In pure X-linked recessive disease, the expected incidence of the disease in female individuals is less than 1%, which is clearly much lower than the occurrence of LHON. Women were affected and transmitted the carrier state to their daughters more frequently than could be accounted for by X-linked recessive inheritance. Based on this complicated picture, Wallace [9] concluded, "A cursory examination of an affected family gives one the impression of a sex-linked inheritance; closer study suggests cytoplasmic inheritance; still more detailed analysis leads to confusion." Wallace and others [9, 11–14] emphasized that nonchromosomal maternal factors were important. Specifically, several authors suspected that a slow viruslike substance was transferred to the maternal ooplasm or reached the embryo transplacentally [9, 11–14]. Wallace [9], in 1970, concluded that the "pure pattern of maternal inheritance argues strongly in favor of vertical transmission of an infective agent."

Because Leber's disease is not lethal, there have been no opportunities to study the histopathological changes that accompany the acute loss of vision. Several reports have described histopathological changes of axonal degeneration in patients with long-standing optic neuropathy from LHON [15, 16]. One report described an inflammatory infiltrate in the meningeal tissues [16]. There are no histopathological confirmations of pathological adhesions in the leptomeninges.

Environmental factors also were believed to be contributory. In 1965, Wilson [15] correlated the severity of visual loss in LHON with tobacco smoking and suggested a defect in cyanide metabolism. Later studies by Berninger and associates [17] identified a patient with elevated blood levels of cyanide during the acute phase of visual loss; the cyanide level normalized after the acute phase, and 12 other patients with long-standing optic atrophy also had normal levels.

■ Clinical Characteristics

The clinical characteristics of LHON have been studied in numerous large pedigrees. Early series may have included patients with other diseases, and therefore some of what is described here as being phenotypical may turn out to be untrue when only genetically proved cases are considered.

Incidence and Onset

LHON causes an acute or subacute failure of visual acuity in both eyes, although usually not simultaneously. There is a clear sex predilection. Leber [1] recognized that the disease affected men nine times more often than women. In studies of whites from the United States, Canada, Australia, and Europe, 80% to 90% of affected individuals are male [6, 8, 9, 18–24]. In the most recent series, Newman and associates [20] found that 59 of 72 (82%) genetically proved cases of LHON from forty-nine different pedigrees occurred in men. The preponderance of males is somewhat less marked in Japanese series [25, 26].

The onset is typically between adolescence and age 30 years. In the series by Newman and co-workers [20], the age range was 8 to 60 years, with a mean of 27.6 years. Nearly 70% of patients were between ages 16 and 37. Cases have been reported in other series from age 1 to 70 years [6, 8, 19, 24, 25], but none of these is genetically proved. Within the same pedigree, it seems that women will develop the disease at an older age than men, but the age at which initial symptoms occur can vary widely even among siblings.

The second eye is usually involved within weeks or months. In the series by Newman's group [20] the average time was 1.8 months, with a range from simultaneous presentation (which occurred in 55% of cases) to 9 months. Many of the allegedly simultaneous cases likely represent sequential involvement of the eyes in which the attack in the first eye was not recognized. In one series, 2 patients in a well-documented pedigree had only monocular involvement after 12 and 14 years, respectively [19].

Symptoms

Patients present with symptoms that are typical of a subacute optic neuropathy. There is loss of central vision and dyschromatopsia. In many instances, dyschromatopsia is the initial deficit [19, 27, 28]. Pain is typically absent, although headache occasionally occurs. The presentation with headache has been suggested as supporting concurrent meningeal inflammation. Transient worsening of vision associated with exercise or heat (Uhthoff's sign) has been reported in LHON [2, 20, 28]. Visual acuity typically is approximately 5/200 to 20/200 and rarely is depressed to the level of hand movements or light perception. Total blindness from LHON is exceedingly rare. Visual field testing shows a central or centrocecal scotoma in virtually all cases [20].

Ophthalmoscopic Findings

The importance of the classic ophthalmoscopic appearance in patients with acute LHON was initially emphasized by Smith and colleagues [2] in 1973. In fact, Leber [1] commented on tortuosity of vessels and "white-striated opacity" in the peripapillary region. The findings also include circumpapillary telangiectatic microangiopathy, pseudoedema or swelling with hyperemia of the nerve fiber layer around the disc, and the absence of true edema or staining of the disc on fluorescein angiography. The hyperemic or swollen appearance of the disc had been described previously, but the pathognomonic value of the triad of findings was first emphasized in this report. Duke-Elder [29] described an acute phase of papillitis characterized by swelling and obscuration of the disc margin without hemorrhages or exudates. Lauber [30] and van Heuven [31] were actually first to recognize the importance of the retinal microangiopathy in the diagnosis of LHON.

The significance of these ophthalmoscopic findings is threefold. First, if these features are identified, the physician can diagnose LHON confidently and spare the patient additional invasive testing. Second, the findings imply an optic neuropathy as opposed to atrophy and suggest that the disease might be a manifestation of a microvascular disorder that secondarily causes axonal dysfunction. Finally, these findings can possibly be used to identify patients within a family at risk for developing the disease as they are present in a subset of patients who are in the preclinical phase [19, 28, 32]. Newman and associates [20] found that in six of the nineteen pedigrees with genetically proved LHON, at least one other family member demonstrated the characteristic funduscopic appearance. In one series, 68% of the male and 38% of the female offspring of women in one pedigree had characteristic funduscopic changes; none of the descendants of men within the pedigree had these changes [32]. In a follow-up series of 9 patients, Nikoskelainen and associates [23, 33] examined the funduscopic appearance and fluorescein angiographic characteristics in the presymptomatic and acute phases of LHON. Nerve fiber layer hemorrhages were identified in 2 patients. Arteriovenous shunting in the telangiectatic vascular bed were seen prior to the onset of symptoms. These authors concluded that the presymptomatic and acute changes were so characteristic that their "absence should exclude Leber's disease" and that the disease is a "vascular neuroretinopathy." The strength in these observations is the fact that they were made in a prospective fashion in several cases as they evolved. All LHON patients subsequently go on to develop some form of optic atrophy, regardless of the acute appearance of the fundus. Some cases are associated with cupping [34].

In many cases, the acute nerve fiber layer and vascular changes are absent [20, 34–36]. Later, after the onset of optic atrophy, it can be even more difficult to identify patients with LHON. When Trobe and co-workers [34] showed fundus photographs of nine different categories of optic atrophy to ophthalmologists, the diagnostic accuracy in the 16 cases of LHON ranged from 0% to 38%. Therefore, because the acute changes are often absent and the late changes are not diagnostic, the diagnosis of LHON should never be dismissed solely on the basis of the appearance of the nerve.

The local changes at the optic nerve head have led many to conclude that there are unique features that place the intraocular, and perhaps even only the papillomacular bundle, ganglion cells at greatest risk for damage in LHON. However, the disease's curious association with other conditions and results of ancillary testing suggest alternatively that more may be occurring than is seen with the ophthalmoscope. In a patient with slowly progressive visual loss from LHON, ultrasonography of the orbit revealed distended and fluid-filled optic nerve sheaths [36]. Magnetic resonance imaging (MRI), particularly with short-time inversion recovery (STIR) sequences, demonstrated abnormal signals in at least one of the optic nerves in all 8 patients studied with this technique [37]. The brains in all these patients were normal. However, nonspecific white matter lesions have been reported on the MRI scans of affected individuals [20]. Cerebrospinal fluid analysis, electroretinography, and electroencephalography are not helpful. Auditory evoked potentials were abnormal in 7 of 11 affected individuals in one series [38]. Visual evoked responses showed prolonged latency and reduced amplitude and have been reported to be abnormal also in some asymptomatic relatives of LHON patients [19, 27]. Abnormalities of mitochondrial metabolism have been demonstrated, by phosphorus 31 magnetic resonance spectroscopy, in the occipital lobes and skeletal muscles in patients with LHON spectroscopy [39, 40]. This is not a clinically important test, but brains in these patients were shown, by the same technique, to have abnormal energy reserves. Finally, reduced activity of NADH-coenzyme Q oxidoreductase was found in the platelets of 4 men with LHON [41].

Associated Conditions

Various neurological abnormalities, cardiac conduction defects, and skeletal deformities have been associated with LHON. Leber [1] reported patients with syncope and palpitations. Subsequently, abnormal electrocardiograms (ECGs) and, more specifically, conduction abnormalities have been convincingly demonstrated in various pedigrees. Rose and associates [42] reported 2 cases with abnormal Q and R waves. Nikoskelainen and associates [21, 33, 43] found preexcitation syndromes in all 10 families in which ECGs were obtained. Wolff-Parkinson-White and Lown-Ganong-

Levine syndromes were the most common abnormalities found. ECG abnormalities were seen in 51% of the descendants of female carriers in the pedigree [21]. Other ECG abnormalities included Q waves, atrial fibrillation, bundle branch blocks, and ventricular hypertrophy. In 11 subjects studied by electrocardiography, 5 showed evidence of cardiomyopathy. In Newman's series [20], 17 patients had ECGs, 14 of which were normal and 1 each of which exhibited supraventricular tachycardia, premature ventricular contractions, and a short Q-T interval. It is important to recognize that cardiac disease is often asymptomatic and can be found in patients with no evidence of optic neuropathy. Skeletal deformities including pes cavus, talipes equinovarus, kyphoscoliosis, congenital hip dislocation, arachnodactyly, arched palate, and spondyloepiphyseal dysplasia have been found in patients with LHON [9, 44–47].

Neurological disease associated with LHON was recognized by Ferguson and Critchley [44] in 1928 in a case associated with disseminated sclerosis. In this case there was associated pyramidal tract degeneration, ataxia, and loss of proprioception. The authors concluded that LHON was related to the heredofamilial ataxias. Other families with Charcot-Marie-Tooth disease have been found to have optic neuropathy and visual loss in a pattern consistent with LHON [48, 49]. Similar cases of LHON associated with dystonia and basal ganglia lesions have been reported [50–52].

Wallace [9] reported a large pedigree of patients with optic atrophy, encephalitis, and movement disorders. In another series, two-thirds of the LHON patients had minor neurological abnormalities that were similar to those found in multiple sclerosis, including cerebellar symptoms [53]. A disease very similar to, or the same as, multiple sclerosis has been reported also by others to occur with LHON [28, 53–55]. In Newman's series [20], 3 of 72 LHON patients had a peripheral neuropathy, and a case of LHON associated with hereditary motor sensory neuropathy has been reported as well [56].

Visual Acuity

The visual acuity nadir in LHON can be as good as 20/20 and as bad as no light perception. Improvement of vision is not rare. Nikoskelainen and associates [23] reported improvement in 32% of their patients. This number is somewhat high because these investigators examined both symptomatic and asymptomatic cases and therefore found cases of remitting, recurring, and monocular visual loss. Other studies found rates of visual recovery of 12% [57], 29% [58], and 25% [6]. Bird and McEachern [18] reported recovery in 9 of 11 patients in one pedigree. Lessell and associates [59] reported a series of 5 young men with LHON type presentations, all of whose vision dramatically improved after a period of 4 to 21 months. These authors believed that the absence of the characteristic microvascular fundus changes of LHON at presentation may correlate with recovery. In

Newman's series [20], of the patients with the 11778 mutation, visual acuity improved to 20/40 or better in only 4 of 109 eyes.

■ Mitochondrial Genetics

Mendelian inheritance occurs when nuclear DNA sequences are transmitted to the offspring and result in most of our genetically determined normal characteristics. When altered, they can result in inherited disease. Since we receive half of our nuclear genes from our mother and half from our father, the expected frequencies of various traits carried on nuclear genes can be accurately predicted. In LHON, it became clear that no affected male individual ever had an affected descendant, which was incompatible with mendelian inheritance. Instead, the gene is transmitted vertically from an affected mother to all her offspring. Mitochondrial inheritance was the most plausible explanation. Mitochondria are intracytoplasmic organelles, and because the oocyte contributes virtually all the cytoplasm of the developing zygote, all mitochondria are inherited from the mother. It follows that only daughters will pass on the mitochondria to their descendants.

Mitochondria are unique among cellular organelles because they contain their own DNA. The mitochondrial matrix, in addition to containing enzymes and an apparatus for transcription and translation, has two to ten copies of a double-stranded circular DNA of approximately 16.5 kilobases, which contain 37 genes that are essential to the respiratory chain. This genetic material represents only a fraction of a percent of the cell's genetic material. Thirteen of these genes encode for essential proteins in the respiratory chain. Specifically, they encode for two subunits of adenosine triphosphatase, three subunits of cytochrome c oxidase, one subunit of ubiquinol-cytochrome c oxidoreductase, and seven subunits of NADH dehydrogenase [60–62]. The other twenty-four genes encode for the transfer and ribosomal RNA molecules required for production of the respiratory chain proteins. The mitochondria contain ribosomes and therefore are completely self-sufficient in terms of the ability to synthesize the proteins encoded by their DNA. The other proteins and cofactors, which are actually the majority of those required for oxidative phosphorylation, are encoded for by the nuclear DNA and are subsequently transported into the mitochondria. Because of the symbiotic relationship between the mitochondria and the cell, "mitochondrial disease" can result from defects in either the mtDNA or the nuclear DNA. Possible defects in nuclear DNA include abnormalities in the nuclear regulation of mitochondrial genes, in the additional nuclear proteins required for oxidative phosphorylation, and in those required for the synthesis or transport of these proteins to the mitochondria.

mtDNA differs from nuclear DNA in that it contains very few noncoding sequences and often there is overlap of neighboring genes. The mtDNA has a unique method of replication and transcription. In addition, it has a slightly different genetic code that alters the reading of a stop codon employed by nuclear DNA. Therefore, the transcription apparatus for each nuclear DNA and mtDNA is separate and distinct.

Through a series of random events called *replicative segregation,* any particular molecule of mtDNA can be found in very disparate amounts in daughter cells. That is, mtDNA replicates randomly within the mitochondria. Mitochondria subsequently divide unequally without regard to the amount of mtDNA [60, 63]. During cell division, mitochondria, as all cytoplasmic organelles, are divided randomly between the two daughter cells. This series of events can be used to explain some of the clinical characteristics and inheritance patterns of LHON (see section on Heteroplasmy, page 161).

The mtDNA Mutation Associated with LHON

Examination of the mitochondrial genome in patients with LHON led to the discovery of a point mutation by Wallace and associates [3] in 1988. For the mutation to be considered responsible for the condition, it would have to (1) change a highly evolutionarily conserved amino acid, (2) be present in multiple LHON pedigrees, (3) not be found in normal individuals, and (4) alter, not eliminate, the respiratory function of the NADH subunit. These criteria are all met by the 11778 mutation that occurs in a sequence of mtDNA that is highly conserved and is more than 85% homologous in mouse, cow, and human. A mutation satisfying these criteria was found in nine of eleven pedigrees and in none of 45 unrelated control individuals [3]. The guanine-to-adenine substitution results in a subtle change of the basic amino acid arginine to histidine. The result is an abnormal subunit 4 of the NADH dehydrogenase, which is the first enzyme in the pathway of oxidative phosphorylation.

Affected individuals were identified using the polymerase chain reaction and restriction endonuclease SfaNI. The mutation of guanine to adenine in LHON patients eliminates a normal cleavage point of SfaNI. Since this test is dependent on a negative result or on cleavage not occurring, there is a small chance of a false-positive result. That is, since the mtDNA mutates at five to ten times the rate of nuclear DNA, the possibility exists that a false-positive result will occur because of harmless polymorphism. Alternatively, other restriction endonucleases, specifically *Mae* III, cleave only mutated LHON mtDNA that contains the guanine-to-adenine switch, thereby reducing the false-positive results and making the test 100% specific for the disease [64]. Newer methods of detecting the mutation, requiring only polymerase chain reactions without endonuclease cleavage, have been reported and will eventually lead to more widespread availability of the test [65]. The 11778 mutation has subsequently been identified in ten of nineteen pedigrees from Finland [66], in Asian families [67–69], and in pedigrees from France [70] and England [71]. Wallace's laboratory has identified forty-nine different pedigrees with the mutation [20].

These seemingly unrelated pedigrees and the sporadic, nonfamilial occurrence of LHON (twenty-eight of forty-nine pedigrees are singleton cases in Wallace's laboratory [20]) suggest that the mutation has arisen spontaneously on more than one occasion. Further proof of this is in the work of Singh and associates [4], who studied mtDNA markers on an American black pedigree and compared it with markers from European pedigrees. They found that the 11778 mutation was associated with two different mtDNA polymorphisms and sequence variants and concluded that the mutation must have arisen twice independently. Vilkki and associates [66] reported a pedigree in which only the 2 affected members demonstrated the mutation, suggesting that it was of recent origin.

However, the 11778 mutation alone is not a sufficient explanation for all cases of LHON. Alone, it does not explain the variable occurrence of the disease within the same pedigree, its wide spectrum of phenotypical expression, and the susceptibility of male offspring. Only approximately half of the pedigrees with clinically diagnosed LHON have the 11778 mutation [61, 62, 66, 69, 71–75]. In the series of nineteen Finnish pedigrees, nine did not have the mutation, and these nine seemed to have low penetrance of the phenotypical expression of optic atrophy, whereas those with the mutation seemed to have a high rate of optic atrophy in maternal offspring [66]. Later, a second mutation was identified in three Finnish pedigrees [76]. In these unrelated families, a transition of guanine to adenine occurs at position 3460, resulting in an amino acid change of alanine to threonine in subunit 1 of NADH dehydrogenase. Other NADH complex I mtDNA mutations in LHON have been identified by Howell and colleagues [77], Johns and Berman [78], and Brown and colleagues [79]. A series of patients with multiple NADH complex III mutations, with normal complex I genome, has also been identified [80].

Basis for the Phenotypical Expression of the mtDNA Mutation

The variable phenotypical expression of the mtDNA mutation is as yet unexplained, but three theories have been advanced: heteroplasmy, a second genetic factor (possibly on the X chromosome), and environmental factors. Most likely, all of these factors contribute to the phenotypical expression of the disease [62].

Heteroplasmy *Heteroplasmy* refers to the coexistence of mutant and normal mtDNA. Since the mutated mtDNA is still capable of normal replication and the division of mitochondria to daughter cells is random, any percentage of the thousands of mtDNA molecules in each daughter cell can be represented by mutant DNA. At each division, the fraction of mutated DNA can drift toward or away from a totally normal or totally mutant state [54, 62, 63]. Thus, the phenotype will vary depending on the percentage of mutant DNA. When a certain threshold is reached, dysfunction will occur. This dysfunction would be more likely when the metabolic needs of the cell are greatest. Heteroplasmy for the 11778 mutation has been demonstrated in affected and unaffected individuals [20, 72, 73, 81, 82]. In some pedigrees, the percentage of mutant mtDNA remains constant throughout different members and generations [72, 82]. Lott and co-workers [81] reported a pedigree in which the amount of mutant mtDNA increased from one generation to the next and correlated with increased phenotypical expression. They also found proportions of mutant DNA in the blood different from those found in the hair of the same individual. Lott's group [81] emphasized that the detection and quantification of heteroplasmy is of great importance in the diagnosis and counseling of these patients and may also be an important factor in determining phenotypical expression. Two other studies have recently correlated the proportion of mutant DNA to disease severity [83, 84]. Meiotic segregation can also result in heteroplasmy in children of the same affected woman. Heteroplasmy has been offered as an explanation for phenotypical variability in other mitochondrially inherited disease as well [85, 86].

Most patients with LHON are homoplasmic for the mutation, with a single population of mutant mtDNA [87]. Vilkki and associates [66] found that all individuals in families with LHON were homoplasmic for the mutation regardless of their disease status. Even homoplasmic LHON individuals are born with the ability to see. It is only after a period of time that the axons in their optic nerves begin to malfunction. Therefore, the mutation alone cannot explain the loss of vision.

A Second Genetic (X-Chromosome) Factor Because of the predominance of affected male individuals, attempts were made to link the disease to X-chromosome factors. Chen and associates [88] were unable to demonstrate an X-linked gene by linkage analysis. However, their data were analyzed without consideration of the mtDNA mutation as the primary cause of LHON. Vilkki and colleagues [89] convincingly demonstrated linkage of optic atrophy in patients with and without the 11778 mutation to the proximal Xp chromosome. They pointed out that other X-linked eye conditions (Norrie disease, congenital stationary night blindness, and X-linked retinitis pigmentosa) are linked to the same region of the X chromosome. Bu and Rotter [90] postulated involvement of the X chromosome based on segregation analysis of the available pedigrees. Other possible genetic determinants of phenotypical expression include other identified mtDNA mutations [77, 78] and nuclear-encoded factors that can alter mitochondrial function. In this situation of multiple genetic defects, it may be an overall decrease in cell energy production that causes disease, as opposed to a specific enzyme defect [79].

Environmental Factors Final consideration should therefore be given to tissue-specific factors and environmental contributions to optic atrophy. The nerve cells of the eye and central nervous system are most dependent on mitochondrial adenosine triphosphate. Mitochondrial function may decrease with age [91] and may have different reserves in men and women. Optic nerve axons may have a critical point at which energy is insufficient to run cellular pumps and allow for adequate protein synthesis. External factors, such as cyanide poisoning, alcohol, and environmental toxins, that could damage oxidative phosphorylation may contribute to the onset of visual loss. None of these factors reliably accompanies the acute visual deterioration in affected individuals, but it seems feasible that they can alter the genetically programmed cell death in a given individual.

■ Treatment

There is no known effective prophylaxis or treatment for the visual loss that occurs with LHON. Steroids, cyanide antagonists, and hydroxocobalamin have been tried without effect [2, 17, 23, 28, 92]. Imachi and associates [25, 93] have reported neurosurgical lysis of arachnoidal adhesions in patients in Japan with good results. Although this seemed promising in the early 1970s, there has been no subsequent report from these or other authors on the usefulness of the procedure. It is difficult to imagine how chiasmal arachnoiditis could be responsible for the funduscopic changes of LHON unless they are unrelated and both are epiphenomena of the same disease process. Some physicians recommend that family members in LHON pedigrees and patients affected in one eye with LHON avoid tobacco and heavy use of alcohol [62, 75]. Finally, in other diseases that affect mitochondrial energy production some success has been reported with the use of cofactors such as succinate and coenzyme Q [94–96]. Caigianut and associates [97] have emphasized the importance of diet in patients with defects in the respiratory chain. The role of these various therapies in treating or preventing of LHON remains to be proved.

■ Conclusion

Discovery of the mtDNA mutation responsible for LHON has raised as many questions as it answered. Clearly, the implications for clinical practice are profound. The test is highly specific, with no false-positive outcomes. Definitive molecular genetic diagnosis can help to avoid the emotional pain and expense of extensive diagnostic evaluations and treatment in patients with LHON. This can be particularly helpful in sporadic cases. Unfortunately, the identification of the 11778 mutation may be associated with a poor prognosis of visual recovery [20, 66, 73]. Knowing the specific defect in energy production may help in developing specific therapies aimed at bypassing or lessening the impact of the defect. Genetic counseling can be offered if the mutation is identified and, as the significance and ability to quantitate heteroplasmy are better understood, there may be some hope for maternal descendants in LHON pedigrees. Precise genetic testing will help us to define more exactly the clinical profile of LHON patients. Finally, the discovery of the mutation in LHON will serve as a model for investigation of other diseases suspected of being transmitted by mtDNA [98].

The unexplained issues are numerous and have wide implications. Clinically, the gender difference, variability among members of the same pedigree, timing of onset of visual loss, factors that contribute to recovery in some patients, role of the environment, and isolation of the disease to the eye remain unexplained by the single mtDNA mutation. Geneticists and ophthalmologists must continue to work together to understand these seemingly inexplicable phenomena.

■ References

1. Leber T. Ueber hereditare und congenital angelegte Sehnervenleiden. Albrecht Von Graefes Arch Klin Exp Ophthalmol 1871;17:249–291
2. Smith JL, Hoyt WF, Susac JO. Ocular fundus in acute Leber optic neuropathy. Arch Ophthalmol 1973;90:349–354
3. Wallace DC, Singh G, Lott MT, et al. Mitochondrial DNA mutation associated with Leber's hereditary optic neuropathy. Science 1988;242:1427–1430
4. Singh G, Lott MT, Wallace DC. A mitochondrial DNA mutation as a cause of Leber's hereditary optic neuropathy. N Engl J Med 1989;320:1300–1305
5. Von Graefe A. Ein ungewohhnlicher Fall von hereditare Amaurose. Arch Fr Ophthalmol 1858;4:266–268
6. van Senus AHC. Leber's disease in the Netherlands. Doc Ophthalmol 1963;17:1–162
7. Seedorff T. Leber's disease. Acta Ophthalmol (Copenh) 1968;46:4–25
8. Seedorff T. The inheritance of Leber's disease: a genealogical follow-up study. Acta Ophthalmol (Copenh) 1985;63:135–145
9. Wallace DC. A new manifestation of Leber's disease and a new explanation for the agency responsible for its unusual pattern of inheritance. Brain 1970;93:121–132
10. Waardenburg PJ. Some remarks on the clinical and genetic puzzle of Leber's optic neuritis. J Genet Hum 1969;17:479–495
11. Erickson RP. Leber's optic atrophy, a possible example of maternal inheritance. Am J Hum Genet 1972;24:348–349
12. Harper PS. Mendelian inheritance or transmissible agent? The lesson of Kuru and the Australia antigen. J Med Genet 1977;14:389–398
13. Wallace DC. Leber's optic atrophy: a possible example of vertical transmission of a slow virus in man. Australas Ann Med 1970;19:259–262

14. Colenbrander MC. Observations on the heredity of Leber's disease. Ophthalmologica 1962;144:446–450

15. Wilson J. Leber's hereditary optic atrophy—some clinical and aetiological considerations. Brain 1963;86:347–362

16. Adams JH, Blackwood W, Wilson J. Further clinical and pathological observations on Leber's optic atrophy. Brain 1966;89:15–26

17. Berninger TA, Meyer LV, Siess E, et al. Leber's hereditary optic atrophy: further evidence for a defect of cyanide metabolism? Br J Ophthalmol 1989;73:314–316

18. Bird A, McEachern D. Leber's hereditary optic atrophy in a Canadian family. Can Med Assoc J 1949;61:376–383

19. Carroll WM, Mastaglia FL. Leber's optic neuropathy: a clinical and visual evoked potential study of affected and asymptomatic members of a six generation family. Brain 1979;102:559–580

20. Newman NJ, Lott MT, Wallace DC. The clinical characteristics of pedigrees of Leber's hereditary optic neuropathy with the 11778 mutation. Am J Ophthalmol 1991;111:750–762

21. Nikoskelainen EK, Savontaus M-L, Wanne OP, et al. Leber's hereditary optic neuroretinopathy, a maternally inherited disease: a genealogical study in four pedigrees. Arch Ophthalmol 1987;105:665–671

22. Lundsgaard R. Leber's disease: a genealogic, genetic and clinical study of 101 cases of retrobulbar optic neuritis in 20 Danish families. Acta Ophthalmol (Copenh) 1944;22(suppl 21):1–306

23. Nikoskelainen E, Hoyt WF, Nummelin K. Ophthalmoscopic findings in Leber's hereditary optic neuropathy: II. The fundus findings in the affected family members. Arch Ophthalmol 1983;101:1059–1068

24. Bell J. Eugenetics laboratory memoirs: XXVI. The treasury of human inheritance, vol 2, part 4. Cambridge, Engl: Cambridge University Press, 1931:324–423

25. Imachi J. Neuro-surgical treatment of Leber's optic atrophy and its pathogenetic relationship to arachnoiditis. Prog Neuro-ophthalmol 1969;2:121–127

26. Yamanaka H. The mode of inheritance of Leber's disease. Acta Soc Ophthalmol Jpn 1971;75:1930–1936

27. Livingstone IR, Mastaglia FL, Howe JW, Aherne GES. Leber's optic neuropathy: clinical and visual evoked response studies in asymptomatic and symptomatic members of a 4-generation family. Br J Ophthalmol 1980;64:751–757

28. Nikoskelainen E, Sogg RL, Rosenthal AR, et al. The early phase in Leber hereditary optic atrophy. Arch Ophthalmol 1977;95:969–978

29. Duke-Elder S. System of ophthalmology, vol 12. St Louis: Mosby, 1971:108–111

30. Lauber H. Eine Fall con familiarer retrobulbarer Neuritis. Wien Klin Wochenschr 1902;15:1264–1265

31. van Heuven GJ. Die Diagnose der hereditaren Leberschen Sehnervenatrophie. Klin Monatsbl Augenheilkd 1924;73:252–253

32. Nikoskelainen E, Hoyt WF, Nummelin K. Ophthalmoscopic findings in Leber's hereditary optic neuropathy: I. Fundus findings in asymptomatic family members. Arch Ophthalmol 1982;100:1597–1602

33. Nikoskelainen E, Hoyt WF, Nummelin K, Schatz H. Fundus findings in Leber's hereditary optic neuroretinopathy: III. Fluorescein angiographic studies. Arch Ophthalmol 1984;102:981–989

34. Trobe JD, Glaser JS, Cassady JC. Optic atrophy: differential diagnosis by fundus observation alone. Arch Ophthalmol 1980;98:1040–1045

35. Lopez PF, Smith JL. Leber's optic neuropathy: new observations. J Clin Neuro Ophthalmol 1986;6:144–152

36. Smith JL, Tse DT, Byrne SF, et al. Optic nerve sheath distention in Leber's optic neuropathy and the significance of the "Wallace mutation." J Clin Neuro Ophthalmol 1990;10:231–238

37. Kermode AG, Moseley IF, Kendall BE, et al. Magnetic resonance imaging in Leber's optic neuropathy. J Neurol Neurosurg Psychiatry 1989;52:671–674

38. Mondelli M, Rossi A, Scarpini C, et al. BAEP changes in Leber's hereditary optic atrophy: further confirmation of multisystem involvement. Acta Neurol Scand 1990;81:339–343

39. Cortelli P, Montagna P, Avoni P, et al. Mitochondrial metabolism in Leber's hereditary optic neuropathy. Neurology 1990;40(suppl 1):310

40. Cortelli P, Montagna P, Avoni P, et al. Leber's hereditary optic neuropathy: genetic, biochemical, and phosphorus magnetic resonance spectroscopy study in an Italian family. Neurology 1991;41:1211–1215

41. Parker WD Jr, Oley CA, Parks JK. A defect in mitochondrial electron-transport activity (NADH-coenzyme Q oxidoreductase) in Leber's hereditary optic neuropathy. N Engl J Med 1989;320:1331–1333

42. Rose FC, Bowden AN, Bowden PMA. The heart in Leber's optic atrophy. Br J Ophthalmol 1970;54:388–393

43. Nikoskelainen E, Wanne O, Dahl M. Pre-excitation syndrome and Leber's hereditary optic neuropathy. Lancet 1985;1:696

44. Ferguson FR, Critchley M. Leber's optic atrophy and its relationship with the heredo-familial ataxias. J Neurol Psychopathol 1928;9:120–132

45. Merritt HH. Hereditary optic atrophy (Leber's disease). Arch Neurol Psychiatry 1930;24:775–781

46. Kwittken J, Barest HD. The neuropathology of hereditary optic atrophy (Leber's disease): the first complete anatomic study. Am J Pathol 1958;34:185–207

47. Hodess AB, Harter DH. Leber's optic atrophy associated with spondyloepiphyseal dysplasia. Neurology 1974;24:1082–1085

48. McCluskey DJ, O'Connor PS, Sheehy JT. Leber's optic neuropathy and Charcot-Marie-Tooth disease: report of a case. J Clin Neuro Ophthalmol 1986;6:76–81

49. McLeod JG, Low PA, Morgan JA. Charcot-Marie-Tooth disease with Leber optic atrophy. Neurology 1978;28:179–184

50. Novotny EJ Jr, Singh G, Wallace DC, et al. Leber's disease and dystonia: a mitochondrial disease. Neurology 1986;36:1053–1060

51. Bruyn GW, Went LN. A sex-linked heredo-degenerative neurological disorder associated with Leber's optic atrophy: I. Clinical studies. J Neurol Sci 1964;1:59–80

52. Bruyn GW, Vielvoye GJ, Went LN. Hereditary spastic dystonia: a new mitochondrial encephalopathy? Putaminal necrosis as a diagnostic sign. J Neurol Sci 1991;103:195–202

53. De Weerdt CJ, Went LN. Neurological studies in families with Leber's optic atrophy. Acta Neurol Scand 1971;47:541–554

54. Lees F, MacDonald A-ME, Turner JW. Leber's disease with symptoms resembling disseminated sclerosis. J Neurol Neurosurg Psychiatry 1964;27:415–421

55. Palan A, Stehouwer A, Went LN. Studies on Leber's optic neuropathy III. Doc Ophthalmol 1989;71:77–87

56. Weiller C, Ferbert A. Hereditary motor and sensory neuropathy (HMSN) and optic atrophy (HMSN type VI, Vizioli). Eur Arch Psychiatry Neurol Sci 1991;240:246–249

57. Brunette J-R, Bernier G. Study of a family of Leber's optic atrophy with recuperation. Prog Neuro-ophthalmol 1969;2:91–97

58. Holloway TB. Leber's disease. Arch Ophthalmol 1933;9:789–800

59. Lessell S, Gise RL, Krohel GB. Bilateral optic neuropathy with remission in young men: variation on a theme by Leber? Arch Neurol 1983;40:2–6

60. Shoffner JM IV, Wallace DC. Oxidative phosphorylation diseases: disorders of two genomes. Adv Hum Genet 1990;19:267–330

61. Newman NJ, Wallace DC. Mitochondria and Leber's hereditary optic neuropathy. Am J Ophthalmol 1990;109:726–730

62. Newman NJ. Leber's hereditary optic neuropathy. Ophthalmol Clin North Am 1991;4:431–447
63. Wallace DC. Mitochondrial genes and disease. Hosp Pract 1986;21:77–87, 90–92
64. Stone EM, Coppinger JM, Kardon RH, Donelson J. *Mae* III positively detects the mitochondrial mutation associated with Type I Leber's hereditary optic neuropathy. Arch Ophthalmol 1990;108:1417–1420
65. Norby S, Lestienne P, Nelson I, Rosenberg T. Mutation detection in Leber's hereditary optic neuropathy by PCR with allele-specific priming. Biochem Biophys Res Commun 1991;175:631–636
66. Vilkki J, Savontaus M-L, Nikoskelainen EK. Genetic heterogeneity in Leber hereditary optic neuroretinopathy revealed by mitochondrial DNA polymorphism. Am J Hum Genet 1989;45:206–211
67. Yoneda M, Tsuji S, Yamauchi T, et al. Mitochondrial DNA mutation in a family with Leber's hereditary optic neuropathy. Lancet 1989;1:1076–1077
68. Hiida Y, Mashima Y, Oguchi Y, et al. Mitochondrial DNA analysis of Leber's hereditary optic neuropathy. Jpn J Ophthalmol 1991;35:102–106
69. Fujiki K, Hotta Y, Hayakawa M, et al. A mutation of mitochondrial DNA in Japanese families with Leber's hereditary optic neuropathy. Jpn J Hum Genet 1991;36:143–147
70. Johns DR. Improved molecular-genetic diagnosis of Leber's hereditary optic neuropathy. N Engl J Med 1990;323:1488–1489
71. Poulton J, Deadman ME, Bronte-Stewart J, et al. Analysis of mitochondrial DNA in Leber's hereditary optic neuropathy. J Med Genet 1991;28:765–770
72. Bolhuis PA, Bleeker-Wagemakers EM, Ponne NJ, et al. Rapid shift in genotype of human mitochondrial DNA in a family with Leber's hereditary optic neuropathy. Biochem Biophys Res Commun 1990;170:994–997
73. Holt IJ, Miller DH, Harding AE. Genetic heterogeneity and mitochondrial DNA heteroplasmy in Leber's hereditary optic neuropathy. J Med Genet 1989;26:739–743
74. Phillips CI, Gosden CM. Leber's hereditary optic neuropathy and Kearns-Sayre syndrome: mitochondrial DNA mutations. Surv Ophthalmol 1991;35:463–472
75. Morris MA. Mitochondrial mutations in neuro-ophthalmological diseases: a review. J Clin Neuro Ophthalmol 1990;10:159–166
76. Huoponen K, Vilkki J, Aula P, et al. A new mtDNA mutation associated with Leber hereditary optic neuroretinopathy. Am J Hum Genet 1991;48:1147–1153
77. Howell N, Kubacka I, Xu M, McCullough DA. Leber hereditary optic neuropathy: involvement of the mitochondrial ND1 gene and evidence for an intragenic suppressor mutation. Am J Hum Genet 1991;48:935–942
78. Johns DR, Berman J. Alternative, simultaneous complex I mitochondrial DNA mutations in Leber's hereditary optic neuropathy. Biochem Biophys Res Commun 1991;174:1324–1330
79. Brown MD, Voljavec AS, Lott MT, et al. Mitochondrial DNA complex I and III mutations associated with Leber's hereditary optic neuropathy. Genetics 1992;130:163–173
80. Johns DR, Neufeld MJ. Cytochrome b mutations in Leber hereditary optic neuropathy. Biochem Biophys Res Commun 1991;181:1358–1364
81. Lott MT, Voljavec AS, Wallace DC. Variable genotype of Leber's hereditary optic neuropathy patients. Am J Ophthalmol 1990;109:625–631
82. Vilkki J, Savontaus M-L, Nikoskelainen EK. Segregation of mitochondrial genomes in a heteroplasmic lineage with Leber hereditary optic neuroretinopathy. Am J Hum Genet 1990;47:95–100
83. Isashiki Y, Nakagawa M. Clinical correlation of mitochondrial DNA heteroplasmy and Leber's hereditary optic neuropathy. Jpn J Ophthalmol 1991;35:259–267
84. Zhu DP, Economou EP, Antonarakis SE, Maumenee IH. Mitochondrial DNA muta-

tion and heteroplasmy in type I Leber hereditary optic neuropathy. Am J Med Genet 1992;42:173–179

85. DiMauro S, Bonilla E, Zaviani M, et al. Mitochondrial myopathies. Ann Neurol 1985;17:521–538

86. Rosing HS, Hopkins LC, Wallace DC, et al. Maternally inherited mitochondrial myopathy and myoclonic epilepsy. Ann Neurol 1985;17:228–237

87. Johns DR. The molecular genetics of Leber's hereditary optic neuropathy. Arch Ophthalmol 1990;108:1405–1407

88. Chen JD, Cox I, Denton MJ. Preliminary exclusion of an X-linked gene in Leber optic atrophy by linkage analysis. Hum Genet 1990;82:203–207

89. Vilkki J, Ott J, Savontaus ML, et al. Optic atrophy in Leber hereditary optic neuro-retinopathy is probably determined by an X-chromosomal gene closely linked to DXS7. Am J Hum Genet 1991;48:486–491

90. Bu XD, Rotter JI. X chromosome-linked and mitochondrial gene control of Leber hereditary optic neuropathy: evidence from segregation analysis for dependence on X chromosome inactivation. Proc Natl Acad Sci USA 1991;88:8198–8202

91. Trounce I, Byrne E, Marzuki S. Decline in skeletal muscle mitochondrial respiratory chain function: possible factor in ageing. Lancet 1989;1:637–639

92. Miller NR. The hereditary optic neuropathies: monosymptomatic hereditary optic neuropathy. In: Miller N, ed. Walsh and Hoyt's clinical neuro-ophthalmology, ed 4, vol 1. Baltimore: Williams & Wilkins, 1982:311–317

93. Imachi J, Nishizaki K. The patients of Leber's optic atrophy should be treated brain-surgically. Folia Ophthalmol Jpn 1970;21:209–217

94. Bresolin N, Bet L, Binda A, et al. Clinical and biochemical correlations in mitochondrial myopathies treated with coenzyme Q10. Neurology 1988;38:892–899

95. Shoffner JM, Lott MT, Voljavec AS, et al. Spontaneous Kearns-Sayre/chronic external ophthalmoplegia plus syndrome associated with a mitochondrial DNA deletion: a slip-replication model and metabolic therapy. Proc Natl Acad Sci USA 1989;86:7952–7956

96. Wallace DC. Mitochondrial DNA mutations and neuromuscular disease. Trends Genet 1989;5:9–13

97. Cagianut B, Schnebli HP, Rhyner K, Furrer J. Decreased thiosulfate sulfur transferase (rhodanese) in Leber's hereditary optic neuropathy. Klin Wochenschr 1984; 62:850–854

98. Parker WD Jr. Preclinical detection of Parkinson's disease: biochemical approaches. Neurology 1991;41(suppl 2):34–37

MELAS Syndrome: A Mitochondrially Inherited Disorder

Edward M. Stroh, M.D.

Jacqueline M. S. Winterkorn, M.D., Ph.D.

Alex E. Jalkh, M.D.

Simmons Lessell, M.D.

Encephalomyopathies caused by mutations in mitochondrial DNA (mtDNA) constitute a growing group of disorders with prominent ophthalmic manifestations [1–10]. These include Kearns-Sayre syndrome (KSS), characterized by progressive external ophthalmoplegia, retinopathy, and cardiomyopathy [7]; MERRF, a syndrome of *myoclonus*, *epilepsy*, and *ragged red fibers* [11]; and MELAS, a syndrome of *myopathy*, *encephalopathy*, *lactic acidosis*, and *strokelike* episodes [12]. Leber's hereditary optic neuropathy, another mitochondrially inherited disorder, is characterized by sequential bilateral visual loss without myopathy. Several mitochondrial mutations have been identified in Leber's hereditary optic neuropathy [13]. The ophthalmic manifestations of MELAS have not been well recognized or characterized. We have documented their presence in patients and relatives from a single family who harbor the prevalent mitochondrial point mutation of the disorder.

Clinical and Laboratory Findings in MELAS

Patients with MELAS are typically short but otherwise develop normally until the onset of sensorineural deafness, headaches, episodic vomiting, seizures, and strokelike episodes, resulting in hemiparesis, hemianopia, and cortical blindness [1]. Early motor and cognitive development are normal. The first manifestation of MELAS is usually a growth disturbance. The average age of onset of reported cases is 5.2 years (range, birth to 15 years); the average age of first "stroke" is 14.7 years (range, 7 to 33 years). Male patients outnumber female patients by more than 2:1.

Magnetic resonance imaging (MRI) shows multifocal areas of hyperintense signal on T_2-weighted images in the cortex of the cerebrum, cerebellum, and immediately adjacent white matter [14]. Laboratory evaluation typically shows lactic acidosis and an elevated cerebrospinal fluid (CSF) lactate level.

MELAS patients generally have normal findings in the following tests: complete blood cell count, blood chemistries, renal and hepatic function tests, pH, pCO_2, and bicarbonate, triglycerides, cholesterol, amino acids, endocrine function, and immunological function. Serum and urine lactic acid and pyruvate levels are usually elevated. CSF fluid is normal except for a mildly elevated protein level, with a normal electrophoretic pattern.

Light microscopy of long-muscle specimens show ragged red fibers in modified Gomori's trichrome stain. Electron microscopy shows increased numbers of large mitochondria in the sarcolemmal region. Neuropathological workup of patients with KSS, MERRF, and MELAS shows a similar underlying spongiform degeneration in the brain [2].

Oxidation rates and adenosine triphosphate (ATP) production are diminished in muscle homogenate. Single enzyme activities are generally normal except for succinate c oxidoreductase, which is diminished.

■ Cases

Patient 1

A 33-year-old white man was referred for neuro-ophthalmic evaluation. His childhood development had been normal except for short stature (63 inches) and slight build in comparison with his father (73 inches). He was a cigarette smoker. At age 18, he developed proteinuria, and a renal biopsy revealed sclerotic changes in arterioles, consistent with a vasculitis. He continued to work as a fireman until his midtwenties, when he developed a sensorineural hearing deficit that progressed to profound deafness over several years. At age 27, he complained of severe headaches accompanied by nausea and vomiting. Computerized tomography (CT) scanning demonstrated a right occipital infarct and basal ganglia calcifications. He subsequently developed tonic-clonic seizures, which were treated with phenobarbital and phenytoin. Within the next 6 months, his intellectual function deteriorated until he became demented and combative. Another CT scan confirmed the old right parietooccipital infarct and demonstrated a new left temporoparietooccipital infarct.

The patient underwent a comprehensive evaluation at 30 years of age. Visual acuity at distance without correction was 16/100 in each eye, improving with pinhole to 16/40. Pupils and ocular motility were normal. Visual fields could not be tested adequately owing to the patient's dementia. Slit-lamp examination revealed no abnormality in the anterior segment. Indirect ophthalmoscopy of the fundus showed alternating areas of hyperpigmentation and hypopigmentation, especially in the posterior pole. Mul-

Table 1 *Electroretinographic Results of Patient 1*

Parameter	OD	OS	Normal Range
Blue (0.5 Hz)	82.4 μV	82.4 μV	100–275 μV
White (0.5 Hz)	305.8 μV	270.5 μV	350–700 μV
White (30 Hz)	41.1 μV	57.1 μV	50–125 μV
White (30 Hz) Implicit time	32 msec	32 msec	25–32 msec

OD = right eye; OS = left eye.

tiple subretinal deposits at the level of the retinal pigment epithelium (RPE) blocked fluorescence throughout the study, without late staining. Dark adaptation could not be performed because of poor cooperation. Electroretinography (ERG) showed decreased cone and rod function in each eye with normal implicit times, compatible with a mild disturbance of the RPE (Table 1). On three different days, serum lactic acid concentrations were 4.1, 1.9, and 4.1 μg/L, respectively (normal, 0.5 to 2.2 μg/L). The CSF protein level was 63 mg/dl. The CSF lactic acid level was not measured. The ragged red fibers of a mitochondrial myopathy were seen on light microscopy of a muscle biopsy, suggesting the diagnosis of MELAS syndrome.

When examined at 33 years of age, the patient was demented, belligerent, and abusive. He was taking carbamazepine and phenobarbital and had been free of seizures for 2 years. Neurological examination showed rigidity of the upper and lower extremities and ataxia.

On neuro-ophthalmic examination, the best-corrected visual acuity attained on a near card was 20/70 in each eye. Testing the patient's visual field by confrontation revealed a left homonymous hemianopia. Ductions were full, but pursuit was saccadic. The patient was uncooperative to voluntary testing of saccades. Optokinetic nystagmus (OKN) testing showed poorly formed OKN following to the right and intact right-beating OKN following to the left. Ptosis was present bilaterally. Examination of the fundus revealed a cup-to-disc ratio of 0.3 in each eye with mild optic atrophy. The vessels were mildly tortuous and narrowed. Alternating areas of hyperpigmentation and hypopigmentation were present in the posterior pole, and the subretinal deposits appeared to enlarge and coalesce. There were several areas of dot hyperpigmentation with surrounding halos of hypopigmentation. Along the arcades were patches of hypopigmentation.

Patient 2

The 66-year-old mother of Patient 1 had no neurological complaints. Her neurological examination, including the electromyogram (EMG), was normal. She was well except for a history of mild osteoarthritis and angina pectoris. This patient was short (62 inches). Her best visual acuity was

20/25 in each eye with normal color vision. Visual fields were full on the Humphrey visual field 30-2 threshold test. Pupils were normal, and ocular motility was intact. There was ptosis in each eye with palpebral fissures of 8 mm in the right and 7.5 mm in the left eye. Levator excursions were 14 mm bilaterally, and orbicularis function was normal. Slit-lamp examination revealed no abnormality in the anterior segment. Examination of the fundus showed normal optic nerves but areas of alternating hyperpigmentation and hypopigmentation in the macula.

Patient 3

The 36-year-old sister of Patient 1 had developed insulin-dependent diabetes mellitus 2 years previously. She had no neurological complaints. Her neurological examination, including an EMG, was normal. Visual acuity was 20/20 in each eye while wearing extended-wear soft contact lenses for myopia. Color vision was intact, and visual fields were full on Humphrey visual field 30-2 threshold test. Pupils and eye movements were normal. The patient had severe bilateral ptosis, with palpebral fissures of 6 mm in the right and 6.5 mm in the left eye. Levator excursions were 14 mm bilaterally, and orbicularis function was normal. Because of her ptosis, the patient maintained a chin-up posture. Slit-lamp examination revealed no abnormality in the anterior segment, and examination of the fundus revealed normal optic nerves. Multiple areas of alternating hyperpigmentation and hypopigmentation were seen in the posterior pole. There were several areas of dot hyperpigmentation with surrounding halos of hypopigmentation.

■ Laboratory Investigation

Mitochondrial DNA was extracted from blood buffy coat from all 3 patients and analyzed by Dr. John M. Shoffner at the Emory Molecular Diagnostics Laboratory, Atlanta, GA. Patients 2 and 3 refused muscle biopsy for analysis. The APAI restriction and Southern blot analysis confirmed a point mutation in the $tRNA^{Leu(UUR)}$ gene of mtDNA in each of the 3 family members [3]. Analysis revealed an A to G transition at nucleotide 3,243 of the mtDNA.

■ The Mitochondrion

Mitochondria are intracytoplasmic organelles that function in oxidative phosphorylation. They are unique among organelles in that they contain their own DNA. In 1964, Schatz and co-workers [15] found DNA in yeast mitochondria, suggesting that they might be self-replicating. Each mitochondrion contains two to ten copies of circular double-stranded DNA.

Mitochondrial DNA encodes for mitochondrial proteins of the electron transport chain. These genes are conserved in animals, plants, fungi, and parasites. The human mtDNA has 16,569 base pairs, representing less than 0.5% of the total DNA in each mammalian cell [16].

The mitochondrial genome encodes for thirty-seven genes. Of these, thirteen encode for essential polypeptides that are part of the respiratory complexes. Transfer RNAs are encoded by twenty-two genes, and ribosomal RNA molecules are encoded by two genes. The remaining fifty subunits of the respiratory complexes are encoded by nuclear DNA and are transported into each mitochondrion. In nuclear DNA, three of the possible codons represent stop sequences; the remaining sixty-one codons encode for the twenty amino acids, requiring thirty-two transfer RNAs. In the mtDNA, only twenty-two transfer RNAs are required. Mitochondrial DNA also has a slightly different genetic code, which may explain why accidental transfer to nuclear DNA does not occur [17].

Human mtDNA is inherited exclusively from the mother [5]. During cell division, mitochondria are randomly distributed to the daughter cells. Most human sperm mitochondria are in the tail, providing energy for motility, and do not enter the egg. Recently, some paternal mtDNA has been found to be transmitted to the offspring in mice and *Drosophila*, but this is limited to at most $10^{-4}\%$ [18–21]. Mutant as well as normal mitochondria replicate in cells. As cell division and organ formation take place, the mitochondria may have to pass a developmental bottleneck, which determines the percentage of mutant mitochondria that passes to the progeny [22] or that exists in individual organs themselves [23]. The varying proportions of normal versus mutant mitochondria in different organs is called *heteroplasmy*.

How a deleted molecule can eventually dominate any mitochondrion is not well understood. One possibility is that a smaller genome may be able to replicate faster than a larger genome [24]. A second possibility is that a feedback loop that normally acts to increase energy production in cells may actually give a replicative advantage to defective mitochondria [6]. If mitochondria are stimulated by nuclear factors to divide in response to subnormal function, mitochondria containing mutant DNA molecules would be stimulated to divide disproportionately [25]. The variable expression of mitochondrial encephalopathies may be related to heteroplasmy and to the background nuclear genotype. In one pedigree, family members with up to 34% mutant mtDNA in leukocytes were phenotypically normal, whereas members with more than 82% mutant mtDNA had the phenotypical disease of neuropathy, ataxia, and retinitis pigmentosa (NARP) [26].

■ Clinical and Genetic Patterns

Our patient with MELAS (Patient 1) had all the features for which the syndrome is named: myopathy, encephalopathy, lactic acidosis, and strokelike episodes. He also exhibited other characteristic features including short stature, sensorineural hearing loss, headaches, and seizures. His mother (Patient 2) and sister (Patient 3), who also carry the MELAS mutation, exhibited only ophthalmic findings. Diabetes mellitus, which was present in the sister, has been reported in KSS but not in MELAS and may be an unrelated finding [4]. However, it could reflect an abnormal mitochondrial population in the pancreas.

Mutations in mtDNA are responsible for various diseases traditionally defined by their supposedly unique combination of component symptoms and signs, which include short stature, sensorineural hearing loss, weakness, dementia, ragged red fibers, optic atrophy, and ophthalmoplegia. The boundaries between these clinical entities are not sharp; "overlap" syndromes are common [27]. Symptoms and signs in mitochondrial myopathies are probably caused by deficiencies in mitochondrial oxidative phosphorylation enzymes, and ocular signs occur when there are deficiencies in ocular tissues. Different mutations clearly can result in different phenotypical expressions (Table 2).

A pattern of inheritance consistent with maternal transmission of MELAS has been observed in families with more than 1 affected member. No male-to-male transmission has been reported [5]. There are deficiencies of mitochondrial respiratory complexes I and IV and an A to G transition at nucleotide 3,243 of the mitochondrial DNA in MELAS [3, 28]. The 3,243 point mutation was found in 21 of 23 patients with phenotypical MELAS and in 12 of 14 asymptomatic family members [29]. An alternative mutation for MELAS has been hypothesized for the 20% of MELAS patients (8 of 40) who do not have the 3,243 point mutation [30]. Recently, a new family with a mitochondrial myopathy was found to have a T to C transition at nucleotide 3,250 of the mtDNA—just seven nucleotides away from the MELAS mutation [31]. Thus, it begins to appear that these dis-

Table 2 *Several Diseases with Mitochondrial Mutations*

Phenotypical Name	Mutations Identified	Coding Respiratory Complex
MELAS	3,243 A to G (91%); unknown (9%)	Complexes I and IV
Leber's hereditary optic neuropathy	11,778 G to A, 4,160, and 3,460	Subunit 4 of complex I
MERRF	8,344 A to G	Complexes II, III, and IV
New myopathy	3,250 T to C	Complexes I and IV
NARP	8,993 T to G	Subunit 6 of complex I
Kearns-Sayre syndrome	Large variable deletions up to 7 kb	Involve origins of both H and L strand replication

MELAS = a syndrome of myopathy, encephalopathy, lactic acidosis, and strokelike episodes; MERRF = a syndrome of myoclonus, epilepsy, and ragged red fibers; NARP = a syndrome of neuropathy, ataxia, and retinitis pigmentosa.

eases should be defined by their underlying mitochondrial mutations, not by their symptom complexes.

Typically, patients with KSS have variably large deletions of muscle mtDNA [32, 33] rather than specific point mutations in tRNAs as have been described in MELAS and MERRF [34]. Deficiencies of complexes II, III, and IV have also been described in MERRF [35], as well as an A to G transition at nucleotide 8,344 in the tRNA gene [23]. The mitochondrial myopathies result from deficiencies in mitochondrial oxidative phosphorylation enzymes, yet different mutations clearly result in different phenotypical expressions. Leber's optic neuropathy is also a mitochondrially inherited disorder associated with one of several simple point mutations in the mtDNA encoding complex I (associated with point mutations in subunit 4 of complex I, with a point mutation at nucleotide 11,778 [36], 4,160 [37], or 3,460 [38]). Interestingly, despite Leber's optic neuropathy being mitochondrially inherited, there is no associated myopathy.

The ophthalmic findings of ptosis, ophthalmoplegia, optic atrophy, and RPE degeneration have not been considered typical of MELAS [4] and are more commonly found in KSS [7–9]. However, our Patient 1 lacked such important features of KSS as heart block and elevated CSF protein and had features found in MELAS but not in KSS, including strokelike episodes, seizures, and adult onset of disease. Some patients with features intermediate between KSS and MELAS have been shown to have deletions typical of KSS [10]. There have also been families in which MELAS developed in one sibling and MERRF in another and patients who evolved from a MERRF to a MELAS phenotype. The presence of the diagnostic 3,243 base pair mutation in all 3 family members presented here, however, is strong evidence to support the diagnosis of MELAS [24]. Therefore, this family is an example of a MELAS mutation with clinical expression of ophthalmic findings, even in nonmyopathic family members. Pavlakis (personal communication), who originally defined the MELAS syndrome, has observed similar ophthalmic abnormalities in 5 of 59 (8.5%) MELAS patients.

■ Treatment of MELAS

Treatment of MELAS is aimed at minimizing the energy demands on the mitochondria. Thiamine was temporarily beneficial in 1 case [39], and coenzyme Q_{10} was beneficial in 2 [40, 41]. Patients should avoid extremes of temperature, high glucose loads, drugs that cause acidosis, and drugs that interfere with the respiratory chain (chloramphenicol, tetracycline, phenytoin, and cigarettes). There has also been a report of clinical improvement with corticosteroids [42]. However, the variable natural course of MELAS makes it difficult to assess the therapeutic efficacy of any regimen.

■ Comments

Awareness of this group of disorders is advancing rapidly. Diagnostic tests are becoming available that will allow us to define the mitochondrial myopathies by their underlying mitochondrial mutations. A complete examination of the patient and all available family members can contribute to correct diagnosis, accurate genetic counseling, possible treatment, and our further understanding of the spectrum of expression of mitochondrial encephalomyopathies and other inherited disorders. A thorough ophthalmic examination is an essential part of such an evaluation.

■ References

1. Pavlakis SG, Phillips PC, DiMauro S, et al. Mitochondrial myopathy, encephalopathy, lactic acidosis, and stroke-like episodes: a distinctive clinical syndrome. Ann Neurol 1984;16:481–488
2. DiMauro S, Bonilla E, Zeviani M, et al. Mitochondrial myopathies. Ann Neurol 1985;17:521–538
3. Goto Y, Nonaka I, Horai S. A mutation in the tRNA$^{Leu(UUR)}$ gene associated with the MELAS subgroup of mitochondrial encephalomyopathies. Nature 1990;348: 651–653
4. Pavlakis SG, Rowland LP, DeVivo DC, et al. Mitochondrial myopathies and encephalopathies. In: Plum F, ed. Advances in contemporary neurology. Philadelphia: Davis, 1988:95–133
5. Shoffner JM IV, Wallace DC. Oxidative phosphorylation diseases: disorders of two genomes. Adv Hum Genet 1990;19:267–330
6. Clarke A. Mitochondrial genome: defects, disease, and evolution. J Med Genet 1990;27:451–456
7. Kearns TP, Sayre GP. Retinitis pigmentosa, external ophthalmoplegia, and complete heart block: unusual syndrome with histologic study in one of two cases. Arch Ophthalmol 1958;60:280–289
8. McKechnie NM, King M, Lee WR. Retinal pathology in the Kearns-Sayre syndrome. Br J Ophthalmol 1985;69:63–75
9. Bosche J, Hammerstein W, Neuen-Jacob E, Schober R. Variation in retinal changes and muscle pathology in mitochondriopathies. Graefes Arch Clin Exp Ophthalmol 1989;227:578–583
10. Zupanc ML, Moraes CT, Shanske S, et al. Deletion of mitochondrial DNA in patients with combined features of Kearns-Sayre and MELAS syndromes. Ann Neurol 1991;29:680–683
11. Wallace DC, Zheng XX, Lott MT, et al. Familial mitochondrial encephalomyopathy (MERRF): genetic, pathophysiological, and biochemical characterization of a mitochondrial DNA disease. Cell 1988;55:601–610
12. van Hellenberg Hubar JLM, Gabreels FJM, Ruitenbeek W, et al. MELAS syndrome: report of two patients, and comparison with data of 24 patients derived from the literature. Neuropediatrics 1991;22:10–14
13. Phillips CI, Gosden CM. Leber's hereditary optic neuropathy and Kearns-Sayre syndrome: mitochondrial DNA mutations. Surv Ophthalmol 1991;35:463–472
14. Mathews PM, Tampieri D, Berkovic SF, et al. Magnetic resonance imaging shows specific abnormalities in the MELAS syndrome. Neurology 1991;41:1043–1046

15. Schatz G, Haslbrunner E, Tuppy H. Deoxyribonucleic acid associated with yeast mitochondria. Biochem Biophys Res Commun 1964;15:127–132
16. Anderson S, Bankier AT, Barrell BG, et al. Sequence and organization of the human mitochondrial genome. Nature 1981;290:457–465
17. Wallace DC. Structure and evolution of organelle genomes. Microbiol Rev 1982; 46:208–240
18. Gyllensten U, Wharton D, Josefsson A, et al. Paternal inheritance of mitochondrial DNA in mice. Nature 1991;352:255–257
19. Matsuura ET, Fukuda H, Chigusa SI. Mitochondrial DNA heteroplasmy maintained in natural populations of *Drosophila simulans* in reunion. Genet Res 1991; 57:123–126
20. Avise JC. Evolution. Matriarchal liberation (news;comment). Nature 1991;358:192
21. Hoeh WR, Blakley KH, Brown WM. Heteroplasmy suggests limited biparental inheritance of *Mytilus* mitochondrial DNA. Science 1991;251:1488–1490
22. Bolhuis PA, Bleeker-Wagemakers EM, Ponne NJ, et al. Rapid shift in genotype of human mitochondrial DNA in a family with Leber's hereditary optic neuropathy. Biochem Biophys Res Commun 1990;170:994–997
23. Obermaier-Kusser B, Muller-Hocker J, Nelson I, et al. Different copy numbers of apparently identically deleted mitochondrial DNA in tissues from a patient with Kearns-Sayre syndrome detected by PCR. Biochem Biophys Res Commun 1990; 169:1007–1015
24. Wallace DC. Mitochondrial DNA mutations and neuromuscular disease. Trends Genet 1989;5:9–13
25. Grossman LI. Mitochondrial DNA in sickness and in health. Am J Hum Genet 1990;46:415–417
26. Holt IJ, Harding AE, Petty RKH, Morgan-Hughes JA. A new mitochondrial disease associated with mitochondrial DNA heteroplasmy. Am J Hum Genet 1990;46: 428–433
27. Berenberg RA, Pellock JM, DiMauro S, et al. Lumping or splitting? Ophthalmoplegia plus or Kearns-Sayre syndrome. Ann Neurol 1988;1:37
28. Kobayashi Y, Momoi MY, Tominaga K, et al. Respiration-deficient cells are caused by a single point mutation in the mitochondrial tRNA-Leu (UUR) gene in mitochondrial myopathy, encephalopathy, lactic acidosis, and stroke like episodes (MELAS). Am J Hum Genet 1991;49:590–599
29. Ciafaloni E, Ricci E, Shanske S, et al. MELAS: clinical features, biochemistry, and molecular genetics. Ann Neurol 1992;31:391–398
30. Goto Y, Nonaka I, Horai S. An alternative mutation in the mitochondrial tRNA-LEU (UUR) gene associated with MELAS. Am J Hum Genet 1991;49(suppl):190
31. Goto Y, Tojo M, Tohyama J, et al. A novel point mutation in the mitochondrial tRNA$^{Leu(UUR)}$ gene in a family with mitochondrial myopathy. Ann Neurol 1992; 31:672–675
32. Holt IJ, Harding AE, Morgan-Hughes JA. Deletions of muscle mitochondrial DNA in patients with mitochondrial myopathies. Nature 1988;331:717–719
33. Moraes CT, DiMauro S, Zeviani M, et al. Mitochondrial DNA deletions in progressive external ophthalmoplegia and Kearns-Sayre syndrome. N Engl J Med 1989; 320:1293–1299
34. Shoffner JM, Lott MT, Lezza AMS, et al. Myoclonic epilepsy and ragged-red fiber disease (MERRF) is associated with a mitochondrial DNA tRNA^{Lys} mutation. Cell 1990;61:931–937
35. Byrne E, Trounce I, Marzuki S, et al. Functional respiratory chain studies in mitochondrial cytopathies: support for mitochondrial DNA heteroplasmy in myoclonus epilepsy and ragged-red fibers (MERRF) syndrome. Acta Neuropathol 1991;81: 318–323

36. Singh G, Lott MT, Wallace DC. A mitochondrial DNA mutation as a cause of Leber's hereditary optic neuropathy. N Engl J Med 1989;320:1300–1305
37. Howell N, Kubacka I, Xu M, et al. Leber hereditary optic neuropathy: involvement of the mitochondrial ND1 gene and evidence for an intragenic suppressor mutation. Am J Hum Genet 1991;48:935–942
38. Huoponen K, Vilkki J, Aula P, et al. A new mtDNA mutation associated with Leber hereditary optic neuroretinopathy. Am J Hum Genet 1991;48:1147–1153
39. Shapira Y, Cederbaum SD, Cancilla A, et al. Familial poliodystrophy, mitochondrial myopathy, and lactate acidemia. Neurology 1975;25:614–621
40. Kishi M, Yamamura Y, Kurihara T, et al. An autopsy case of mitochondrial encephalomyopathy: biochemical and electron microscopic studies of the brain. J Neurol Sci 1988;86:31–40
41. Goda S, Hamada T, Ishimoto S, et al. Clinical improvement after administration coenzyme of Q_{10} in a patient with mitochondrial encephalomyopathy. J Neurol 1987;234:62–63
42. Gubbay SS, Hankey GJ, Tan NTS, Fry JM. Mitochondrial encephalomyopathy with corticosteroid dependence. Med J Aust 1989;151:103–108

The Oculocerebrorenal Syndrome of Lowe

C. William Lavin, M.D.

Craig A. McKeown, M.D.

The oculocerebrorenal syndrome of Lowe (OCRL), or Lowe's syndrome, is an X-linked recessive disease involving the eyes, central nervous system, and kidneys. The clinical features include growth retardation, severe mental retardation, areflexia, hypotonia, noninflammatory joint swelling of unknown cause, and renal tubular dysfunction (Fanconi's syndrome). The ocular findings include cataracts (100%), glaucoma (65%), and corneal keloids. The patients often exhibit an unusual facial appearance with frontal bossing, chubby cheeks, and a fair complexion (Fig 1). Therapy consists mainly of management of the ophthalmological complications, as well as replacement of renal losses from the Fanconi's syndrome. The primary biochemical defect is unknown, but investigations have explored mitochondrial dysfunction, proteoglycan synthesis, and nucleoside pyrophosphate activity. Recently, the location of the gene has been mapped to the long arm of the X chromosome in the region of the Xq25 locus.

OCRL was first described in 1952 by Lowe, Terrey, and MacLachlan [1], but it was not until 1965 that the disease was convincingly demonstrated, by Richards and co-workers [2], to be X-linked recessive. No biochemical clues were available at the time to help with the diagnosis, and recognition of lens opacities in female carriers was not appreciated until the 1970s.

Untreated infants with Lowe's syndrome generally appear to be blind by the age of 6 months. Nystagmus develops, and the child may hold his or her hands in front of the eyes and move them quickly in an attempt to elicit visual input. Ocular trauma from oculodigital stimulation is also common, and the child may develop ecchymotic lesions from this activity.

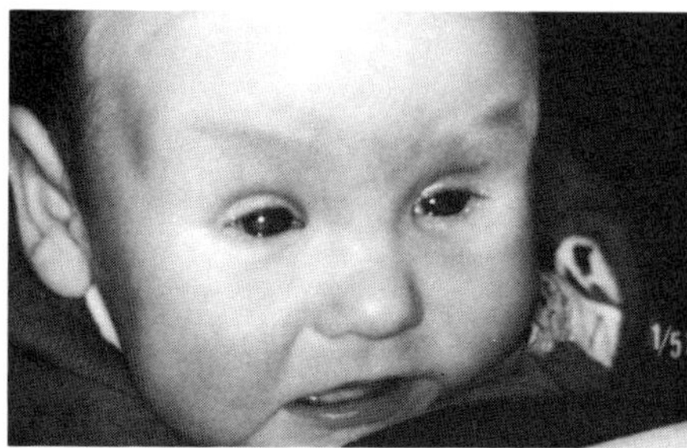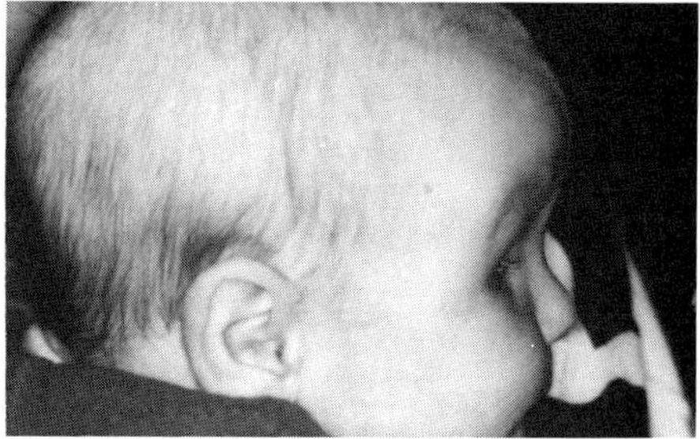

Figure 1 *Facial appearance of child with oculocerebrorenal syndrome of Lowe, with frontal bossing, deep-set eyes, chubby cheeks, and fair complexion.*

■ Clinical Findings

The systemic manifestations of OCRL were recently reviewed in detail by Charnas and Gahl [3]. The major findings are summarized here and in Table 1.

Neurological Manifestations

Individuals with Lowe's syndrome are generally mentally retarded, and an accurate assessment of their status may be impaired by the visual limitation [4]. There are, however, exceptional individuals with OCRL who have less severely limited intellectual abilities and who attend regular school classes. The number of such cases is small and probably biased, since some children with Lowe's syndrome are so severely handicapped

Table 1 *Major Clinical Manifestations of Lowe's Syndrome*

Ocular
Cataracts
Glaucoma
Miosis
Corneal keloids

Neurological
Mental retardation
Growth retardation
Hypotonia
Seizures

Renal
Fanconi's syndrome
Metabolic acidosis
Aminoaciduria
Proteinuria
Hyperphosphaturia

that they require institutionalization and do not come to the attention of community practitioners.

Areflexia and hypotonia are features of the disease, but their origin is unknown. Some studies have noted slowed nerve conduction velocities and evidence of denervation by electromyography (EMG) [5], whereas biopsies have shown significant fiber loss and axonal degeneration. However, other studies have reported normal EMGs and biopsies. Just as the mild peripheral neuropathy is not considered to explain the areflexia seen in these children [6], the chronic renal disease is not believed to be responsible for the peripheral neuropathy. Other diseases in which Fanconi's syndrome occurs, such as cystinosis, exhibit intact reflexes and no clinical evidence of neuropathy on examination or biopsy.

Seizures may occur in OCRL, with generalized tonic seizures being the most common [7]. The electroencephalogram (EEG) is abnormal in the case of patients who exhibit seizure activity [8]. Magnetic resonance imaging (MRI) studies have demonstrated white matter changes [9], which were not related to the degree of mental retardation and were believed to be related to a marked increase in cellularity from gliosis rather than demyelination.

Patients with Lowe's syndrome also have been characterized as exhibiting self-abusive behavior, such as head banging and biting, as well as episodic outbursts known as *Lowe tantrums* [10]. Treatment of these behavioral outbursts has included neuroleptics, stimulants, and carbamazepine, but none of these agents has proved satisfactory.

Histological studies on the brains of patients with OCRL have not identified any consistent changes [11]. Ventriculomegaly and mild cerebral edema have been described. There is some evidence of an abnormal proliferation of filaments in astrocytes and reduced cerebroside levels in patients with the Lowe's syndrome.

Renal Manifestations

Renal involvement in OCRL is due to impairment of tubular as well as glomerular functions. The disorder is characterized by tubular proteinemia and failure to resorb water, phosphorus, glucose, amino acids, carnitine, and other small molecules. This results in Fanconi's syndrome, which may also be seen in galactosemia, tyrosinemia, Wilson's disease, and type 1 glycogen storage disease [12].

Patients with OCRL exhibit mild polyuria with a urine osmolality of 400 mosm/kg. A metabolic acidosis results from wasting of bicarbonate as well as impaired ammonia production [13].

Although serum calcium levels are usually normal, the mean functional excretion of phosphorous is 24% (normal, 10% to 22%). Bone resorption from long-term loss of phosphorous may lead to rickets, which, in OCRL, is not due to vitamin D deficiency or metabolic acidosis but to renal phosphate loss [3].

Despite normal amino acid levels in plasma and cerebrospinal fluid, a variety of laboratory tests verify aminoaciduria, though it is less marked than that seen in cystinosis [13, 14]. Research has focused on whether the amino acid loss is generalized or selective, but the results are inconclusive. Fibroblasts from patients with OCRL have shown normal glycine and lysine uptake. Proteinuria is in the range of 1 g/m^2/day, and protein electrophoresis shows a pattern consistent with tubular loss, exhibiting electrophoretic bands in the gamma globulin zone.

The glomerular filtration rate ranges from 17 to 130 ml/min/1.73 m^2 [15]. By the age of 15, serum creatinine rises sharply, partially explaining the abbreviated life span of patients with advanced renal disease.

Histopathological examination of kidney specimens shows both glomerular and tubular abnormalities, although tubular changes are more consistent. Proximal and distal tubular epithelial cells are atrophic, with interstitial fibrosis predominating (Fig 2) [11]. Electron microscopy shows a thickening of the basement membrane and cast formation.

Musculoskeletal Manifestations

Scoliosis, joint contractures, hypermobility, and dislocated hips are found in patients with OCRL [16]. Hypotonia contributes to joint hypermobility, whereas decreased movement results in the development of limb

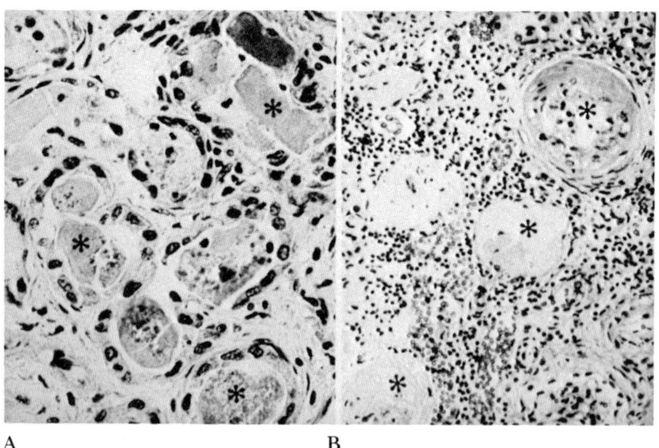

A   B

Figure 2 *Renal changes in specimen from patient with Lowe's syndrome. (A) Interstitial fibrosis and segmentally dilated renal tubules containing granular and hyaline casts* (asterisks) *(× 500). (B) Glomerular hyalinization* (asterisks) *and a chronic inflammatory reaction (× 266). (Reprinted with permission from Tripathi et al [19].)*

contractures. Recurrent fractures from osteopenia are believed to be due to inadequately treated rickets.

Sexual Development

Although the onset of puberty in patients with OCRL is at the appropriate age, fertility may be reduced due to peritubular fibrosis and azoospermia [11]. One study showed that 40% of patients with Lowe's syndrome had either unilateral or bilateral cryptorchidism, which may also be related to infertility [17].

Ocular Involvement

Ocular manifestations of Lowe's syndrome include congenital cataracts in 100% and glaucoma in 65% of affected male patients. Miosis, corneal opacities, and enophthalmos are also prominent signs. The presence of cataracts is essential for the diagnosis. With proper management of the cataract and glaucoma, the best visual outcome is generally in the range of 20/100. The earliest lens changes have been described in a 24-week fetus [3]. Although the lens was of normal size, the posterior capsule showed lenticonuslike changes. No glaucomatous changes were noted at this stage of development.

Lens changes seen in histopathological studies have consistently shown the lenses to be small and discoid, with the absence of a demarcation line between the nucleus and the cortex (Figs 3, 4) [18, 19]. Lens fibers appear immature, which may contribute to the small size of the lens. The lack of demarcation signifies a defect in early embryogenesis. It is believed that either the primary fibers in the posterior pole of the lens grow initially but then rapidly degenerate, or there is failure of growth of the primary lens fibers. With subsequent ingrowth of the secondary lens fibers, no demarcation line forms between the nucleus and the cortex. Failure of the primary fibers to elongate would also lead to the discoid shape of the lens. The posterior capsule of the lens has been noted to be irregular, with wartlike excrescences that indicate abnormal function of the posterior lens epithe-

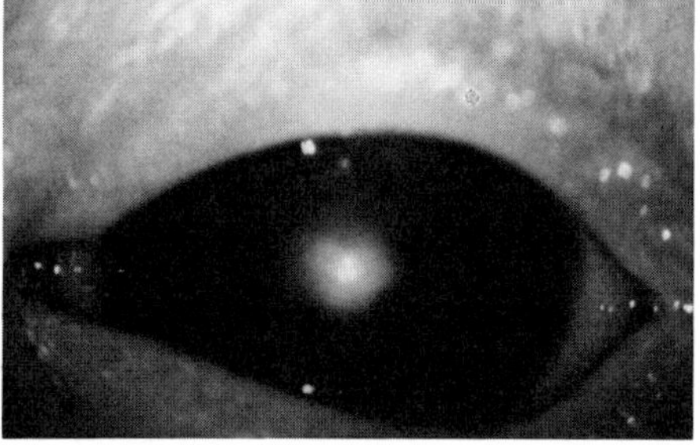

Figure 3 *External photograph of left eye of newborn infant with bilateral congenital cataracts shows dense, central lens opacity. The right eye had a similar cataract. The infant was later found to have Lowe's syndrome.*

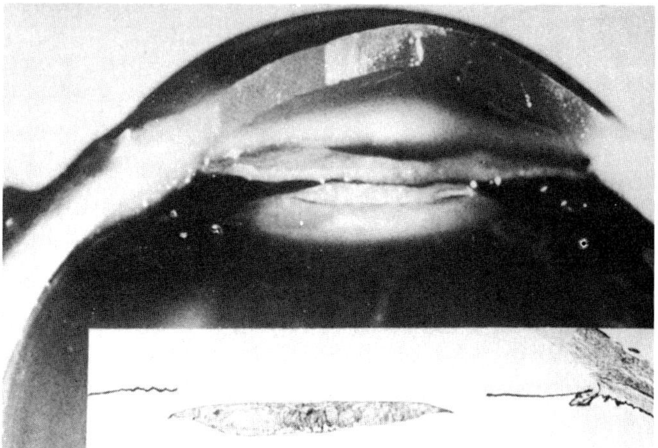

Figure 4 *Macrophotograph of culotted globe shows characteristic small, discoid, cataractous lens of Lowe's syndrome. Microphotograph (inset) shows sectional view of lens. (Reprinted with permission from Tripathi et al [19].)*

lium (Fig 5). Proliferation of the lens epithelium results from degeneration of the primary lens fibers. The excessive formation of lens material may lead to posterior lenticonus, which has been described in OCRL patients.

Lens Changes in the Carrier State

Lenticular opacities appear to be the only consistent finding in female carriers of Lowe's syndrome [20]. The opacities appear gray-white, are punctate, and vary in size from micrometers up to several millimeters (Fig 6). They are found only in the cortex of the lens and not in the nucleus, indicating their formation in adult life. The punctate opacities are typically found in wedge-shaped zones. Since OCRL is X-linked recessive, the focal lens changes in wedge-shaped zones may be explained by the Lyon hypothesis of selective X-chromosome inactivation. Punctate opacities are not specific for the carrier state of OCRL, but the number of opacities and wedge-shaped zones are characteristic. All obligate carriers of the Lowe gene in one study showed 4+ (too many to count) opacities, whereas 0 to 2+ (16 to 80) opacities were seen in control eyes [21]. Typically, the opacities in female carriers are seen just outside the nucleus and extend into the superficial cortical layers. It is not understood why fetal lens cells of carrier females do not show the opacities.

In addition to the characteristic lens opacities in female carriers, investigators have found other manifestations as well. Psychomotor retardation, generalized hypotonia, and absent deep tendon reflexes have been noted, as well as mild aminoaciduria in several female carriers.

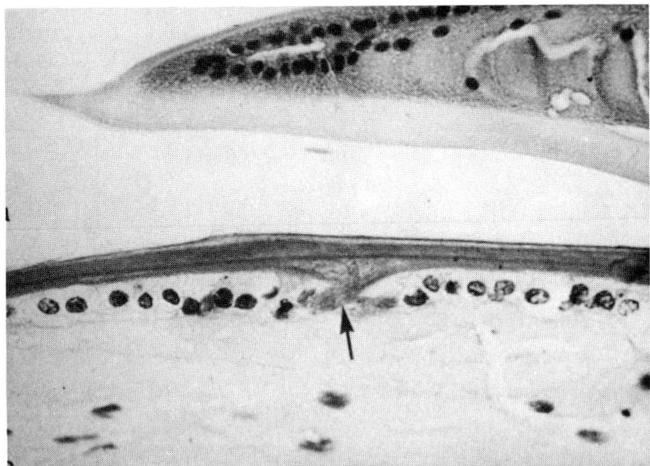

Figure 5 *(Top) Flattened cataractous lens shows sharply angulated profile in equatorial region and prominent thickening of post-equatorial capsule (× 600). (Bottom) Irregular thickening of lens capsule with wartlike excrescences* (arrow) *(× 375). (Reprinted with permission from Tripathi et al [19].)*

Glaucoma

Glaucoma develops in approximately two-thirds of patients with Lowe's syndrome. The elevated intraocular pressure may lead to a cloudy, edematous cornea, and persistently elevated pressures may result in chronic corneal leukomas. Visualization of the posterior pole is difficult, if not impossible, when this occurs. Microscopical examination shows embryonic-appearing angle structures. The iris inserts anteriorly and is partially attached to the base of the trabecular meshwork. Ciliary processes have been noted arising from the posterior peripheral iris, whereas others are

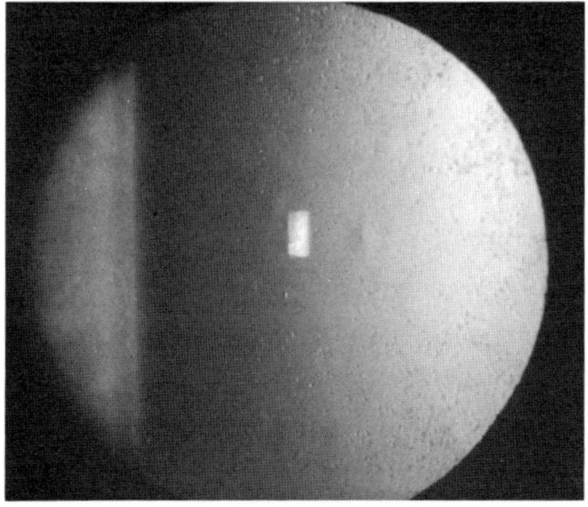

Figure 6 *Gray-white, punctate cortical lens opacities in female carrier of Lowe's syndrome. The wedge-shaped distribution of the opacities with relatively normal appearing cortex between the wedges is characteristic of the carrier state of Lowe's syndrome and probably represents a manifestation of Lyon's hypothesis.*

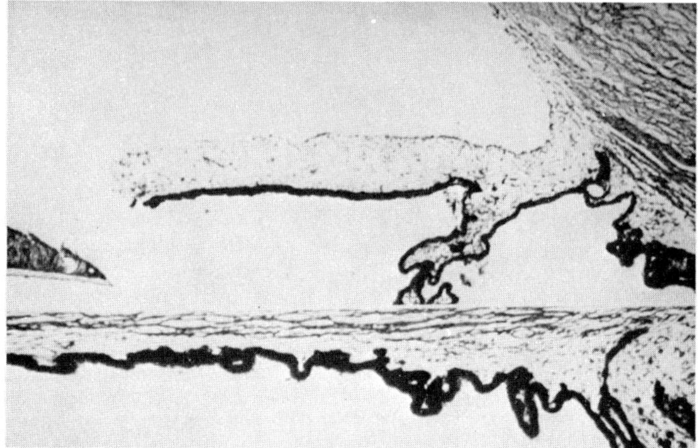

Figure 7 *Photomicrograph of autopsy globe from 5¹/₂-year-old boy with Lowe's syndrome shows embryonic anterior chamber angle and anteriorly displaced ciliary processes, with some arising directly from the posterior aspect of the iris where the dilator muscle is lacking (× 37.5). Inset (below) shows rudimentary character of ciliary processes in region of pars plicata (× 60). (Reprinted with permission from Tripathi et al [19].)*

rudimentary and displaced anteriorly (Fig 7) [19]. The dilator pupillae muscle is hypoplastic, which may be the cause of the chronically miotic pupil.

The cause of glaucoma in OCRL is unknown, but its appearance is similar to that in primary congenital glaucoma. The treatment is also similar, consisting of surgical attempts to decrease the pressure with goniotomy as well as other procedures. However, the response to therapy often is poor.

■ Diagnosis

Prior to recent advances in genetic investigations, the diagnosis of Lowe's syndrome could be made only postnatally by clinical examination and urinary studies. The cardinal features of cataract, glaucoma, and hypotonia are usually readily apparent. The diagnosis is further supported by the characteristic frontal bossing in a child who is usually of fair complexion and blonde. Laboratory testing, in addition to the DNA linkage analysis studies described later, should include a 24-hour urine for total protein excretion. Spot screening of the urine is often normal [22]. Laboratory tests that support the diagnosis of OCRL include elevated creatinine phosphokinase, serum glutamic oxaloacetic transaminase, lactate dehydrogenase, and alpha$_2$-globulin levels.

■ Management of the Patient

The ophthalmologist should be a member of a multidisciplinary team that cares for the child with OCRL. The team often includes a general pediatrician, a pediatric nephrologist, and a geneticist. The ophthalmologist should optimize the visual potential by prompt removal of significant congenital cataracts, ideally in the first 6 weeks of life, before intractable amblyopia and nystagmus develop from sensory deprivation. Although glaucoma develops in two-thirds of patients with OCRL, this problem is not always present at birth. Therefore, frequent evaluation of the intraocular pressure is necessary. The progression of limb contractures is often slowed by physical therapy. Fanconi's syndrome is managed by replacement of citrate, sodium, and potassium [3]. Phosphate, as either the sodium or potassium salt, and vitamin D are given to prevent the onset of rickets.

■ Molecular Genetics

With the application of molecular genetic techniques to chromosome mapping, the location of genes on specific chromosomes can be either precisely determined or approximated. In a landmark paper on mapping of the Lowe's syndrome gene, Silver and colleagues [23], in 1987, localized the gene to the q24-q26 region on the long arm of the X chromosome by utilizing restriction fragment length polymorphisms (RFLPs).

A brief description of RFLPs may be appropriate here. Individuals within a family have unique genetic sequences on each of their maternal and paternal chromosomes. Naturally occurring differences within the chromosome are due to dissimilarities in intervening DNA segments between and within genes. The genetic fingerprint may be further altered when genetic errors (mutations) are present. The RFLP technique identifies the differences between chromosomes by cutting the DNA into fragments using highly specific DNA-cleaving enzymes known as *restriction endonucleases*. Naturally occurring variations and mutations may disrupt the cleavage process for certain endonucleases, resulting in differences in the length of the DNA fragments between different individuals, even within the same family. The DNA fragments are separated by gel electrophoresis and then hybridized by the Southern blot method to specific radiolabeled or fluorescent-labeled nucleotide sequences known as *probes,* which correspond to known areas on the chromosome.

The gene for OCRL was known, by pedigree analysis, to be located on the X chromosome. Silver and colleagues [23] used radionucleotide probes

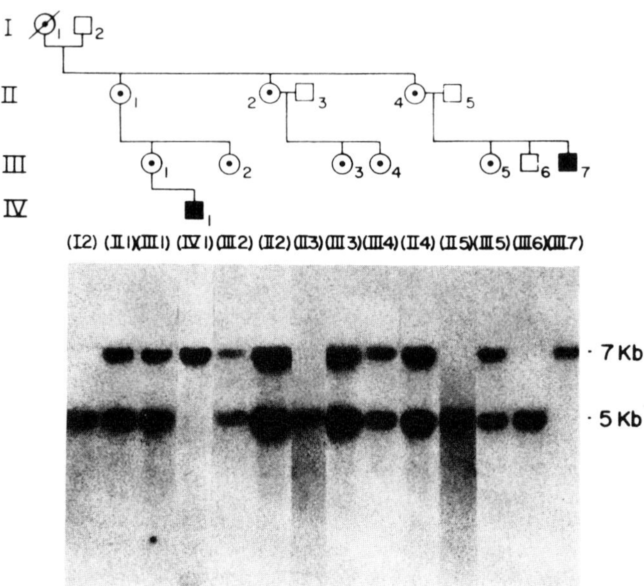

Figure 8 *Segregation of restriction fragment length polymorphism alleles in 1 family with Lowe's syndrome at DXS10 locus. The pattern of 7.0-kb and/or 5.0-kb alleles in Taq I digested DNA is shown directly under the symbol for the corresponding member of the pedigree. ■ = affected male; ⊙ = carrier female; □ = unaffected male. (Reprinted with permission from Silver et al [23].)*

specific for certain known regions of the X chromosome to search for the location of the Lowe's syndrome gene. After digestion with specific endonucleases, hybridization was performed using different probes. Figure 8, reprinted from Silver's article, shows the segregation of RFLP alleles in 1 family at the DXS10 locus. Unaffected male subjects showed a single 5-kilobase (kb) segment of DNA, and male subjects with Lowe's syndrome, a single 7-kb segment. Female carriers had both the 5-kb (normal) and 7-kb (abnormal) sequences corresponding to their one normal and one abnormal X chromosome containing Lowe's gene. Linkage analysis was performed on the eight X-chromosomal loci tested. An *LOD score,* which is the logarithm of the odds of the maximum likelihood of recombination between the Lowe gene and the genetic marker tested, was assigned at each locus (Table 2). For DXS42, which corresponds to the Xq24-q26 position, the LOD score was 5.087, and for DXS10, which corresponds to the Xq26 position, the LOD score was 6.450. This indicated tight linkage of the gene to these two loci and placed the location of the Lowe's syndrome gene between Xq24 and Xq26.

An additional study by the same authors showed tight linkage of markers DXS10 and DXS42 in 6 families with OCRL [24]. This paper also

Table 2 *Linkage Analysis of Eight X-Chromosomal Loci with the Lowe Oculocerebrorenal Syndrome*

Locus Number	Chromosome Location	No. of Informative Families	Recombination Distance	lod
DXS3	Xq21.3-q22	4	0.325	0.492
DXS17	Xq21.3-q22	3	0.325	0.386
DXS42	Xq24-q26	3	0.000	5.087
DXS10	Xq26	3	0.000	6.450
HPRT	Xq26	4	0.100	3.160
DXS51	Xq27	1	0.125	0.757
Factor IX	Xq27	1	0.000	3.116
DXS52	Xq28	4	0.450	0.010

lod = logarithm of the odds of the maximum likelihood of recombination between the Lowe gene and the genetic marker tested.

Reprinted with permission from Silver et al [23].

reported three additional polymorphisms as well as a female patient with Lowe's syndrome. Karyotyping of this patient showed a translocation of a portion of the distal long arm of the X chromosome beyond the Xq25 locus with chromosome 3. Hybrid somatic cell lines were produced, and each derivative chromosome was isolated away from its normal counterpart. Probes for the long arm of the X chromosome were utilized, as in the prior study. DXS42 was mapped to the derivative X chromosome containing Xpter-q25, and DXS10 was mapped to the derivative chromosome 3 containing Xq25-qter. This evidence provided support for the Xq25 position as the possible site for the Lowe's syndrome gene. The study also compared the sensitivity of slit-lamp examination for lens opacities in female carriers of the Lowe gene with genetic analysis of these carriers' X chromosome. Twenty-eight female subjects with a 50% risk of carrying the OCRL gene underwent genetic analysis as well as lens examinations. Fifteen were identified by linked markers DXS10 or DXS42, or both. Thirteen of the 15 carriers were also identified by lens evaluation. Two subjects positive by linkage analysis had normal eye examinations. One of these, a 6-year-old, was informative only for DXS10, and the other, a 25-year-old was informative only for DXS42. The analysis showed an OCRL gene penetrance of 87% (13 of 15).

The existence of well-defined markers on the X chromosome linked to the Lowe's syndrome gene may allow for prenatal diagnosis. A sampling of fetal tissue from the female carrier can be subjected to RFLP analysis and the results compared with other family members. Such work was reported by Gazit and associates [25]. A woman known by pedigree analysis to be a carrier for the OCRL gene was pregnant with a second child. The first child had Lowe's syndrome. Chorionic villus sampling was performed in the ninth week of gestation. DNA analysis for the Lowe's syndrome gene was performed on the fetal sample as well as on the peripheral blood leukocytes of other family members. A probe specific for Xq26 (DXS10) was used. The segregation of the restriction fragments was similar to the unaffected family members and clearly different from those of the female carrier and the affected sibling. A healthy male infant was born at term.

■ Future Studies

The future of research in OCRL includes refinement of laboratory techniques for prenatal diagnosis and identification of the Lowe's syndrome gene. Eventually, the gene may be sequenced and the fundamental biochemical defect causing Lowe's syndrome discovered. Identification of the biochemical defect may help clinicians explore other tissues and organs that are affected by the disease. Finally, a better understanding of the syndrome will help families affected by this incapacitating and lethal condition cope with the despair that is universally sensed when a severe inherited disease is passed from one generation to the next.

■ References

1. Lowe CU, Terrey M, MacLachlan EA. Organic aciduria, decreased renal ammonia production, hydrophthalmos and mental retardation: a clinical entity. Am J Dis Child 1952;83:164–184
2. Richards W, Donnell GN, Wilson WA, et al. The oculo-cerebro-renal syndrome of Lowe. Am J Dis Child 1965;109:185–203
3. Charnas LR, Gahl WA. The oculocerebrorenal syndrome of Lowe. Adv Pediatr 1991;38:75–107
4. Fenichel GM. Clinical pediatric neurology: a signs and symptoms approach. Philadelphia: Saunders, 1988
5. Kornfeld M, Snyder RD, MacGee J, Appenzeller O. The oculo-cerebral-renal syndrome of Lowe: neuromuscular components. Arch Neurol 1975;32:103–107
6. Charnas L, Bernar J, Pezeshkpour GH, et al. MRI findings and peripheral neuropathy in Lowe's syndrome. Neuropediatrics 1988;19:7–9
7. Charnas LR. Seizures in the oculocerebrorenal syndrome of Lowe. Neurology 1989;39(suppl 1):276
8. Illig RV, Dumermuth G, Prader A. Das oculo-cerebro-renale syndrom (Lowe), klinische, metabolische und elektroencephalographische Befunde bei 3 Fallen. Helv Paediatr Acta 1963;18:173–202
9. Charnas L, Choudhry U, Patronas N, Gahl WA. Range of nervous system involvement in patients and heterozygotes for the oculocerebrorenal syndrome of Lowe. Am J Hum Genet 1988;43(suppl):A42
10. Lowe Syndrome Association Comprehensive Survey. Preliminary results on behavior. West LaFayette, IN: The Lowe Syndrome Association, 1989
11. Matin MA, Sylvester PE. Clinicopathological studies of oculocerebrorenal syndrome of Lowe, Terrey and MacLachlan. J Ment Defic Res 1980;24:1–16
12. Schwartz R, Hall PW III, Gabuzda GJ Jr. Metabolism of ornithine and other amino acids in the cerebro-oculo-renal syndrome. Am J Med 1964;36:778–786
13. Hambraeus L, Pallisgaard G, Kildeberg P. The Lowe syndrome: observations on

the amino acid metabolism in a 2-year-old affected boy. Acta Paediatr Scand 1970;59:631–636

14. Bartsocas CS, Levy HL, Crawford JD, Thier SO. A defect in intestinal amino acid transport in Lowe's syndrome. Am J Dis Child 1969;117:93–95
15. Bickel H, Thursby-Pelham DC. Hyperamino-aciduria in Lignac-Fanconi disease, in galactosaemia and in obscure syndrome. Arch Dis Child 1954;29:224–231
16. Holtgrewe JL, Kalen V. Orthopedic manifestations of the Lowe (oculocerebrorenal) syndrome. J Pediatr Orthop 1986;6:165–171
17. Abbassi V, Lowe CU, Calcagno PL. Oculo-cerebro-renal syndrome: review. Am J Dis Child 1968;115:145–168
18. Tripathi RC, Cibis GW, Tripathi BJ. Pathogenesis of cataracts in patients with Lowe's syndrome. Ophthalmology 1986;93:1046–1051
19. Tripathi RC, Cibis GW, Tripathi BJ. Lowe's syndrome. Trans Ophthalmol Soc UK 1980;100:132–139
20. Fagerholm P, Anneren G, Wadelius C. Lowe's oculocerebrorenal syndrome— variation in lens changes in the carrier state. Acta Ophthalmol (Copenh) 1991; 69:102–104
21. Cibis GW, Waelttermann JM, Whitcraft CR, et al. Lenticular opacities in carriers of Lowe's syndrome. Ophthalmology 1986;93:1041–1045
22. Charnas LR, Bernardini I, Rader D, et al. Clinical and laboratory findings in the oculocerebrorenal syndrome of Lowe, with special reference to growth and renal function. N Engl J Med 1991;324:1318–1325
23. Silver DN, Lewis RA, Nussbaum RL. Mapping the Lowe oculocerebrorenal syndrome to Xq24-q26 by use of restriction fragment length polymorphisms. J Clin Invest 1987;79:282–285
24. Silver Reilly D, Lewis RA, Ledbetter DH, Nussbaum L. Tightly linked flanking markers for the Lowe oculocerebrorenal syndrome, with application to carrier assessment. Am J Hum Genet 1988;42:748–755
25. Gazit E, Brand N, Harel Y, et al. Prenatal diagnosis of Lowe's syndrome: a case report with evidence of de novo mutation. Prenat Diagn 1990;10:257–260

X-Chromosome-Linked Juvenile Retinoschisis: Clinical Aspects and Genetics

Philip M. Falcone, M.D.

Robert J. Brockhurst, M.D.

X-chromosome-linked juvenile retinoschisis (XJR) is a genetic, congenital condition affecting young men. It is characterized by foveal retinoschisis, often with associated peripheral retinoschisis. The disorder is visually disabling and progressive, with eventual visual acuity in the 20/200 range or worse [1]. There is no effective treatment.

Genetic linkage analysis localized the retinoschisis (RS) gene to the distal short arm of the X chromosome, but its precise location has not been determined [2–4]. Current carrier detection has been made possible by the use of electroretinography (ERG) and by analysis of haplotypes using DNA probes [5, 6].

Historical Perspectives

XJR was first described by Haas in 1898 [7]. Pagenstecher [8] documented the first pedigree in 1913. In 1932, Thomson [9] described a familial neuroretinopathy found only in male individuals [9], and this characteristic was later more firmly established by Sorsby and associates [10]. Jager [11] introduced the term *retinoschisis* in 1953, although many other designations have also been used to describe this disease, including *vitreous veils* [12], *congenital vascular veils in the vitreous* [13], *congenital cystic retinal detachment* [14], and still others [15].

Inheritance

In an X-linked recessive disorder, if the father has the disease, all the daughters are obligate carriers and all the sons are spared. If the mother is a carrier, the sons have a 50% chance of inheriting the disease and the daughters have a 50% chance of being carriers. One homozygous woman has been described, the product of an affected man and his second cousin [16].

The gene is said to have 100% penetrance; however, there is variable expressivity, and therefore affected individuals may exhibit a variety of clinical manifestations. The foveal lesion is said to have 100% penetrance [15], which means that all male patients will have foveal pathological findings.

■ Epidemiological Features

XJR has been described primarily in white families, but some pedigrees have been reported in blacks [17], Indonesians [15], and Japanese [18] families as well. It is most frequently seen in Finland and may be the most common X-linked disorder in that country [1].

■ Natural History

Boys, usually aged 5 to 10 years, are typically identified when they fail a vision screening examination in school or when they present with vitreous hemorrhage. The earliest age of diagnosis is 10 weeks in a family with known XJR [19]. The usual visual acuity is in the 20/60 to 20/100 range, possibly worse, although 20/25 vision has been reported [1, 20]. Visual acuity may stabilize in the young adult years, but typically there is a slow deterioration in later life, with legal blindness noted in all patients older than 70 years [1].

■ Patient Evaluation

Clinical Findings

Foveal schisis is said to be present in 100% of cases (Fig 1). It may be the only finding in 50% [15]; however, the fovea may appear to be perfectly normal, in which case retinoschisis is diagnosed only by electrophysiological testing (EL Berson, personal communication). Characteristically, the macula has a stellate, spokelike appearance with microcysts evident on contact lens examination. The foveal schisis is bilateral but may be asymmetrical. If the peripheral schisis involves the macular area, the characteristic macular appearance may be obscured. With age, loss of folds with cyst enlargement is seen, resembling a pseudohole. In middle age, pigmentary changes in the retinal pigment epithelium ensue and, later in life, the appearance resembles dry age-related macular degeneration [1].

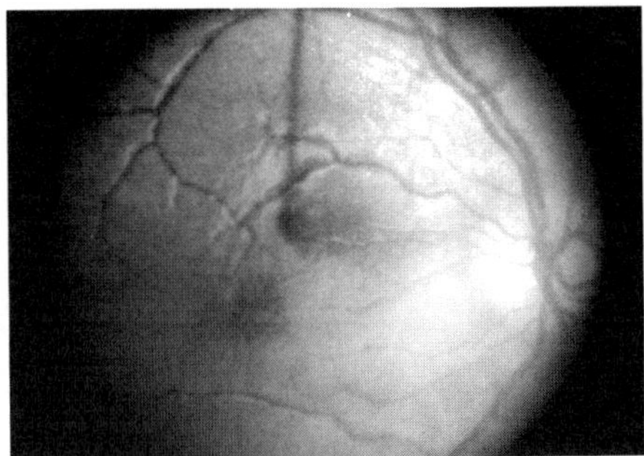

Figure 1 *Typical spokelike appearance of fovea with microcysts in X-linked juvenile retinoschisis.*

Peripheral retinoschisis is seen in approximately 50% of cases, most commonly in the inferotemporal quadrant (96%) [21], although other quadrants may be involved. The condition may be unilateral or bilateral. The superficial inner layer schisis cavity is thin, bullous, and often has large oval holes within it. Vessels may bridge from the inner schisis layer to the outer layer (Fig 2). With vitreal traction, these vessels may bleed and cause vitreous hemorrhage. In later years, the peripheral bullous schisis cavities tend to flatten, and often only a rim of the inner retinal layer remains (Fig 3).

The retinal periphery may manifest other changes including silver-gray spots, dendriform or corkscrew vascular change, and perivascular silver-gray cuffs that resemble sheathing [15]. In end-stage disease, severe pigmentary abnormalities can occur with large areas of chorioretinal atrophy. Demarcation lines can occur in the absence of true retinal detachment, marking the boundary of the schisis cavity with normal retina [22]. Avascular or vascular vitreous veils are seen in approximately 50% of patients. The veils may be attached to the disc but, as a rule, are seen in the periphery. Separation of these membranes can result in a vitreous hemorrhage or may be without sequelae. Vitreous hemorrhage has an incidence of 4% in these patients and may occur within schisis cavities.

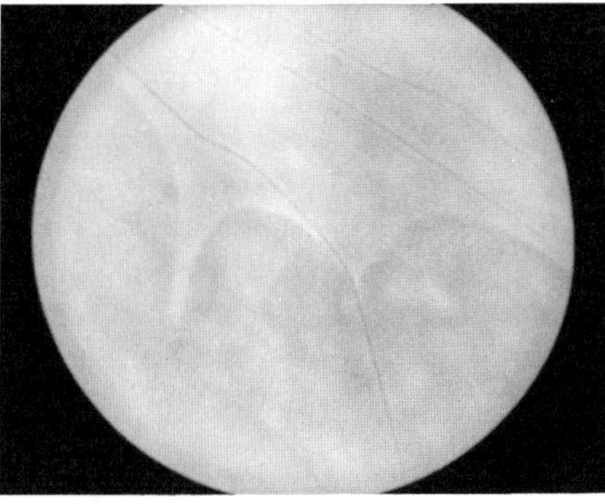

Figure 2 *Vessels bridging from inner to outer retinal layers in peripheral juvenile retinoschisis.*

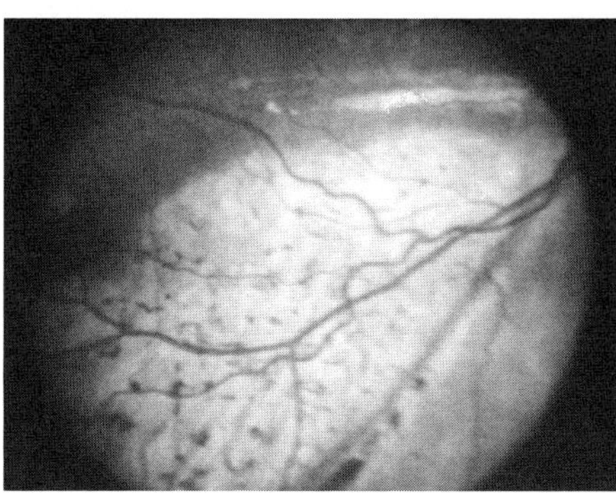

Figure 3 *Residual rim of schisis cavity with peripheral retinal atrophic and pigmentary change. (Courtesy of Dr. John Loewenstein.)*

It usually resolves without therapeutic intervention, although pars plana vitrectomy may be necessary [22].

True retinal detachment in XJR occurs when holes are present in both the inner and outer retinal layers. Deutman [15] believes this to be a rare occurrence, but others have claimed an incidence as high as 11% [21]. The differential diagnosis may be difficult to make. Diagnostic photocoagulation through the elevated retinal tissue is probably the most helpful procedure [22]. In a true retinal detachment, one will not see the bright white photocoagulation burn that is seen in the outer layer of a schisis cavity. Scleral depression techniques may also be helpful in differentiating between the two. If pigment cells are seen in the vitreous, rhegmatogenous retinal detachment is the more likely diagnosis. Most cases occur at a young age and respond to scleral buckling techniques, although recurrence rates of 40% have been reported [21, 23].

Pathological Findings

In 1968, Yanoff and co-workers [24] discovered that the retinoschisis cavity in XJR resulted from splitting in the sensory retina, predominantly in the nerve fiber layer. This is unlike the senile form, in which the retinoschisis occurs primarily in the outer plexiform layer. They postulated that a Müller cell abnormality could explain the pathological retinal splitting seen in these patients.

Diagnostic Tests

Color-vision testing in XJR may yield normal findings or, more often, a mild dyschromatopsia, usually red-green, becomes evident [15, 25]. The visual field will reveal an absolute scotoma in the area of schisis involvement, in contrast to a true retinal detachment where a relative scotoma exists.

The A-wave in ERG is typically normal, with a subnormal B-wave and an abnormal B/A-wave ratio (less than 1). As the disease progresses, there is more widespread peripheral retinal change, with decreased A- and B-wave responses. However, the amplitude ratio will remain less than normal [15, 20]. The electroretinograph is usually normal in young XJR individuals but may not be useful in later years when the light peak–dark trough ratio deteriorates [20, 26]. The visual evoked response exhibits delayed peak times consistent with abnormal macular function.

As a rule, there is no leakage or staining of the macula on fluorescein angiography (i.e., the cystoid spaces do not leak). This may be extremely helpful in differentiating XJR from other entities that may cause cystoid macular edema [26–28]. If macular atrophy and retinal pigment epithelial changes ensue, one may see corresponding areas of hypofluorescence or hyperfluorescence. Peripheral areas of nonperfusion may also be seen.

Associated Ocular Findings

Most XJR patients described are hyperopic with astigmatic errors. Strabismus and nystagmus occur frequently [15]. Stellate posterior cataracts may evolve, usually beginning in the third decade of life [26]. Iridocorneal angle abnormalities have been described along with abnormal insertion of the iris root [15, 29].

Associated Systemic Findings

To date, there have been no systemic disorders reportedly associated with XJR.

Differential Diagnosis

The following entities should be considered in the differential diagnosis of XJR but usually can be excluded with a comprehensive history, physical examination, and ancillary testing:

Goldmann-Favre disease
Wagner's vitreoretinal dystrophy
Cystoid macular edema
Familial foveal retinoschisis [30]
Familial foveal retinoschisis associated with rod-cone dystrophy [31]
Autosomal dominant hereditary retinoschisis [32]
Congenital retinoschisis with night blindness [33]
Peripheral retinoschisis (cystoid/reticular)
Stargardt's disease
Eales's disease
Inferior dialysis of the young [15]
Retinoblastoma
Foveal choroidal folds [26]
Retinoschisis secondary to intermediate uveitis

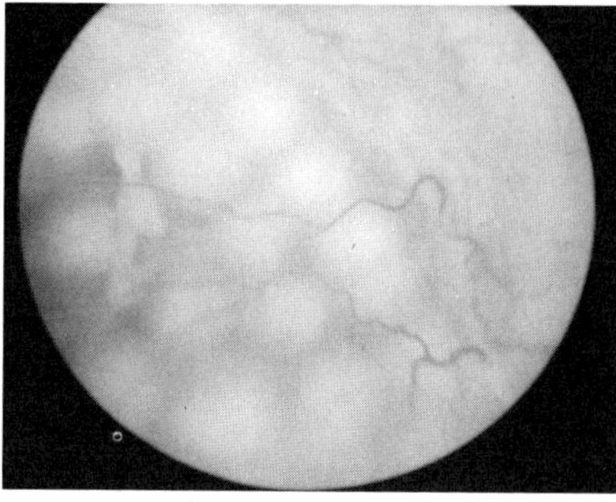

Figure 4 *Laser photocoagulation to an area of retinoschisis.*

■ Treatment

The treatment of retinoschisis has been a source of debate and controversy. Laser photocoagulation has been tried in an attempt to flatten schisis cavities and to provide a barrier against advancement (Fig 4). Other authors have used combinations of cryotherapy, scleral buckling, and vitrectomy, without demonstrable improvement in visual acuity. It is now generally accepted that surgical attempts to flatten schisis cavities is of no benefit and may, in fact, result in retinal detachment [23, 34].

■ Genetic Research

Recombinant DNA technology has enabled genetic mapping to be performed to identify specific gene loci. DNA restriction enzymes recognize DNA sequences, catalyze cleavage sites, and leave behind DNA fragments of defined lengths. The differences in these restriction fragment length polymorphisms (RFLPs) are recognized by their altered mobility on electrophoresis, and they are separated by molecular size. The DNA sequence can be detected by hybridization techniques using radioactive probes. Thereby, variants within a specific region of the genome can be identified using fragments of human DNA [35–37].

Genetic Detection of XJR

Preliminary work in 1970 linked the RS gene to the Xg locus at the distal end of the X chromosome [38]. In 1983, Wieacker and colleagues [39] used a cloned DNA sequence, RC8 (DX59 locus), from the short arm of the X chromosome to study linkage relationships. Using RFLPs and blood samples from 2 affected families in Italy and Germany, these investigators were able to suggest a linkage of the RS gene to the DX59 locus and to provide an approximate location of the RS gene on the distal X-chromosomal Xp21 segment.

Alitalo and co-workers [2] examined 231 Finnish families with 88 affected male members and confirmed the close linkage of the RS gene to the marker loci DXS43, DXS16, DXS207, and DXS41, all located on the distal Xp22.1-p.22.3 segment. Sieving and associates [4] looked at the linkage patterns of the RS gene and found no evidence of heterogeneity, a contradictory finding given the variable phenotypical presentation of XJR. Modifying genes, genetic mutations, or environmental factors are believed to be the cause of the polymorphic clinical presentation.

Alitalo's group [3] further refined the location of the RS gene as lying between DXS207/DXS43 and DXS274 loci [3]. The locus DXS274 represents a new marker closely linked to the RS gene. The genetic distance between the closest markers flanking the gene was estimated at 7 centimorgans (cM).

At present, the precise location of the RS gene is unknown. The search for closer genetic markers continues. The current locus order is as follows:

> DXS16-DXS207-DXS43—RS—DXS274-DXS41-DXS92
> DXS43—7cM—DXS274
> Xp22.2—Xp22.1
> Distal X chromosome

Carrier Detection

Unlike other ocular X-linked recessive disorders, no ophthalmoscopically detectable abnormalities have been consistently described in heterozygous carriers of XJR. Therefore, the female carrier has been identifiable only after the birth of an affected son.

However, recent work using DNA probes and the observation of abnormal rod-cone interaction in female carriers may allow proper genetic counseling prior to conception.

Linked DNA Probes Using RFLPs, Dahl and Pettersson [6] compared the haplotype of a 1-year-old male infant with his brother, who was known to be affected with XJR. The brothers displayed the same haplotype at five linked markers, which extended between the DXS164 and DXS85 loci, encompassing the RS locus. With identical haplotypes, a diagnosis of XJR was made genetically and was subsequently confirmed by clinical and ERG testing.

Dahl's group [6] also provided genetic counseling for a pregnant woman who had a brother with XJR. Her haplotype was different from her brother's at three linked loci that flanked the RS gene; therefore, she was excluded as a carrier (99% probability) and it was determined that the fetus was unlikely to inherit the RS gene.

Reliability is not 100% (93% to 95%) because of the risks of single- or double-recombination events during meiosis, and risk calculations can be based only on well-defined genetic distances. However, in families with male members affected with XJR, those members' serum can be used to provide genetic markers, and predictions can be made with a high degree of certainty about female carrier status, or a DNA-based diagnosis can be made complementing the clinical and ERG findings [6].

Loss of Rod-Cone Interaction   Normal individuals have a suppressive rod-cone interaction—that is, the ability of the photopic system to detect flicker becomes impaired as the rods adapt to dark conditions. This rod-cone interaction is most likely the result of postsynaptic feedback, possibly from the horizontal cells, onto the cone photoreceptors. In conditions of photoreceptor disease, rod-cone interaction can still be demonstrated. In contrast, in conditions where postsynaptic abnormalities appear to be the primary disturbance, the rod-cone interaction is absent. Recent work implicating Müller cells as a migration determinant for retinal development and neuronal interconnections would explain the absence of this phenomenon in XJR [5].

Arden and colleagues [5] looked at 11 obligate female heterozygous carriers of the RS gene, all of whom had complete loss of normal rod-cone interaction but who otherwise exhibited normal findings on funduscopic and functional testing. In a study of potential carriers, 2 lacked rod-cone interaction, identifying them as probable RS carriers. Larger study size and prospective testing are necessary to establish the reliability and specificity of this method. However, this selective loss of rod-cone interaction may allow carrier detection of an individual independently, without requiring DNA analysis [5].

■ References

1. Forsius H, Krause U, Helve J, et al. Visual acuity in 183 cases of X-chromosomal retinoschisis. Can J Ophthalmol 1973;8:385–393
2. Alitalo T, Forsius H, Karna J, et al. Linkage relationships and gene order around the locus for X-linked retinoschisis. Am J Hum Genet 1988;43:476–483
3. Alitalo T, Kruse T, de la Chapelle A. Refined localization of the gene causing X-linked juvenile retinoschisis. Genomics 1991;9:505–510
4. Sieving PA, Bingham EL, Roth MS, et al. Linkage relationship of X-linked juvenile retinoschisis with Xp22.1-p.22.3 probes. Am J Hum Genet 1990;47:616–621
5. Arden GB, Gorin MB, Polkinghorne PJ, et al. Detection of the carrier state of X-linked retinoschisis. Am J Ophthalmol 1988;105:590–595
6. Dahl N, Pettersson U. Use of linked DNA probes for carrier detection and diagnosis of X-linked juvenile retinoschisis. Arch Ophthalmol 1988;106:1414–1416
7. Haas J. Ueber das Zusammenvorkommen von Veranderungen der Retina und Chorioidea. Arch Augenheilkd 1898;37:343–348
8. Pagenstecher HE. Ueber eine unter dem Bilde der Netzhautablosung verlaufende, erbliche Erkrankung der Retina. Arch Ophthalmol 1913;86:457–462

9. Thomson E. Memorandum regarding a family in which neuroretinal disease of an unusual kind occurred only in males. Br J Ophthalmol 1932;16:681–686

10. Sorsby A, Klein M, Gann JH, et al. Unusual retinal detachment, probably sex-linked. Br J Ophthalmol 1951;35:1–10

11. Jager GM. A hereditary retinal disease. Trans Ophthalmol Soc UK 1953;73: 617–619

12. Condon GP, Brownstein S, Wang N, et al. Congenital hereditary (juvenile X-linked) retinoschisis: histopathologic and ultrastructural findings in three eyes. Arch Ophthalmol 1986;104:576–583

13. Balian JV, Falls HF. Congenital vascular veins in the vitreous: hereditary retinoschisis. Arch Ophthalmol 1960;63:92–101

14. Juler F. Unusual form of retinal detachment (?cystic) in children. Trans Ophthalmol Soc UK 1948;67:83–96

15. Deutman AF. Vitreoretinal dystrophies. In: Krill AE, ed. Hereditary retinal and choroidal diseases, vol 2. Hagerstown, MD: Harper & Row, 1977:1043–1062

16. Forsius H, Vainio-Mattila BA, Eriksson AW. X-linked hereditary retinoschisis. Br J Ophthalmol 1962;46:678–681

17. Constantaras AA, Dobbie JG, Choromokes EA, et al. Juvenile sex-linked recessive retinoschisis in a black family. Am J Ophthalmol 1972;74:1166–1178

18. Saito T, Satoh Y, Seimiya T, Koda N. A family with juvenile retinoschisis (Japanese). Jpn J Clin Ophthalmol 1971;25:849–856

19. Arkfeld DF, Brockhurst RJ. Vascularized vitreous membranes in congenital retinoschisis. Retina 1987;7:20–23

20. Hirose T, Wolf E, Hara A. Electrophysiological and psychophysical studies in congenital retinoschisis of X-linked recessive inheritance. Doc Ophthalmol 1977;13: 173–184

21. Kellner U, Brummer S, Foerster MH, Wessing A. X-linked congenital retinoschisis. Graefes Arch Clin Exp Ophthalmol 1990;228:432–437

22. Brockhurst RJ. Photocoagulation in congenital retinoschisis. Arch Ophthalmol 1970;84:158–165

23. Greven CM, Moreno RJ, Tasman W. Unusual manifestations of X-linked retinoschisis. Trans Am Ophthalmol Soc 1990;88:211–226

24. Yanoff M, Rahn EK, Zimmerman LE. Histopathology of juvenile retinoschisis. Arch Ophthalmol 1968;79:49–53

25. Helve J. Colour vision in X-chromosomal juvenile retinoschisis. Mod Probl Ophthalmol 1990;11:122–129

26. Lewis RA. Juvenile hereditary macular dystrophies. In: Newsome DA, ed. Retinal dystrophies and degenerations. New York: Raven Press, 1988:115–134

27. Ewing CC, Cullen AP. Fluorescein angiography in X-chromosomal maculopathy and retinoschisis (juvenile hereditary retinoschisis). Can J Ophthalmol 1972;7: 19–28

28. Green JL, Jampol LM. Vascular opacification and leakage in X-linked (juvenile) retinoschisis. Br J Ophthalmol 1979;63:368–373

29. Sabates FN. Juvenile retinoschisis. Am J Ophthalmol 1966;62:683–688

30. Lewis RA, Lee GB, Martonyi CL, et al. Familial foveal retinoschisis. Arch Ophthalmol 1977;95:1190–1196

31. Noble KG, Carr RE, Siegel IM. Familial foveal retinoschisis associated with a rod-cone dystrophy. Am J Ophthalmol 1978;85:551–557

32. Yassur Y, Nissenkorn I, Ben-Sira I, et al. Autosomal dominant inheritance of retinoschisis. Am J Ophthalmol 1982;94:338–343

33. Hirose T, Schepens CL, Brockhurst RJ, et al. Congenital retinoschisis with night blindness in two girls. Ann Ophthalmol 1980;12:848–856

34. Turut P, François P, Castier P, Milazzo S. Analysis of results in the treatment of

peripheral retinoschisis in sex-linked congenital retinoschisis. Graefes Arch Clin Exp Ophthalmol 1989;227:328–331

35. Botstein D, White RL, Davis RW, Skolnick M. Construction of a genetic linkage map in man using restriction fragment length polymorphisms. Am J Hum Genet 1980;32:314–331

36. Drayna D, White R. The genetic linkage map of the human X-chromosome. Science 1985;230:753–758

37. Orkin SH. Molecular genetics and inherited human disease. In: Scriver CR, et al, eds. The metabolic basis of inherited disease, ed 6. New York: McGraw-Hill, 1989:165–177

38. Ives EJ, Ewing CC, Innes R. X-linked juvenile retinoschisis and Xg linkage in five families (abstr). Am J Hum Genet 1970;22:17–18

39. Wieacker P, Wienker TF, Dallapiccola B, et al. Linkage relationships between retinoschisis, Xg, and a cloned DNA sequence from the distal short arm of the X chromosome. Hum Genet 1983;64:141–145

Clinical Methods for Detecting the Carrier State of X-Chromosome-linked Retinal Disorders

Kenneth J. Wald, M.D.
Tatsuo Hirose, M.D.

Many disorders of the visual system are inherited through an X-chromosome-linked mode of transmission. This mode of inheritance has implications for genetic counseling as well as for prognostication of the clinical course. The X-linked genotype is often the most severely affected of a disease phenotype. The most widely available and simplest methods for recognizing the X-linked genotype are family pedigree analysis and examination of female relatives for manifestations of the usually clinically silent heterozygote, or carrier state. Molecular genetic analysis eventually will support and perhaps supplant current diagnostic methods. Correlations between clinical and electrophysiological data and specific gene defects also will be important.

■ The X Chromosome

One X chromosome is randomly inactivated in each cell of a female individual, leaving each cell with its complement of active X-chromosome genes from either maternal or paternal origin [1]. It follows that an X-linked gene defect is present in approximately one-half of all female cells. The normal X chromosome usually protects a female individual from full expression of the gene defect, resulting in a carrier state. Variable expressivity of the gene defect at the cellular level may result in a phenotypical mosaic. Clinical manifestations of this mosaicism may be recognized and can be useful as a marker for the X-chromosome-linked inheritance pattern.

X-linked recessive diseases affect male individuals much more severely than female individuals for a given age. There is no male-to-male transmission. All female offspring of an affected man are carriers. Half of the sons of a female carrier are affected, and half of the daughters of a female carrier are carriers.

The clinical methods for carrier detection of the following X-linked disorders will be reviewed: retinitis pigmentosa, albinism, choroideremia, cone dystrophy, congenital stationary night blindness, juvenile retinoschisis, and blue cone monochromatism.

■ X-Chromosome-linked Retinitis Pigmentosa

Affected Male Individual

X-chromosome-linked disease is typically the most severe form of retinitis pigmentosa. Visual acuity of less than 20/50 by age 20 to 39 years, onset of night blindness by age 20 years, and myopia of greater than − 2.00 are significantly more prevalent in X-chromosome-linked retinitis pigmentosa than the other inheritance types [2]. An extinguished electroretinogram (ERG) was formerly believed to be characteristic but, with newer techniques of electronic filtering and computer averaging of signals, amplitudes of less than 1 μV have been recorded [3].

Female Carrier

An asymptomatic female individual from a family with an X-linked inheritance pattern of retinitis pigmentosa, with an affected father or son, is an obligate heterozygote. Clinical examination to detect phenotypical expression of the gene defect is confirmatory but not necessary for identification of the carrier state. Women with a family pedigree consistent with X-linked inheritance but without an affected father or son are considered *presumed* heterozygotes and must be investigated for the clinical stigmata of the carrier state to determine whether they are genetic heterozygotes.

The sensitivity of ophthalmoscopic examination in recognizing the carrier state of X-linked retinitis pigmentosa is not established. Berson and co-workers [4] found *diagnostic* signs of the carrier state in 61% of obligate carriers (14 of 23). Among women of childbearing age (15 to 40 years), only 43% (3 of 7) had a diagnostic fundus abnormality [4]. Fishman and colleagues [5] reported peripheral pigmentary changes and tapetal reflex in 87% of presumed carriers (40 of 46). Bird [6] reported peripheral pigment epithelial alterations (with or without fluorescein angiography), intra-retinal pigment migration, or a tapetal reflex in 100% of obligate heterozygotes (19 of 19). It is unclear whether subtle retinal pigment epithelial changes can be considered diagnostic for the carrier state. The tapetal reflex has traditionally been considered a hallmark of the carrier fundus

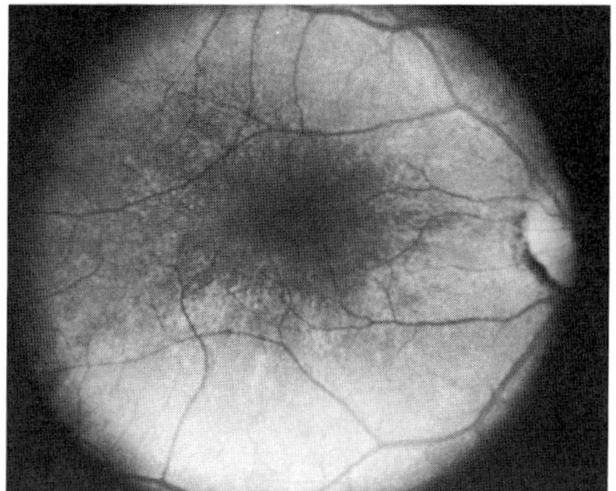

Figure 1 *Fundus photograph demonstrating the golden tapetal reflex seen in carriers of X-linked retinitis pigmentosa.*

[7], but there is considerable disagreement among investigators regarding the utility of this finding (Fig 1). Berson and co-workers [4] found tapetal reflexes in 23% of female obligate heterozygotes (3 of 13), and Krill [8] observed it in 14% of carriers (2 of 14). Fishman and associates [5] found tapetal reflexes in more than 50% of presumed carriers (24 of 46), and this was the only fundus abnormality in 41% (19 of 46). Bird [6] noted the tapetal reflex in several young women in his series but considered it indistinguishable from the normal fundus reflex of young patients; only one older woman had this fundus finding. The association with age was not corroborated by Fishman [5] or Berson [4], who found that 35% (8 of 23) and 67% (2 of 3), respectively, of the female carriers with tapetal reflexes were older than 40 years. Pigmentary changes, including areas of atrophy, pigment clumping, and migration into the sensory retina as bone spicules, are a frequent finding in all series (Fig 2) [4–8]. A spectrum ranging from scattered areas of pigmentary degeneration of the retina with rare spots of intraretinal pigment migration to a more widespread degeneration with attenuated retinal vessels and optic nerve pallor may be found. There is evidence that two distinct genotypes for X-linked retinitis

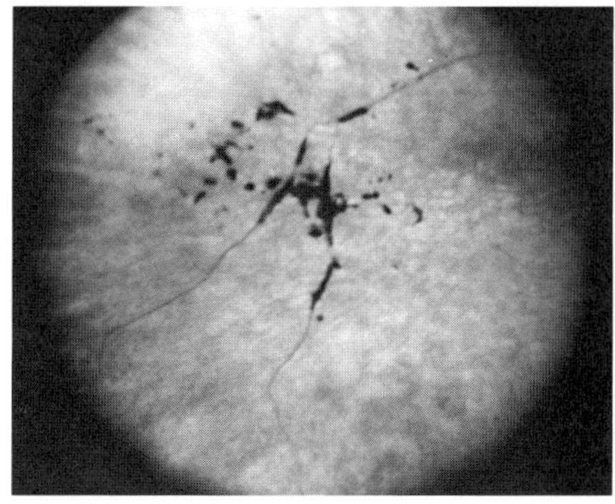

Figure 2 *An isolated island of bone spicule intraretinal pigmentation. The rest of the fundus appeared normal.*

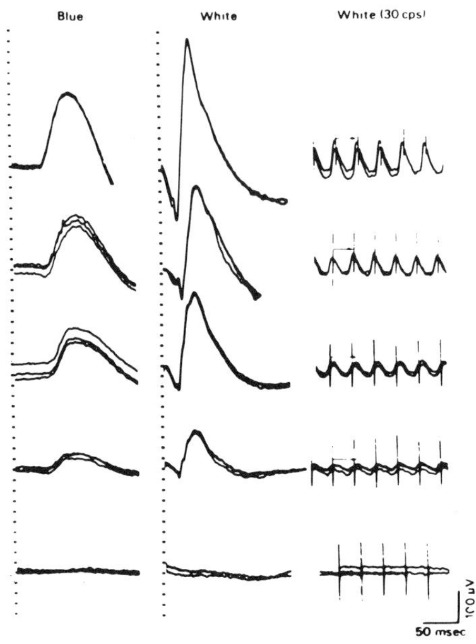

Figure 3 *Electroretinogram of 1 normal and 4 obligate female carriers of X-linked retinitis pigmentosa. Two to three responses to the same stimulus are represented. Stimulus onset is designated by the vertical hatched lines for columns 1 and 2, and vertical shock artifacts for column 3. Arrows in column 3 designate cone B-wave implicit time. There is loss of amplitude to blue and white stimuli in all carriers and prolongation of the implicit time in 3 of 4 carriers. Responses seen in rows 2 and 4 were from patients with normal fundi. (Reprinted with permission from EL Berson et al, Electroretinographic testing as an aid in detection of carriers of X-chromosome-linked retinitis pigmentosa. Am J Ophthalmol 1979;87: 460–468. Copyright © The Ophthalmic Publishing Company.)*

pigmentosa exist, with genetic loci at different segments on the short arm of the X chromosome; the tapetal reflex may be specific for one of the genotypes [9]. There is eye–to–fellow eye as well as interfamilial variability of the fundus appearance [5].

Additional clinical features of the carrier state include moderate to high corneal astigmatism and moderate to high degrees of myopia [5].

Electrophysiological testing can detect abnormalities in female carriers with normal fundi and can be used as an aid in diagnosis. The sensitivity of electrophysiological testing for carrier state detection is high. Reduced amplitudes on the ERG were found in 90% of obligate carriers (27 of 30) in one series [5]. Another report demonstrated that more than 95% of obligate carriers (22 of 23) had an abnormal ERG in at least 1 eye: The abnormality was a decrease in the amplitude of the bright-flash, dark-adapted ERG (less than 350 µV), or a delay of the cone B-wave implicit time, or both (greater than 32 msec) [4] (Fig 3). The early receptor potential, which indicates the functioning of the photoreceptor outer segments, can be diminished in female carriers [10]. A reduced rod flicker sensitivity in female heterozygotes has also been reported [11].

Experimental diagnostic techniques have been described including vitreous fluorophotometry to detect abnormalities of the blood retinal barrier [12] and reflectometry to measure retinal rhodopsin concentration [13].

In summary, the detection of the heterozygote state of retinitis pigmentosa may be accomplished by family analysis alone (obligate heterozygote) or by a combination of pedigree analysis, electroretinography, and ophthalmoscopy; the ERG appears to be the most sensitive diagnostic aid.

■ Choroideremia

Affected Male Individual

Male individuals with choroideremia have symptoms of night blindness beginning in the first decade of life, followed by loss of the peripheral visual field [14–16]. The earliest finding on ophthalmoscopic examination is mottled depigmentation, which may be detected as early as the first year of life [14]. Later, choroidal and retinal pigment epithelial atrophy begin in the midperiphery and then extend both anteriorly and posteriorly. Sparing of the central macular area until late in the disease course is typical. The ERG is abnormal early in life and becomes extinguished later [14–16].

Female Carrier

The visual acuity of the female carrier occasionally may be mildly decreased or, rarely, severely diminished [14]. Loss of visual field may occur in elderly carriers [15]. A subjective abnormality in dark adaptation can be elicited in one-third of female carriers [14]. Fundus changes, including pigmentary mottling and areas of depigmentation, are most common in the midperiphery but may also involve the macular region. Pigmentary granules of an irregular, squared-off appearance and variable size are often oriented in irregular bands radiating toward the peripheral retina [16], or they may be clumped, especially in the equatorial region, and may be clustered in dotlike shapes of varying sizes [8] (Figs 4, 5). The macular pigmentary changes, when present, usually consist of a fine mottling [8]. Areas of choroidal atrophy, such as that seen in affected male individuals, may be seen in the periphery, the macula, or the peripapillary region [8]. Progression of funduscopic changes has been documented, beginning with

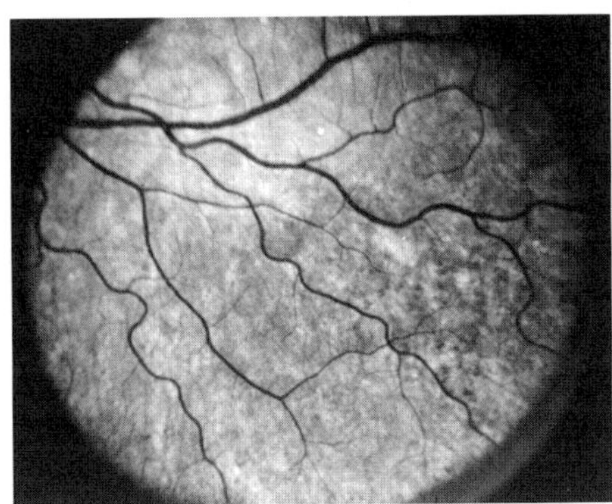

Figure 4 *Fundus photograph of female carrier with choroideremia. There is a subtle pigmentary abnormality in the midperiphery.*

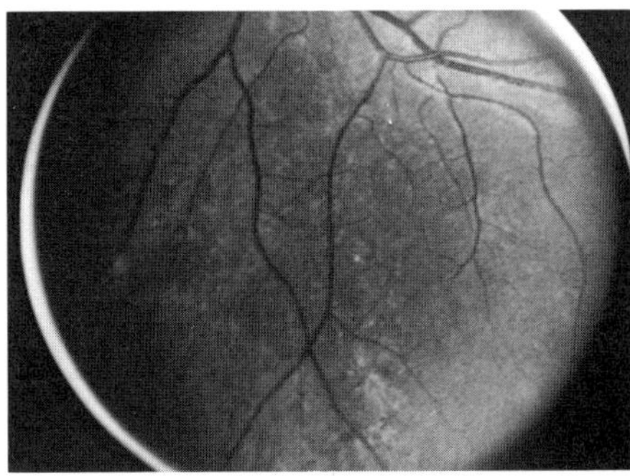

Figure 5 *Fundus photograph of a female carrier with choroideremia. Note clumps of round dotlike pigment granules surrounded by depigmented halos. Also note streaky nature of the pigmentary abnormality.*

subtle pigmentary changes in the midperipheral retina and progressing to marked choroidal atrophy, resembling the fundi of younger affected male patients [14, 17]. Early pigmentary alterations are accentuated by fluorescein angiography. Fluorescein angiography may also demonstrate delayed filling of the choroidal vessels in female carriers with marked fundus changes [17]. A completely normal fundus appearance is rare if the subtle changes are carefully sought [14–17].

A delay in scotopic B-wave implicit time was found in 3 of 10 carriers in one report [8], and the ERG was extinguished in 3 of 20 carriers in another series [14]. A recent series of ERG recordings in obligate female carriers demonstrated an abnormality in 15% (4 of 26). A delay in the cone implicit time was the most frequent finding [18].

Ophthalmoscopy is highly sensitive for recognition of the choroideremia carrier state, but the findings are inconstant, subtle, and nonspecific. The midperipheral fundus is the most frequently affected area. Analysis of the family pedigree is imperative. The combination of ophthalmoscopic findings in a female individual from the choroideremia pedigree is highly specific. In contrast to X-linked retinitis pigmentosa, electrophysiological testing has marginal utility for carrier detection in choroideremia. There are no reported cases in which a normal fundus registers an ERG abnormality.

■ X-Chromosome-linked Ocular Albinism (Nettleship-Falls Type)

Affected Male Individual

Male patients with X-linked ocular albinism present with nystagmus soon after birth. High refractive errors and strabismus are common. The skin and hair coloration are usually normal, but there may be areas of cutaneous hypopigmentation. The iris is usually blue but may be dark brown, with radial transillumination defects seen on biomicroscopy [19–21]. Transillumination defects are not present in blacks with this disorder

[19]. The irides of blacks with this disorder may demonstrate a pigment mosaicism, with alternating spokes of dark and light pigment [22]. (Transillumination defects are due to defects in the pigment of the posterior epithelial layer of the iris, whereas iris color is contributed by the iris stroma [21].) Visual acuity is diminished [19–21, 23, 24]. The fundus has variable pigmentation, with normal or light pigmentation at the macular area and depigmentation of the periphery, with clear visibility of the choroidal vessels [21]. Fundus pigmentation may appear normal in blacks [20]. Foveal hypoplasia is present [21, 24].

Pathological study of clinically normal skin reveals giant pigment granules in the dermis and epidermis (more than 15 per 5 mm). The granules stain with the Fontana-Masson stain and are dopa-oxidase positive. Silver stains may increase the sensitivity of skin biopsy specimens. On electron microscopy, the giant pigment granules are seen to be single large melanosomes within melanocytes and keratocytes. Their size averages 1.75 to 4.3 μm, up to a maximum of 12 μm. Normal melanosome size is usually approximately 0.5 μm in diameter, with a maximum of just over 1 μm. The abnormal melanogenesis affects the pigment epithelium of the iris, ciliary body, and retina (neuroectoderm), but the uveal stroma (neural crest) contains normal-sized melanosomes. (The biochemical pathways responsible for melanin synthesis are the same in all melanin-producing cells.) The pigment epithelial layers have fewer melanosomes than normal [21].

Female Carrier

The female heterozygote is asymptomatic, has normal visual acuity, and does not have nystagmus. Rarely, female heterozygotes are affected as severely as male patients [23]. The iris may demonstrate mild radial transillumination defects [24], but the macula is normally developed [21, 24]. A recent literature review noted that 87% of female carriers have mottling of the retinal pigment epithelium in the midperiphery and posterior pole [24]. The peripheral fundus can appear as alternating stripes of hypopigmentation and normal pigmentation (Figs 6, 7). Biopsy of clinically

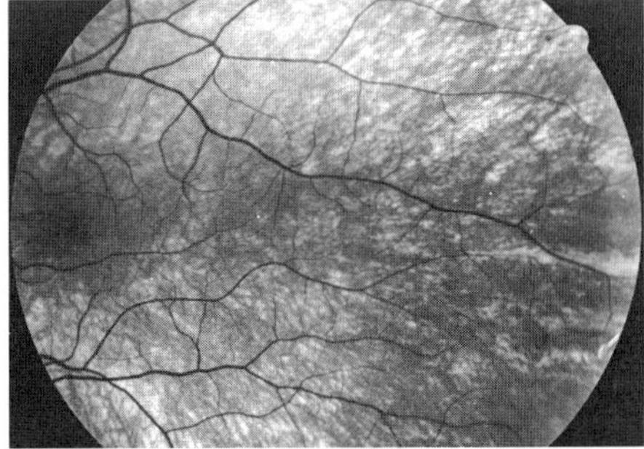

Figure 6 *Macula and temporal midperiphery of a female carrier of X-linked ocular albinism. Note streaky areas of depigmentation in the midperipheral fundus and tiny wreaths of depigmentation surrounding a darker center. (Courtesy of Dr. RA Lewis and Larry Merin.)*

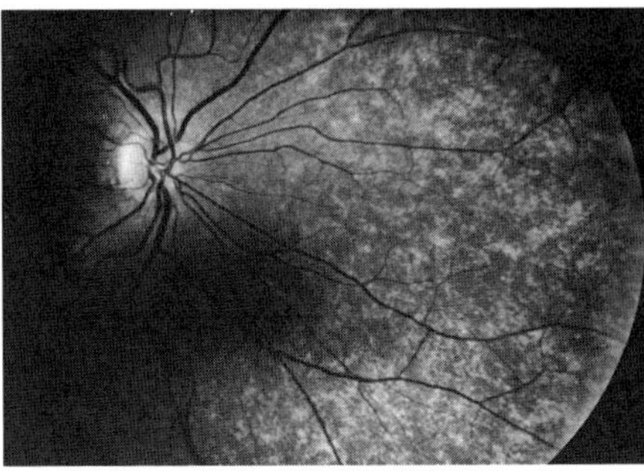

Figure 7 *Nasal retina of a female carrier of X-linked ocular albinism. Note more pronounced wreathlike depigmented areas deep to the retina than in Figure 6. In contrast to the choroideremia carrier, there is no pigmentary clumping or hyperpigmentation. (Courtesy of Dr. RA Lewis and Larry Merin.)*

normal skin reveals giant melanosomes identical to those in affected male patients but less numerous (up to 5 per 5 mm) [21].

In summary, female carriers have normal-appearing skin, hair, and ocular coloration. Subtle transillumination defects in a brown (or blue) iris must be sought in female relatives of ocular albinos. The funduscopic abnormality of variable areas of depigmentation also may be inconspicuous. Random-area skin biopsy is a useful adjunct but is not pathognomonic for this disorder.

■ Cone Dystrophy

Affected Male Individual

There is progressive but gradual decline of central visual function with cone dystrophy [25, 26]. Patients may not become symptomatic until the fourth decade of life [26]. Photosensitivity and central scotoma are the earliest complaints, and color vision is impaired [26]. The ophthalmoscopic findings are nonspecific and evolve with advancing age. During youth, the macular retinal pigment epithelium may appear granular, and a loss of the foveal reflex may become apparent. Progressive atrophic changes occur. A bull's-eye pattern of degenerative change, which is accentuated by fluorescein angiography, is seen later in the course. Temporal pallor of the optic nerve may be seen [26]. A peripheral retinal sheen, which may disappear with dark adaptation (Mizuo-Nakamura phenomenon), has been reported [25]. The diagnosis is confirmed by electrophysiological testing, which demonstrates a highly abnormal cone-mediated ERG [25–27].

Female Carrier

The obligate carrier state of cone dystrophy can be determined by pedigree analysis, as in other X-linked disorders; in fact, this may be the only means of detection. Heterozygotes are asymptomatic, and visual acuity is normal [26]. Fundus findings are infrequent and may include macular pigmentary granularity and mild temporal pallor of the optic nerve [25, 26]. Peripheral tapetal sheen has also been reported [25]. Abnormal color vision may be seen in patients with ophthalmoscopic findings [26]. Electrophysiological testing may reveal an abnormality of the photopic ERG (decreased B-wave amplitude) or a diminished response to a 30-Hz flicker (Fig 8) [26, 27]. One pedigree demonstrated a diminished response to red-light stimuli [27]. ERG findings occur in some female heterozygotes with normal fundus findings [25–27].

Analysis of the current methodology suggests that clinical detection of the carrier state of this disorder is unreliable. Careful ophthalmoscopy and ERG testing may detect some carriers.

■ Congenital Stationary Night Blindness

Affected Male Individual

Male patients with congenital stationary night blindness have diminished night vision and a mild to moderate decrease in Snellen acuity (20/40 to 20/120) [28]. Moderate to severe myopia (-3.5 to -14.5) is present

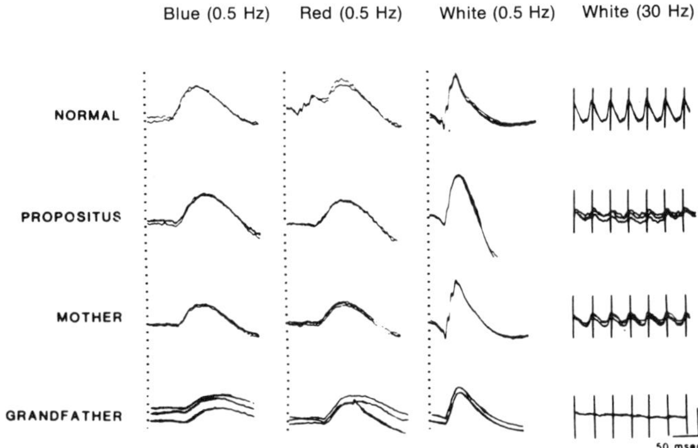

Figure 8 *Full-field electroretinographic responses from a normal subject, the propositus, his mother, and his maternal grandfather from a family with X-linked cone degeneration with predominant loss of red-cone function. The obligate carrier (mother of propositus) demonstrates a loss of the cone contribution to the B-wave elicited by a red stimulus and diminished responses to 30-Hz flicker. Her response to blue stimuli is normal, consistent with normal rod function. Stimulus onset is designated by the vertical hatched lines in columns 1 to 3 and the vertical lines in column 4. (Reprinted with permission from E Reichel et al, An electroretinographic and molecular genetic study of X-linked cone degeneration. Am J Ophthalmol 1989;108:540–547. Copyright © The Ophthalmic Publishing Company.)*

[28]. Nystagmus, which is horizontal and may be fine or coarse, is frequent (two-thirds of patients) [28]. The bright-stimulus, dark-adapted ERG is electronegative; there is a normal A-wave and a low-amplitude B-wave, which has a normal or shortened peak latency (implicit time) [28]. The early oscillatory components in response to long-wavelength suprathreshold light are often reduced, and the corneal positive response to short-wavelength suprathreshold light is absent [29]. Dark adaptation is monophasic, lacking a rod contribution [28].

Female Carrier

In the female carrier, Snellen acuity, night vision, and visual field are normal [30]. The amplitudes of the A- and B-waves in the single-flash ERG, the amplitude of the scotopic and photopic B-waves, and the peak time of the oscillatory potentials also are normal. The summation of the oscillatory potential amplitudes was 2 standard deviations below normal in 17 of 22 eyes of 12 female obligate heterozygotes under dark-adapted bright-flash conditions (Fig 9) [30]. Additional studies have confirmed these findings and have suggested that the idea testing conditions to demonstrate the diminished oscillatory potentials of this disorder are dark adaptation with a blue-flash stimulus [31].

In summary, the clinical features are not helpful in detecting the carrier state of congenital stationary night blindness. However, a unique ERG feature of this disease, the diminished amplitude of the oscillatory potentials, has proved useful in evaluating the carrier state.

■ Juvenile Retinoschisis

Affected Male Individual

Characteristic foveal schisis is seen soon after birth in all juvenile retinoschisis patients; peripheral schisis is seen in 50%. The visual acuity is diminished in the first decade of life to the 20/40 to 20/60 range and then deteriorates progressively so that by the seventh decade the acuity is rarely better than 20/200 [32]. The ERG demonstrates an intact A-wave with a subnormal B-wave [33].

Female Carrier

There are no definitive ophthalmoscopic findings for the carrier state in juvenile retinoschisis. One report described wrinkling of the internal limiting membrane around the fovea of 1 eye of the mother of an affected male child [34]. There was no evidence of foveal schisis, and this has not been demonstrated in other cases. Arden and colleagues [35] reported an electrophysiological study in which abnormal rod-cone interaction was demonstrated in carriers. There was a lack of the usual derangement in

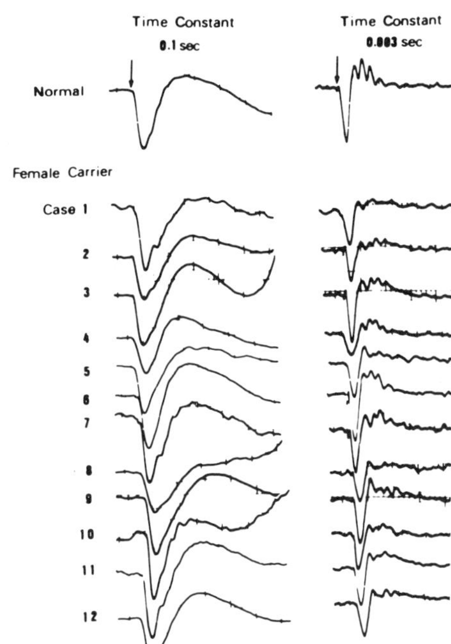

Figure 9 *The dark-adapted bright-flash electroretinogram of 1 normal and 12 obligate carriers of X-linked congenital stationary night blindness. There is a decrease in the sum of the oscillatory potentials compared with normals. (Reprinted with permission from Y Miyake and Y Kawase, Reduced amplitude of oscillatory potentials in female carriers of X-linked recessive congenital stationary night blindness. Am J Ophthalmol 1984;98:208– 215. Copyright © The Ophthalmic Publishing Company.)*

the photopic flicker response during dark adaptation in 11 of 11 obligate carriers.

Clinical detection of the carrier state is not definitive based on present methods. Electroretinography was useful in one report [35].

■ Blue-Cone Monochromatism

Affected Male Individual

The visual acuity in patients affected with blue-cone monochromatism is in the 20/60 to 20/200 range, and nystagmus, photophobia, and poor color discrimination are present, with a deutanlike axis of confusion on the Farnsworth D-15 panel [36]. Other features are compound myopic astigmatism and a normal fundus appearance, with the exception of a diminished foveal light reflex. The ERG demonstrates normal rod-mediated responses and minimally detectable cone responses to 30-Hz white flicker [37].

Female Carrier

Clinical examination reveals a normal fundus, with normal color vision and dark adaptation, but the cone ERG in carriers may be abnormal [38, 39]. Berson and co-workers [40] reported ERG abnormalities in all obligate

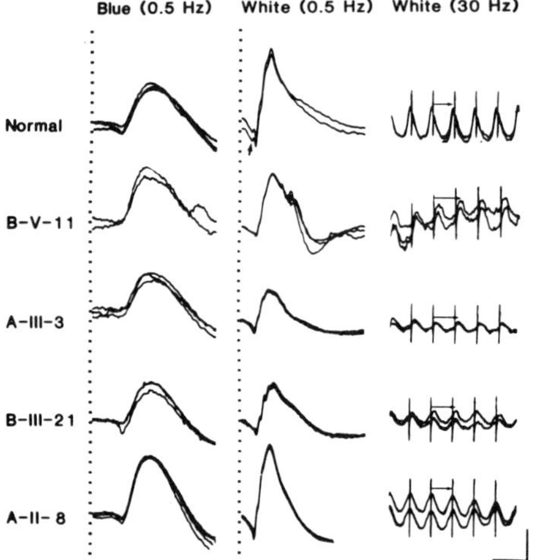

Figure 10 *Full-field electroretinograms of 1 normal and 4 obligate carriers of blue-cone monochromatism. Two or three consecutive responses are illustrated for each stimulus condition. Time of stimulus onset is designated by vertical lines in columns 1 and 2 and vertical shock artifacts in column 3. The arrowhead designates the A_1 oscillation in the normal response; it is absent in the obligate carrier. There is also a delay in the cone B-wave implicit time to a 30-Hz flicker stimulus, seen in column 3. (Reprinted with permission from EL Berson et al, Electroretinogram in carriers of blue-cone monochromatism. Am J Ophthalmol 1986;102:254–261. Copyright © The Ophthalmic Publishing Company.)*

carriers (7 of 7) (Fig 10). Rod-mediated responses were normal. The mixed cone and rod responses exhibited a lack of the A1 oscillation of the A-wave, which is seen in normals. The most commonly occurring abnormality was a delay in the cone B-wave implicit time to a 30-Hz flicker stimulus. Obligate carriers had average cone amplitudes to photopically matched stimuli that were approximately 50% of normal. In another study, 60% of obligate carriers (3 of 5) had ERG abnormalities, including prolongation of the cone implicit time to flicker and to single flashes in the dark-adapted state [41].

■ Genetic Analysis

Advances in human genome analysis eventually will be useful for confirming and diagnosing all genetic diseases. DNA probes (bacterial DNA sequence–specific endonucleases, also called *restriction enzymes*) have been developed for each of the diseases discussed in this chapter, enabling accurate mapping of the X chromosome. Using recombinant DNA methods, identification of heterozygotes has been possible in some pedigrees [27, 42–48]. The gene for choroideremia has recently been identified and cloned [49]. The nature of the translated protein is not yet known. There may be two mutations responsible for blue-cone monochromatism [50]. The first is caused by a mutation in the cone pigment gene; the second mutation causes a defect in a gene necessary for transcription of both the red and green cone pigments [50].

■ References

1. Lyon MF. Gene action in the X-chromosome of the mouse (*Mus musculus L.*). Nature 1961;190:372–373
2. Berson EL, Rosner B, Simonoff E. Risk factors for genetic typing and detection in retinitis pigmentosa. Am J Ophthalmol 1980;89:763–775
3. Andreasson SOL, Sandberg MA, Berson EL. Narrow-band filtering for monitoring low-amplitude cone electroretinograms in retinitis pigmentosa. Am J Ophthalmol 1988;105:500–503
4. Berson EL, Rosen JB, Simonoff EA. Electroretinographic testing as an aid in detection of carriers of X-chromosome-linked retinitis pigmentosa. Am J Ophthalmol 1979;87:460–468
5. Fishman GA, Weinberg AB, McMahon TT. X-linked recessive retinitis pigmentosa: clinical characteristics of carriers. Arch Ophthalmol 1986;104:1329–1335
6. Bird AC. X-linked retinitis pigmentosa. Br J Ophthalmol 1975;59:177–199
7. Falls HF, Cotterman CW. Chorio-retinal degeneration: a sex-linked form in which heterozygous women exhibit a tapetal-like retinal reflex. Arch Ophthalmol 1948;40:685–703
8. Krill AE. Observations of carriers of X-chromosomal-linked chorioretinal degenerations: do these support the "inactivation hypothesis"? Am J Ophthalmol 1967;64:1029–1040
9. Nussbaum RL, Lewis RA, Lesko JG, Farrell R. Mapping X-linked ophthalmic diseases: II. Linkage relationships of X-linked retinitis pigmentosa to X chromosomal short arm markers. Hum Genet 1985;70:45–50
10. Berson EL, Goldstein EB. The early receptor potential in sex-linked retinitis pigmentosa. Invest Ophthalmol 1970;9:58–63
11. Ernst W, Clover G, Faulkner DJ. X-linked retinitis pigmentosa: reduced rod flicker sensitivity in heterozygote females. Invest Ophthalmol Vis Sci 1981;20:812–816
12. Gieser DK, Fishman GA, Cunha-Vaz J. X-linked recessive retinitis pigmentosa and vitreous fluorophotometry: a study of heterozygous females. Arch Ophthalmol 1980;98:307–310
13. Ripps H, Brin KP, Weale RA. Rhodopsin and visual threshold in retinitis pigmentosa. Invest Ophthalmol Vis Sci 1978;17:735–745
14. Kurstjens JH. Choroideremia and gyrate atrophy of the choroid and retina. Doc Ophthalmol 1965;19:1–122
15. McCulloch C. Choroideremia and other choroidal atrophies. In: Newsome DA, ed. Retinal dystrophies and degenerations. New York: Raven Press, 1988:285–295
16. Rubin ML, Fishman RS, McKay RA. Choroideremia: study of a family and literature review. Arch Ophthalmol 1966;76:563–574
17. Forsius H, Hyvarinen L, Nieminen H, Flower R. Fluorescein and indocyanine green fluorescence angiography in a study of affected males and in female carriers with choroideremia: a preliminary report. Acta Ophthalmol (Copenh) 1977;55:459–470
18. Sieving PA, Niffenegger JH, Berson EL. Electroretinographic findings in selected pedigrees with choroideremia. Am J Ophthalmol 1986;101:361–367
19. O'Donnell FE Jr, Green WR, Fleischman JA, Hambrick GW. X-linked ocular albinism in blacks: ocular albinism cum pigmento. Arch Ophthalmol 1978;96:1189–1192
20. Goodman G, Ripps H, Siegal IM. Sex-linked ocular disorders: trait expressivity in males and carrier females. Arch Ophthalmol 1965;73:387–398
21. O'Donnell FE, Hambrick GW Jr, Green WR, et al. X-linked ocular albinism: an oculocutaneous macromelanosomal disorder. Arch Ophthalmol 1976;94:1883–1892

22. Maguire AM, Maumenee IH. Iris pigment mosaicism in carriers of X-linked ocular albinism cum pigmento. Am J Ophthalmol 1989;107:298–299
23. Waardenburg PJ, Van den Bosch J. X-chromosomal ocular albinism in a Dutch family. Ann Hum Genet 1956;21:101–122
24. Lang GE, Rott HD, Pfeiffer RA. X-linked ocular albinism: characteristic pattern of affection in female carriers. Ophthalmic Paediatr Genet 1990;11:265–271
25. Heckenlively JR, Weleber RG. X-linked recessive cone dystrophy with tapetal-like sheen: a newly recognized entity with Mizuo-Nakamura phenomenon. Arch Ophthalmol 1986;104:1322–1328
26. Jacobsen DM, Thompson SH, Bartley JA. X-linked progressive cone dystrophy: clinical characteristics of affected males and female carriers. Ophthalmology 1989; 96:885–895
27. Reichel E, Bruce AM, Sandberg MA, Berson EL. An electroretinographic and molecular genetic study of X-linked cone degeneration. Am J Ophthalmol 1989;108: 540–547
28. Merin S, Rowe H, Auerbach E, Landau J. Syndrome of congenital high myopia with nyctalopia: report of findings in 25 families. Am J Ophthalmol 1970;70:541–547
29. Hill DA, Arbel KF, Berson EL. Cone electroretinograms in congenital nyctalopia with myopia. Am J Ophthalmol 1974;78:127–136
30. Miyake Y, Kawase Y. Reduced amplitude of oscillatory potentials in female carriers of X-linked recessive congenital stationary night blindness. Am J Ophthalmol 1984; 98:208–215
31. Young RSL, Chaparro A, Price J, Walters J. Oscillatory potentials of X-linked carriers of congenital stationary night blindness. Invest Ophthalmol Vis Sci 1989;30: 806–812
32. Forsius H, Krause U, Helve J, et al. Visual acuity in 183 cases of X-chromosomal retinoschisis. Can J Ophthalmol 1973;8:385–393
33. Krill AE. Hereditary retinal and choroidal diseases, vol 2. New York: Harper & Row, 1972
34. Wu G, Cotlier E, Brodie S. A carrier state of X-linked juvenile retinoschisis. Ophthalmic Paediatr Genet 1985;5:13–17
35. Arden GB, Gorin MB, Polkinghorne PJ, et al. Detection of the carrier state of X-linked retinoschisis. Am J Ophthalmol 1988;105:590–595
36. Alpern M, Lee GB, Spivey BE. Cone monochromatism. Arch Ophthalmol 1965; 74:334–337
37. Lewis RA. Juvenile hereditary macular dystrophies. In: Newsome DA, ed. Retinal dystrophies and degenerations. New York: Raven Press, 1988:115–134
38. Spivey BE, Pearlman JT, Burian HM. Electroretinographic findings (including flicker) in carriers of congenital X-linked achromatopsia. Doc Ophthalmol 1964; 18:367
39. Pagon RA, Chatrian GE, Hamer RD, Lindberg KA. Carrier detection in an X-linked recessive cone dysfunction syndrome by electroretinography. Clin Res 1981;29: 116A
40. Berson EL, Sandberg MA, Maguire A, et al. Electroretinogram in carriers of blue cone monochromatism. Am J Ophthalmol 1986;102:254–261
41. Pagon RA, Chatrian G, Hamer RD, Lindberg KA. Heterozygote detection in X-linked recessive incomplete achromatopsia. Ophthalmic Paediatr Genet 1988;9: 43–56
42. Musarella MA. Mapping of the X-linked recessive retinitis pigmentosa gene: a review. Ophthalmic Paediatr Genet 1990;11:77–88
43. Aldridge J, Kunkel L, Bruns GA, et al. Strategy to reveal high-frequency RFLP's along the human X-chromosome. Am J Hum Genet 1984;36:546–564
44. Nussbaum RL, Lewis AL, Lesko JG. Choroideremia is linked to the restriction

fragment length polymorphism DXYS1 at Xq13-21. Am J Hum Genet 1985;37: 473–481

45. Dahl N, Pettersson U. Use of linked DNA probes for carrier detection and diagnosis of X-linked juvenile retinoschisis. Arch Ophthalmol 1988;106:1414–1416

46. Lewis RA, Holcomb JD, Bromley WC, et al. Mapping X-linked ophthalmic diseases: III. Provisional assignment of the locus for blue cone monochromacy to Xq28. Arch Ophthalmol 1987;105:1055–1059

47. Lewis RA, Nussbaum RL, Ferrel R. Mapping X-linked ophthalmic diseases. Provisional assignment of the ocus for choroideremia to Xq13-q24. Ophthalmology 1985;92:800–806

48. Bergen AB, Samann C, Van Dorp DB, et al. Localization of the X-linked ocular albinism gene (OA1) between DXS278/DXS237 and DXS143/DXS16 by linkage analysis. Ophthalmic Paediatr Genet 1990;11:165–170

49. Cremers FPM, van de Pol DJR, van Kerkhoff LPM, et al. Cloning of a gene that rearranges in patients with choroideremia. Nature 1990;347:674–677

50. Nathans J, Davenport CM, Maumenee IH, et al. Molecular genetics of human blue cone monochromacy. Science 1989;245:831–838

Retinitis Pigmentosa and the Rhodopsin Gene

Mohammad T. Shokravi, M.D.

Thaddeus P. Dryja, M.D.

Retinitis pigmentosa names a group of inherited disorders of the retina characterized by night blindness, progressive visual field loss, and abnormal or nonrecordable electroretinograms (ERGs). It is uncertain who was the first to describe the fundus features of retinitis pigmentosa [1]. However, Donders [2] was the first to explain the pathological findings in this disease, and the term *retinitis pigmentosa* is attributed to him [3]. This term has created some confusion because the primary disease process is not believed to be inflammatory.

Retinitis pigmentosa is found worldwide. Its prevalence in the United States, China, and Switzerland is estimated at 1 in 3,500, 1 in 4,016, and 1 in 7,000, respectively [4–7]. Although all cases of retinitis pigmentosa are believed to be genetic, in approximately half of the cases in the United States there is no family history and so these cases are designated as *simplex, isolate,* or *sporadic.* In the remainder of cases, the disease is inherited as an autosomal dominant, autosomal recessive, or X-chromosome-linked recessive trait [4, 8]. Most of the simplex cases are probably autosomal recessive, but some may be due to an X-linked mutation or a new dominant mutation.

■ Classification

Retinitis pigmentosa can be divided into two large groups. In the first group, primary retinitis pigmentosa, there is ocular involvement only. In the second group, the retinitis pigmentosa is associated with extraocular disease. Various classification schemes for primary retinitis pigmentosa are summarized in Table 1 [7–11].

Table 1 *Classification Schemes for Primary Retinitis Pigmentosa (RP)*

I. Anatomical type
  A. Typical
  B. Atypical
    1. RP sine pigmento
    2. Sectoral RP
    3. Unilateral RP
    4. Central RP
    5. RP punctata albescens
II. Electroretinographic findings
  A. Rod-cone RP
  B. Cone-rod RP
III. Age of onset
  A. Leber's congenital amaurosis
  B. Childhood-onset RP
  C. Juvenile-onset RP
  D. Adult-onset RP
  E. Late-onset RP
IV. Functional deficit
  A. Mild progressive
  B. Moderate progressive
  C. Severe progressive
V. Inheritance pattern
  A. Autosomal dominant
    1. Rod-cone RP
    2. Cone-rod RP
    3. Leber's congenital amaurosis (in rare cases)
    4. RP punctata albescens (in rare cases)
  B. Autosomal recessive
    1. Rod-cone RP
    2. Cone-rod RP
    3. Leber's congenital amaurosis
    4. RP punctata albescens
    5. Goldmann-Favre disease
  C. X-linked recessive
    1. Rod-cone RP
    2. Cone-rod RP
  D. Simplex, isolate, or sporadic

■ Diagnosis

The hallmarks of typical retinitis pigmentosa include night blindness, losses of central vision and visual field, fundus changes, and characteristic ERG findings.

Night Blindness

Night blindness is a frequent but not universal initial complaint. If it occurs, it usually begins in the first or second decade of life [7, 8, 12].

Central Vision Loss

Patients with autosomal dominant retinitis pigmentosa are more likely than those with autosomal recessive or X-linked disease to retain visual acuity beyond the age of 60 years [13]. Patients with autosomal recessive or X-linked retinitis pigmentosa usually become legally blind (visual acuity 20/200 or worse) by the age of 30 or 40 years [13]. Central vision can be reduced as a result of ocular abnormalities other than photoreceptor degeneration, such as lens opacities (subcapsular cataracts) [14, 15], diffuse retinal vascular leakage [16], cystoid macular edema [17, 18], and macular preretinal fibrosis [19].

Visual Field Loss

Visual field loss is insidious and progressive and frequently occurs symmetrically in both eyes [20]. In most cases of typical retinitis pigmentosa, it begins in the midperiphery and progresses to create a ring scotoma. Peripheral visual loss is universal in typical retinitis pigmentosa. In most cases, the central field is retained until late in the disease [7, 8, 13, 20–23].

Fundus Changes

The fundus findings in typical retinitis pigmentosa are present bilaterally and symmetrically [20, 23] and include attenuated retinal vessels, granularity of the retinal pigment epithelium and bone spicule pigmentation, waxy pallor of the optic nerve head and, in very advanced cases, prominent large choroidal vessels due to loss of the retinal pigment epithelium and choriocapillaris [7–11].

Electroretinography

The ERG is a valuable and sensitive tool for the diagnosis and evaluation of patients with retinitis pigmentosa. The ERG can identify patients affected with X-linked, autosomal dominant, or autosomal recessive retinitis pigmentosa before any signs or symptoms of the disease occur. There has been no reported case of a patient with a normal ERG at the age of 6 or older who later developed the disease [24–26]. The ERG is also useful in identifying female carriers of X-linked retinitis pigmentosa [27].

ERG evaluation should include stimuli that evoke rod and cone function independently, as well as stimuli that give an overall response. In some cases of retinitis pigmentosa, rods are affected more severely and earlier than cones. However, in advanced stages, all electrical responses are lost. Using computer averaging, it is possible to detect ERG responses that are nonrecordable with conventional techniques and to evaluate the progress of the disease. Berson and colleagues [13, 24–30] have emphasized the importance of rod- and cone-mediated B-wave implicit times in the diagnosis and evaluation of retinitis pigmentosa.

■ Pathological Features

Photoreceptors degenerate early in the disease [31]. In electron-microscopic studies of a 68-year-old patient with autosomal dominant retinitis pigmentosa, only abnormal cone photoreceptors remained [32]. Ultrastructural studies in a 24-year-old patient with X-linked retinitis pigmentosa showed that the foveal cones were reduced 50% in number. The remaining cones had distorted inner segments with twice the normal diameter, and the outer segments were absent or shortened [33].

Concurrent with the photoreceptor degeneration, there is a gradual depigmentation of the retinal pigment epithelium. Pigment cells migrate into the sensory retina where they accumulate in and around the vessel walls and elsewhere. These clumps of pigment cells are responsible for the bone spicules seen in the fundus. The pigmentary changes begin in the equatorial region [31].

In early cases observed clinically, the arteries appear to be narrowed without other histopathological abnormalities. In late cases, the retinal vessels have hyaline thickening of the walls and the lumens are narrow [31]. The ganglion cell and nerve fiber layers may be preserved until late stages. However, in very advanced cases, degeneration of axons and ganglion cells may also occur [31, 34].

■ The Rhodopsin Gene

In 1983, Nathans and Hogness [35] cloned a bovine rod opsin cDNA sequence. They found a coding region of 1,044 base pairs specifying 348 amino acids. The amino acid sequence was identical to that previously determined by others using conventional peptide sequencing [36]. This gene has five exons and four introns [35]. Later, Nathans, Hogness, and colleagues [37, 38] cloned the genes encoding human rod opsin (rhodopsin) as well as the three cone opsins (red, green, and blue). Like the rod opsin gene, the blue opsin gene was found to have five exons interrupted by four introns. The intron-exon arrangement is similar in the red and green opsin genes except for an additional intron dividing exon 1. The proteins encoded by the red and green opsin genes are 364 amino acids long; those encoded by the blue cone and the rod opsin genes have 348 amino acids [37, 38]. Chromosome-mapping studies have localized the rhodopsin gene to human chromosome 3, the red and green pigment genes to the X chromosome, and the blue pigment gene to chromosome 7 [39].

Rhodopsin Mutations

In 1989, McWilliam and co-workers [40] discovered linkage between autosomal dominant retinitis pigmentosa in one large Irish pedigree and a restriction fragment length polymorphism (RFLP) from chromosome 3q named CRI-C17 [40]. A few months later Dryja and colleagues [41] reported a C-to-A transversion in codon 23 of the rhodopsin gene (also on chromosome 3q) in 12% of their unrelated patients affected with autosomal dominant retinitis pigmentosa. This point mutation changed the specificity of codon 23 from proline to histidine. The mutation cosegregated with the disease in the families that carried it and was never found in unaffected individuals. This mutation was therefore believed to be the cause of one form of autosomal dominant retinitis pigmentosa [41, 42].

Since then, several groups have found a number of additional mutations of the rhodopsin gene in patients with autosomal dominant retinitis pigmentosa (Table 2, figure) [43–48]. It is estimated that 25% to 30% of patients with autosomal dominant retinitis pigmentosa have disease due to a mutation in the rhodopsin gene [44, 47]. More recently, Rosenfeld and associates [49] reported a null mutation in the rhodopsin gene in a family with autosomal recessive retinitis pigmentosa. The mechanism(s) by which the mutant rhodopsin alleles cause photoreceptor degeneration is still unknown. Of particular interest is why cones degenerate as a result of a defect in a rod-specific gene.

Retinal Function in Patients with a Rhodopsin Mutation

Berson and colleagues [50] found that patients with autosomal dominant retinitis pigmentosa and a Pro-23-His allele had significantly better visual acuity and larger ERG amplitudes than did patients without this mutation [50]. Two other groups described a number of patients affected with Pro-23-His mutation. They noted that their patients appeared to have a better prognosis for retaining central vision. They also found a regional distribution of pigmentary changes and retinal degeneration in their patients [51, 52].

Berson's group [53] also reported that patients with autosomal dominant retinitis pigmentosa with the point mutation Pro-347-Leu had a significantly smaller visual field area and smaller ERG amplitudes than did patients without this mutation. Fishman and co-workers [54] studied 2 families with autosomal dominant retinitis pigmentosa, one with the mutation Thr-17-Met, and the other with Gly-182-Ser. They found a sectoral distribution of pigmentary changes and larger ERG amplitudes with better visual prognosis in their patients than the average case of autosomal dominant retinitis pigmentosa.

Jacobson and associates [55] studied retinal function and rhodopsin

Table 2 *Rhodopsin Mutations Reported in Autosomal Dominant Retinitis Pigmentosa*

No.	Exon	Codon	Sequence	Amino Acid Change
1	1	17	ACG→ATG	Thr→Met
2	1	23	CCC→CAC	Pro→His
3	1	23	CCC→CTC	Pro→Leu
4	1	45	TTT→TTC	Phe→Leu
5	1	51	GGC→GTC	Gly→Val
6	1	58	ACG→AGG	Thr→Arg
7	1	68–71	Deletion	Leu-Arg-Thr-Pro→del
8	1	87	CTG→CAG	Val→Asp
9	1	89	GGT→GAT	Gly→Asp
10	1	106	GGG→GGT	Gly→Trp
11	2	125	CTG→CGG	Leu→Arg
12	2	135	GGC→TTC	Arg→Leu
13	2	135	GGC→GGT	Arg→Trp
14	2	167	TGC→CGC	Cyc→Arg
15	2	171	CCA→CTA	Pro→Leu
16	2	178	CAT→CGT	Thr→Cys
17	2	181	GAG→AAG	Glu→Lys
18	3	182	GGC→AGC	Gly→Ser
19	3	186	TCG→CCG	Ser→Pro
20	3	188	GGA→AGA	Gly→Arg
21	3	190	GAC→AAC	Asp→Asn
22	3	190	GAC→GGC	Asp→Gly
23	3	211	CAC→CCC	His→Pro
24	4	255	Deletion	Ile→del
25	4	267	CCC→CTC	Pro→Leu
26	4	296	AAG→GAG	Lys→Glu
27	5	344	GAC→GAT	Gln→End
28	5	345	GTG→ATG	Val→Met
29	5	347	CCG→TCG	Pro→Ser
30	5	347	CCG→CTG	Pro→Leu

levels in 20 patients with autosomal dominant retinitis pigmentosa from 6 families with five different point mutations. In a family with a nonsense mutation at the carboxyl end of rhodopsin (Gln-344-End), the young patients were asymptomatic but had slightly reduced rod and normal cone ERG amplitudes. In 3 families with the mutations Arg-135-Leu or Arg-135-Trp, the affected individuals had the characteristic funduscopic findings of retinitis pigmentosa, undetected rod function, no measurable rhodopsin, and variably impaired cone function. In families carrying the mutations Thr-58-Arg or Thr-17-Met, rod and cone functions in the superior retina were less impaired than in the inferior retina.

In another study, Kemp and colleagues [56] showed that the rate of rod dark adaptation varies according to whether a patient has a Pro-23-His, Thr-17-Met, or Thr-58-Arg mutation. These studies indicate that differ-

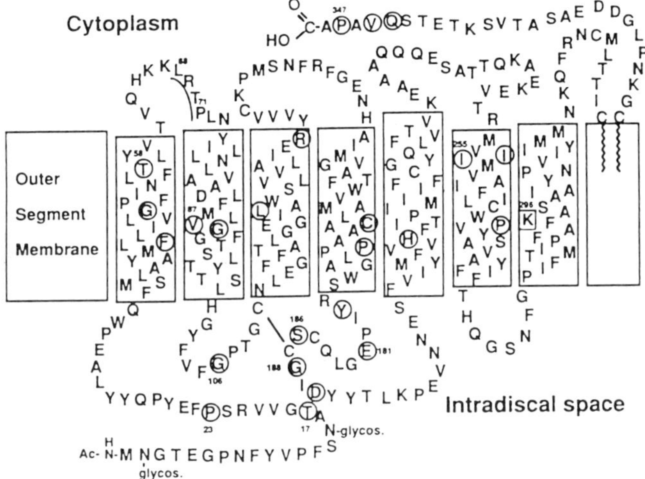

Schematic representation of human rhodopsin showing the amino acids altered by mutations in the rhodopsin gene. These amino acids are circled, except for adjacent curved line for deletion of residues 68–72.

ences in the characteristics of retinitis pigmentosa may correlate, to some extent, with each particular mutation [50–56].

■ Other Genes Causing Dominant Retinitis Pigmentosa

Recently, a few cases of autosomal dominant retinitis pigmentosa were found to be due to mutations in the RDS locus on chromosome 6p [57, 58]. *RDS* is the name given to the human homologue of the murine retinal degeneration slow gene (the rds gene). This gene encodes a membrane-associated glycoprotein that may help to maintain the structure of the outer segment discs [59–61]. A third autosomal dominant retinitis pigmentosa locus has been mapped to the pericentric region of chromosome 8 by linkage in a large American pedigree [62], but the responsible gene has not yet been identified.

■ References

1. Bell J. Retinitis pigmentosa and allied diseases, congenital stationary night-blindness, glioma. In: Pearson K, ed. The treasury of human inheritance, vol 2. London: Cambridge University Press, 1922:1–28
2. Donders FC. Beitrage zur pathologischen Anatomie des Auges: 2. Pigmentbildung in der Netzhaut. Arch Ophthalmol 1857;3(1):139–150

3. Mooren A. De la retinite pigmenteuse. Ann d'Oculistique 1859;T.XLL:21–31
4. Bunker CH, Berson EL, Bromley WC, et al. Prevalence of retinitis pigmentosa in Maine. Am J Ophthalmol 1984;97:357–365
5. Hu DN. Genetic aspects of retinitis pigmentosa in China. Am J Med Genet 1982;12:51–56
6. Ammann F, Klein D, Franceschetti A. Genetic and epidemiological investigations on pigmentary degeneration of the retina and allied disorders in Switzerland. J Neurol Sci 1965;2:183–196
7. Weleber RG. Retinitis pigmentosa and allied disorders. In: Ryan SJ, ed. Retina, vol 1. St Louis: Mosby, 1989:299–420
8. Newsome DA. Retinitis pigmentosa, Usher's syndrome, and other pigmentary retinopathies. In: Newsome DA, ed. Retinal dystrophies and degenerations. New York: Raven Press, 1988:161–194
9. Jimenez-Sierra JM, Ogden TE, Van Boemel GB. Inherited retinal diseases: a diagnostic guide. St Louis: Mosby, 1989:111–173
10. Heckenlively JR. Retinitis pigmentosa. Philadelphia: Lippincott, 1988
11. Benson WE, Grand MG, Green WR, et al. Retina and vitreous. In: Wilson FM, ed. Basic and clinical science course, section 11. San Francisco: American Academy of Ophthalmology, 1991:104–126
12. Tanino T, Ohba N. Studies on pigmentary retinal dystrophy: I. Age of onset of subjective symptoms and the mode of inheritance. Jpn J Ophthalmol 1976;20:474–481
13. Berson EL, Sandberg M, Rosner B, et al. Natural course of retinitis pigmentosa over a three-year interval. Am J Ophthalmol 1985;99:240–251
14. Heckenlively J. The frequency of posterior cataract in the hereditary retinal degeneration. Am J Ophthalmol 1982;93:733–738
15. Fishman GA, Anderson RJ, Lourenco P. Prevalence of posterior subcapsular lens opacities in patients with retinitis pigmentosa. Br J Ophthalmol 1985;69:263–266
16. Newsome DA. Retinal fluorescein leakage in retinitis pigmentosa. Am J Ophthalmol 1986;101:354–360
17. Ffytche TJ. Cystoid maculopathy in retinitis pigmentosa. Trans Ophthalmol Soc UK 1972;92:265–283
18. Fetkenhour CL, Choromokos E, Weinstein J, Shoch D. Cystoid macular edema in retinitis pigmentosa. Trans Am Acad Ophthalmol Otolaryngol 1977;83:OP515–521
19. Hansen RI, Friedman AH, Gartner S, Henkind P. The association of retinitis pigmentosa with preretinal macular gliosis. Br J Ophthalmol 1977;61:597–600
20. Massof RW, Finkelstein D, Starr SJ, et al. Bilateral symmetry of vision disorders in typical retinitis pigmentosa. Br J Ophthalmol 1979;63:90–96
21. Marmor MF. Visual loss in retinitis pigmentosa. Am J Ophthalmol 1980;89:692–698
22. Sunga RN, Sloan LL. Pigmentary degeneration of the retina: early diagnosis and natural history. Invest Ophthalmol 1967;6:309–325
23. Biro I. Symmetrical development of pigmentation: as a feature of the fundus pattern in retinitis pigmentosa. Am J Ophthalmol 1963;55:1176–1179
24. Berson EL. Retinitis pigmentosa and allied retinal diseases: electrophysiologic findings. Trans Am Acad Ophthalmol Otolaryngol 1976;81:OP659–666
25. Berson EL. Retinitis pigmentosa and allied diseases: application of electroretinographic testing. Int Ophthalmol 1981;4:7–22
26. Berson EL. Hereditary retinal disease: classification with the full field electroretinogram. Doc Ophthalmol 1977;13:149–171
27. Berson EL, Rosen JB, Simonoff EA. Electroretinographic testing as an aid in detection of carriers of X-chromosome-linked retinitis pigmentosa. Am J Ophthalmol 1979;87:460–468

28. Andreasson SOL, Sandberg MA, Berson EL. Narrow-band filtering for monitoring low-amplitude cone electroretinograms in retinitis pigmentosa. Am J Ophthalmol 1988;105:500–503
29. Berson EL. Electrical phenomena in the retina. In: Moses RA, Hart WM Jr, eds. Adler's physiology of the eye: clinical application. St Louis: Mosby, 1987:506–567
30. Berson EL, Howard J. Temporal aspects of the electroretinogram in sector retinitis pigmentosa. Arch Ophthalmol 1971;86:653–665
31. Gartner S, Henkind P. Pathology of retinitis pigmentosa. Ophthalmology 1982; 89:1425–1432
32. Kolb H, Gouras P. Electron microscopic observations of human retinitis pigmentosa, dominantly inherited. Invest Ophthalmol 1974;13:487–498
33. Szamier RB, Berson EL, Klein R, Meyers S. Sex-linked retinitis pigmentosa: ultrastructure of photoreceptors and pigment epithelium. Invest Ophthalmol Vis Sci 1979;18:145–160
34. Spencer WH. Ophthalmic pathology, ed 3. Philadelphia: Saunders, 1985:1210–1220
35. Nathans J, Hogness DS. Isolation, sequence analysis, and intron-exon arrangement of the gene encoding bovine rhodopsin. Cell 1983;34:807–814
36. Hargrave PA. Rhodopsin chemistry, structure and topography. In: Osborne NN, Chader GJ, eds. Progress in retinal research, vol 1. Elmsford, NY: Pergamon Press, 1982:1–51
37. Nathans J, Hogness DS. Isolation and nucleotide sequence of the gene encoding human rhodopsin. Proc Natl Acad Sci USA 1984;81:4851–4855
38. Nathans J, Thomas D, Hogness DS. Molecular genetics of human color vision: the genes encoding blue, green, and red pigments. Science 1986;232:193–202
39. Nathans J, Piantanida TP, Eddy RL, et al. Molecular genetics of inherited variation in human color vision. Science 1986;232:203–210
40. McWilliam P, Farrar GJ, Kenna P, et al. Autosomal dominant retinitis pigmentosa (ADRP): localization of an ADRP gene to the long arm of chromosome 3. Genomics 1989;5:619–622
41. Dryja TP, McGee TL, Reichel E, et al. A point mutation of the rhodopsin gene in one form of retinitis pigmentosa. Nature 1990;343:364–366
42. Applebury ML. Insight into blindness. Nature 1990;343:316–317
43. Dryja TP, McGee TL, Hahn LB, et al. Mutations within the rhodopsin gene in patients with autosomal dominant retinitis pigmentosa. N Engl J Med 1990;323:1302–1307
44. Dryja TD, Hahn LB, Cowley GS, et al. Mutation spectrum of the rhodopsin gene among patients with autosomal dominant retinitis pigmentosa. Proc Natl Acad Sci USA 1991;88:9370–9374
45. Keen TJ, Inglehearn CF, Lester DH, et al. Autosomal dominant retinitis pigmentosa: four new mutations in rhodopsin, one of them in the retinal attachment site. Genomics 1991;11:199–205
46. Sheffield VC, Fishman GA, Beck JS, et al. Identification of novel rhodopsin mutations associated with retinitis pigmentosa by GC-clamped denaturing gradient gel electrophoresis. Am J Hum Genet 1991;49:699–706
47. Sung CH, Davenport CM, Hennessey JC, et al. Rhodopsin mutation in autosomal dominant retinitis pigmentosa. Proc Natl Acad Sci USA 1991;88:6481–6485
48. Inglehearn CF, Bashir R, Lester DH, et al. A 3-bp deletion in the rhodopsin gene in a family with autosomal dominant retinitis pigmentosa. Am J Hum Genet 1991;48:26–30
49. Rosenfeld PJ, Cowley GS, McGee TL, et al. A null mutation within the rhodopsin gene as a cause of rod photoreceptor dysfunction and autosomal recessive retinitis pigmentosa. Nature Genetics 1992;1:209–213
50. Berson EL, Rosner B, Sandberg MA, Dryja TP. Ocular findings in patients with

autosomal dominant retinitis pigmentosa and a rhodopsin gene defect (Pro-23-His). Arch Ophthalmol 1991;109:92–101

51. Stone EM, Kimura AE, Nichols BE, et al. Regional distribution of retinitis pigmentosa in patients with the proline to histidine mutation in codon 23 of the rhodopsin gene. Ophthalmology 1991;98:1806–1813

52. Heckenlively JR, Rodriguez JA, Daiger SP. Autosomal dominant sectoral retinitis pigmentosa: two families with transversion mutation in codon 23 of rhodopsin. Arch Ophthalmol 1991;109:84–91

53. Berson EL, Rosner B, Sandberg MA, et al. Ocular findings in patients with autosomal dominant retinitis pigmentosa and rhodopsin, proline-347-leucine. Am J Ophthalmol 1991;111:614–623

54. Fishman GA, Stone EM, Sheffield VC, et al. Ocular findings associated with rhodopsin gene codon 17 and codon 182 transition mutations in dominant retinitis pigmentosa. Arch Ophthalmol 1992;110:54–62

55. Jacobson SG, Kemp CM, Sung CH, Nathans J. Retinal function and rhodopsin levels in autosomal dominant retinitis pigmentosa with rhodopsin mutations. Am J Ophthalmol 1991;112:256–271

56. Kemp CM, Jacobson SG, Roman AJ, et al. Abnormal rod dark adaptation in autosomal dominant retinitis pigmentosa with proline-23-histidine rhodopsin mutation. Am J Ophthalmol 1992;113:165–174

57. Kajiwara K, Hahn LB, Mukai S, et al. Mutations in the human retinal degeneration slow gene in autosomal dominant retinitis pigmentosa. Nature 1991;354:480–483

58. Farrar GJ, Kenna P, Jordan SA, et al. A three-base-pair deletion in the peripherin-*RDS* in one form of retinitis pigmentosa. Nature 1991;354:478–480

59. Connell GJ, Molday RS. Molecular cloning, primary structure, and orientation of the vertebrate photoreceptor cell protein peripherin in the rod outer segment disk membrane. Biochemistry 1990;29:4691–4698

60. Connell G, Bascom R, Molday L, et al. Photoreceptor peripherin is the normal product of the gene responsible for retinal degeneration in the *rds* mouse. Proc Natl Acad Sci USA 1991;88:723–726

61. Travis GH, Sutcliffe JG, Bok D. The *retinal degeneration slow (rds)* gene product is a photoreceptor disc membrane–associated glycoprotein. Neuron 1991;6:61–70

62. Blanton SH, Heckenlively JR, Cottingham AW, et al. Linkage mapping of autosomal dominant retinitis pigmentosa (RP1) to the pericentric region of human chromosome 8. Genomics 1991;11:857–869

Diagnosis and Treatment of Gyrate Atrophy

Michael J. Potter, M.D.
Eliot L. Berson, M.D.

Gyrate atrophy is an inherited degeneration of the choroid and retina associated with myopia, progressive constriction of the visual fields, night blindness, cataracts, and elevated levels of the plasma amino acid ornithine. The disorder was first described by Cutler in 1895 [1]. The name *atrophia gyrata choroideae et retinae* was introduced by Fuchs in 1896 [2]. It is an uncommon autosomal recessive disease that has been reported in many countries, the largest number of patients being of Finnish origin. Significant progress has been made in the past 15 years in detailing the genetics, biochemistry, and molecular biology of gyrate atrophy. This knowledge is currently being applied to potential treatments to slow the progression of the disease.

■ Natural History

In 1981, Takki and Milton [3] reported the natural history of gyrate atrophy in 29 Finnish patients aged 8 to 80 years old who were observed for 2 to 31 years. Seventeen were male and 12 female. Visual acuities were excellent in childhood, with many patients having 20/30 vision. A gradual reduction in visual acuity to 20/200 occurred in many eyes of patients 20 to 30 years old. Poor acuity correlated with macular involvement in 19 eyes and with cataract formation in 10 eyes. Fifty percent of phakic eyes retained visual acuity better than 20/200 to age 42, whereas 50% of aphakic eyes retained this acuity to age 55. These findings suggested that cataract extraction was beneficial.

The visual field becomes constricted with advancing age in gyrate atrophy. Some patients have relatively full fields at age 20, whereas others have marked constriction. By age 40, the majority of patients can be expected to have visual field diameters smaller than 10 degrees [3]. It has been proposed that higher plasma ornithine levels may correlate with faster progression, although this assumption remains to be proved. By age 60, patients are usually virtually blind due to extensive chorioretinal atrophy. Those with good central acuity may be severely handicapped by visual field constriction.

Patients may be asymptomatic and are usually identified during routine fundus examination. All patients are myopes, with refractive errors ranging from −4.00 to −20.00 D. No correlation between the degree of myopia and visual acuity or field loss has been observed [3]. Biomicroscopy of the anterior segment frequently reveals central posterior subcapsular cataracts by midadolescence [4]. The intraocular pressure is normal in most cases.

Gyrate atrophy patients younger than 13 to 15 years tend to have multiple round islands of peripheral chorioretinal atrophy [3, 5]. These areas become fused with one another with increasing age. The fundus lesions progress over a period of several years, and the atrophy gradually moves toward the posterior pole. This process results in a scalloped border between atrophic and normal retina in the midperiphery. Peripapillary atrophy is common. The retinal blood vessels become attenuated. Unlike the finding in retinitis pigmentosa, bone-spicule pigmentation is never seen. Both eyes are usually affected symmetrically, although acuity may differ because of macular involvement or more severe lens changes in one eye.

Fluorescein angiography demonstrates hyperfluorescent areas of peripheral atrophy. Choroidal vessels may be seen where the retina has atrophied. A granular appearance may be observed in the macula before atrophic changes are discernible [5]. A zone of pigmentary changes has been seen angiographically, separating the normal and atrophic areas. These zones may represent abnormally functioning retina and pigment epithelium prior to the stage when atrophy becomes apparent on examination [5].

Final dark-adapted rod thresholds are elevated early in life. Full-field electroretinographic (ERG) testing reveals markedly reduced rod- and cone-mediated responses. In early stages, the rod responses are more severely affected than the cone responses [6, 7]. Some patients also have a delayed implicit time on 30-Hz flicker testing. Patients usually have nondetectable (less than 10 μV) ERG responses in adulthood. Computer averaging with narrow-band filtering has made it possible to detect ERG responses well under 1 μV, allowing objective monitoring of the amount of remaining retinal function in most patients [8].

■ Systemic Manifestations

Electroencephalographic abnormalities have been reported in numerous patients with gyrate atrophy [5, 9]. Kaiser-Kupfer and colleagues [9] have described two types of findings in 7 of 10 patients tested: intermittent theta or sharp wave activity, and diffuse or localized rhythmic theta activity. No abnormalities have been found on neurological examination. Some patients have seizures, and a few have subnormal intelligence [5]. Three patients had diminished hearing [5].

Kaiser-Kupfer's group [9] has described abnormalities of the hair in 10 patients. Fine, straight hair with patches of alopecia were noted. Light- and electron-microscopical studies have revealed abnormal morphological features. The observed dark central core was hypothesized to represent a defect in maturation of the hair [9].

Muscle biopsies revealed tubular aggregates present in type II muscle fibers [9, 10]. In culture of muscle biopsy specimens, a high concentration of ornithine was lethal to specimens from gyrate atrophy patients but not to specimens from normal subjects [9]. These studies imply that muscle tissue from normal patients can metabolize ornithine, whereas specimens from gyrate atrophy patients cannot.

■ Pathological Features

Autopsy eyes from 1 patient with gyrate atrophy have been reported [11]. That patient had the vitamin B_6–responsive form of the disease. The retina posterior to the atrophic zone was intact except for focal areas of photoreceptor atrophy and mitochondrial abnormalities. Swollen mitochondria have been described in iris and liver specimens [4]. These abnormalities together with the hair and muscle findings are presumed to result from the metabolic changes.

■ Biochemical Features

Considerable progress has been made in understanding the biochemical abnormalities in gyrate atrophy since the initial report of increased plasma ornithine by Simmel and Takki in 1973 [12]. In 1974, Takki [5] reported 9 patients with a tenfold to twentyfold increase in plasma ornithine. Urinalysis showed an overflow aminoaciduria consisting only of ornithine. Aqueous humor and cerebrospinal fluid had similarly elevated levels of ornithine. Sengers and co-workers [13] observed a deficiency of ornithine aminotransferase (OAT), also known as *ornithine ketoacid transaminase*, in patients with gyrate atrophy. Valle and associates [14] then reported OAT deficiency in transformed lymphocytes derived from patients with gyrate atrophy. Shih's group [15] also noted OAT deficiency in patients with gyrate atrophy. Ornithine is metabolized via the urea cycle. It is decarboxylated via ornithine decarboxylase and metabolized via OAT to glutamic acid and proline. Normal plasma ammonia levels in affected patients imply that the urea cycle functions normally. It has been postulated that high ornithine concentrations may be directly toxic to the retinal pigment epithelium [16].

Shih and colleagues [15] found decreased or absent levels of OAT in cultured skin fibroblasts of patients and reduced activity in carrier parents. These findings are consistent with the autosomal recessive nature of the disease. Although OAT is synthesized in the nucleus, it is transported to the mitochondria, perhaps accounting for the swollen organelles in liver and iris specimens. As with many enzymes in the biochemical pathways for amino acid synthesis, OAT requires pyridoxal phosphate (vitamin B_6) as a cofactor. One patient with gyrate atrophy had levels of OAT activity that increased significantly in the presence of high concentrations of pyridoxal phosphate [6, 15]. Furthermore, arginine is a precursor of ornithine, and a low-arginine diet can be expected to lower ornithine levels, with possible therapeutic benefit.

■ Treatment Studies

Several attempts have been made to treat patients with gyrate atrophy, under the supervision of a nutritionist, with 300 to 400 mg/day of vitamin B_6 or a low-arginine, low-protein diet supplemented with essential amino acids. Berson and co-workers [6, 17] reported 1 patient whose plasma ornithine level dropped from 870 μmol/L to 400 μmol/L with supplementation with 300 mg/day of pyridoxine hydrochloride. An additive effect of dietary protein (arginine) restriction and vitamin B_6 supplementation was found, with a drop to a lowest level of 177 μmol/L in this patient. Normal values of plasma ornithine are 52 to 102 μmol/L [17]. The 4 other patients reported in the same study were not pyridoxine-responsive, but all showed a significant decrease in ornithine levels to approximately 300 to 400 μmol/L. Even severe dietary restriction to the lowest level these patients could tolerate in the hospital did not normalize ornithine levels in any case. When the same patients were followed for 2 years on an outpatient basis on a modified low-protein, low-arginine diet that reduced ornithine levels to the range of 400 to 600 μmol/L, slight enlargement of the areas of chorioretinal atrophy was evident in all, despite ornithine levels 30% to 50% lower than their baselines [18]. None of these patients exhibited any improvement in visual fields or ERG amplitudes.

Weleber and Kennaway [7] and Kaiser-Kupfer and colleagues [19] reported improvement in electrophysiological tests in adults treated with vitamin B_6 or with severe protein and arginine restriction. Their initial studies were performed on small numbers of patients, and the follow-up times were less than 2 years. It is clear that the majority of patients with gyrate atrophy are not pyridoxine responders. A low-protein, low-arginine diet would therefore be required to lower plasma ornithine levels over a sustained period in most patients. Since maintaining patients on this diet is a severe hardship, a clear treatment benefit should be demonstrated before such treatment can be wholeheartedly recommended. It is the inexorable downhill course of the disease that has led investigators to pursue treatment studies despite this difficulty.

Kaiser-Kupfer and co-workers [20] recently reported results of severe arginine restriction of 2 pairs of siblings younger than 10 years who were followed for 5 to 7 years. The plasma ornithine levels were reduced to approximately the normal range (106 and 121 μmol/L) in one pair of siblings and reached twice the upper limit of normal (251 and 313 μmol/L) in the other pair. Although all patients showed evidence of slight progression by all criteria, the fundus photographs of the 2 younger patients are virtually free of atrophy. These patients had significantly less atrophy than their elder siblings when they reached or approached the same age at which their elders began the diet. The significance of these results is dependent in part on there being little variability in family members with identical OAT mutations. Berson and colleagues [17] described 2 sisters with markedly different fundus appearances and psychophysical test results at ages 12 and 13, suggesting that there may indeed be significant intrafamilial variability. Thus, there is evidence that a low-protein, low-arginine diet may slow progression in very young patients, but only a small number of patients have been studied.

■ Molecular Genetics

The biochemical insights into ornithine metabolism led to cloning of the gene coding for OAT from liver to retinoblastoma cells [21–23]. O'Donnell and co-workers [24] first assigned the OAT structural gene to chromosome 10 in 1985. The gene itself spans 21 kilobases (kb) of DNA. It is transcribed in a unit 2.2 kb long from eleven separate exons (coding regions separated by intervening sequences that do not contribute to the final enzyme). There are related sequences (pseudogenes) on the X chromosome that do not produce functional OAT [25, 26]. At least twenty-six OAT mutations have now been reported, including numerous missense mutations and a nine base-pair deletion [20, 27]. McClatchey and colleagues [27] described an acceptor splicing mutation in a patient of Scandinavian ancestry. The patient had a normal coding region of the OAT gene, but a mutation in the intervening sequence that abnormally spliced out exon 5 of the transcript. The enzyme produced by this mechanism was missing a functional segment that is highly conserved in evolution and apparently required for normal activity.

The pyridoxal phosphate binding site spans exons 8 through 10, so mutations in this region could be expected to reduce the binding affinity for vitamin B_6 [27]. Such patients may require high levels of pyridoxal phosphate in order to restore modest amounts of OAT activity—hence, the vitamin B_6 responsiveness. Ramesh and associates [28] showed that different molecular defects in the OAT gene underlie both the pyridoxine-responsive and the pyridoxine-nonresponsive forms of gyrate atrophy. They reproduced the pyridoxine response in an in vitro expression system using a cloned gene from a patient with the pyridoxine-responsive variant; a pyridoxine nonresponder was used as a control. The ornithine binding site has not yet been identified.

Thus, considerable progress has been made in elucidating the biochemical and genetic bases of gyrate atrophy. The disease is autosomal recessive, so the likelihood of carrier parents of an affected patient having a child with the disorder is 1 in 4. An affected parent's children would all be carriers. It would be extremely unlikely for an affected patient to have a child with gyrate atrophy, since that would require the child's other parent to be a carrier or an affected patient.

■ Differential Diagnosis and Treatment

Usually, the fundus findings of peripheral atrophic islands with a scalloped border are sufficiently characteristic that gyrate atrophy is entertained as the likely diagnosis when patients are examined by indirect ophthalmoscopy. Advanced choroideremia may be confused with gyrate atrophy. The former presents with generalized atrophy of the retinal pigment epithelium and choriocapillaris [29]. The macula may be involved earlier than in gyrate atrophy, and pigment is usually observed in the midperiphery. Choroideremia is an X-chromosome-linked disorder, and carriers can usually be detected by ophthalmoscopy [30]. Examining family members may therefore be useful diagnostically. Plasma ornithine concentrations should be measured to confirm the diagnosis of gyrate atrophy.

Although amino acid analysis is widely available, patients with gyrate atrophy should probably be referred to specialized centers where skin fibroblast cultures can be obtained to test for presence or absence of vitamin B_6 responsiveness and retinal function can be monitored with specialized techniques. The value of lowering ornithine levels is still under investigation, but patients who are pyridoxine responders may benefit from vitamin B_6 supplementation. Until a better-tolerated therapy is developed, a low arginine diet remains the only available treatment for nonresponders. These patients, or their parents, must decide whether the potential benefit to vision outweighs the difficulty of adhering to the diet.

This work was supported in part by a grant from the National Retinitis Pigmentosa Foundation Fighting Blindness, Baltimore, MD.

The authors wish to acknowledge gratefully the assistance of Kevin McDermott in translations from the German.

■ References

1. Cutler CW. Drei ungewöhnliche Fälle von retino-Choroideal-Degeneration. Arch Augenheilkd 1895;30:117–122
2. Fuchs E. Über zwei der retinitis pigmentosa verwandte Krankheiten (Retinitis punctata albescens und atrophia gyrata choroideae et retinae). Arch Augenheilkd 1896; 32:111–116
3. Takki KK, Milton RC. The natural history of gyrate atrophy of the choroid and retina. Ophthalmology 1981;88:292–301
4. Weleber RG. Gyrate atrophy of choroid and retina. In: Heckenlively JR, Arden GB, eds. Principles and practice of electrophysiology of vision. St Louis: Mosby-Yearbook 1991:649–658
5. Takki K. Gyrate atrophy of the choroid and retina associated with hyperornithinaemia. Br J Ophthalmol 1974;58:3–23
6. Berson EL, Schmidt SY, Shih VE. Ocular and biochemical abnormalities in gyrate atrophy of the choroid and retina. Ophthalmology 1978;85:1018–1027
7. Weleber RG, Kennaway NG. Clinical trial of vitamin B_6 for gyrate atrophy of the choroid and retina. Ophthalmology 1981;88:316–324
8. Andréasson SOL, Sandberg MA, Berson EL. Narrow-band filtering for monitoring low-amplitude cone electroretinograms in retinitis pigmentosa. Am J Ophthalmol 1988;105:500–503
9. Kaiser-Kupfer MI, Kuwabara T, Askanas V, et al. Systemic manifestations of gyrate atrophy of the choroid and retina. Ophthalmology 1981;88:302–306
10. McCulloch C, Marliss EB. Gyrate atrophy of the choroid and retina with hyperornithinemia. Am J Ophthalmol 1975;80:1047–1057
11. Wilson DJ, Weleber RG, Green WR. Ocular clinicopathologic study of gyrate atrophy. Am J Ophthalmol 1991;111:24–33
12. Simmel O, Takki K. Raised plasma-ornithine and gyrate atrophy of the choroid and retina. Lancet 1973;1:1031–1033
13. Sengers RCA, Trijbels JMG, Brussaart JH, Deutman AF. Gyrate atrophy of the choroid and retina and ornithine-ketoacid aminotransferase deficiency (abstr). Pediatr Res 1976;10:894
14. Valle D, Kaiser-Kupfer MI, Del Valle LA. Gyrate atrophy of the choroid and retina: deficiency of ornithine aminotransferase in transformed lymphocytes. Proc Natl Acad Sci USA 1977;74:5159–5161
15. Shih VE, Berson EL, Mandell R, Schmidt SY. Ornithine ketoacid transaminase deficiency in gyrate atrophy of the choroid and retina. Am J Hum Genet 1978; 30:174–179
16. Del Monte MA, Hu DN, Maumenee IH, et al. Selective ornithine toxicity of cultured human retinal pigment epithelium. Invest Ophthalmol Vis Sci 1982;22(suppl):173
17. Berson EL, Shih VE, Sullivan PL. Ocular findings in patients with gyrate atrophy on pyridoxine and low-protein, low-arginine diets. Ophthalmology 1981;88:311–315
18. Berson EL, Hanson AH, Rosner B, Shih VE. A two year trial of low protein, low arginine diets or vitamin B6 for patients with gyrate atrophy. Birth Defects 1982;18:209–218
19. Kaiser-Kupfer MI, de Monasterio F, Valle D, et al. Visual results of a long-term trial of a low-arginine diet in gyrate atrophy of choroid and retina. Ophthalmology 1981;88:307–310
20. Kaiser-Kupfer MI, Caruso RC, Valle D. Gyrate atrophy of the choroid and retina, long-term reduction of ornithine slows retinal degeneration. Arch Ophthalmol 1991;109:1539–1548
21. Inana G, Totsuka S, Redmond M, et al. Molecular cloning of human ornithine aminotransferase mRNA. Proc Natl Acad Sci USA 1986;83:1203–1207

22. Ramesh V, Shaffer MM, Allaire JM, et al. Investigation of gyrate atrophy using a cDNA clone for human ornithine aminotransferase. DNA 1986;5:493–501
23. Mitchell GA, Looney JE, Brody LC, et al. Human ornithine aminotransferase cDNA cloning and analysis of the structural gene. J Biol Chem 1988;263:14288–14295
24. O'Donnell J, Cox D, Shows T. The ornithine aminotransferase gene is on human chromosome 10. Invest Ophthalmol Vis Sci 1985;26(suppl):128
25. Barrett DJ, Bateman JB, Sparkes RS, et al. Chromosomal localization of human ornithine aminotransferase gene sequences to 10q26 and Xp11.2. Invest Ophthalmol Vis Sci 1987;28:1037–1042
26. Ramesh V, Eddy R, Bruns GA, et al. Localization of the ornithine aminotransferase gene and related sequences on two human chromosomes. Hum Genet 1987;76: 121–126
27. McClatchey AI, Kaufman DL, Berson EL, et al. Splicing defect at the ornithine aminotransferase [OAT] locus in gyrate atrophy. Am J Hum Genet 1990;47: 790–794
28. Ramesh V, McClatchey AI, Ramesh N, et al. Molecular basis of ornithine aminotransferase deficiency in B-6-responsive and -nonresponsive forms of gyrate atrophy. Proc Natl Acad Sci USA 1988;85:3777–3780
29. Takki K. Differential diagnosis between the primary total choroidal vascular atrophies. Br J Ophthalmol 1974;58:24–35
30. Sieving PA, Niffenegger JH, Berson EL. Electroretinographic findings in selected pedigrees with choroideremia. Am J Ophthalmol 1986;101:361–367.

Familial Exudative Vitreoretinopathy

Eleanore M. Ebert, M.D., M.P.H.

Shizuo Mukai, M.D.

Familial exudative vitreoretinopathy (FEVR) is a hereditary disorder first described in 1969 by Criswick and Schepens [1], who reported 6 cases in two kindreds. These patients had bilateral retinal and vitreous abnormalities similar to those seen in retinopathy of prematurity, but they had no history of premature birth, neonatal oxygen therapy, or birth asphyxia. The authors believed that the condition represented a new entity, which they termed *familial exudative vitreoretinopathy.*

Two years later, Gow and Oliver [2] published a report on the second series of patients with this disorder. Evaluation of a large pedigree identified the inheritance pattern of the condition to be autosomal dominant. The fluorescein angiographic findings in FEVR were first described by Canny and Oliver [3], who noted the presence of areas of capillary nonperfusion anterior to the equator and again emphasized the similarity between FEVR and retinopathy of prematurity.

The disorder has been referred to in the literature by various names, including *Criswick-Schepens syndrome, dominant exudative vitreoretinopathy, autosomal dominant exudative vitreoretinopathy,* and *hereditary exudative vitreoretinopathy.* The genetic defect responsible for this disorder is not known.

Clinical Manifestations

The clinical appearance of FEVR varies greatly from individual to individual, with some patients manifesting only mild abnormalities of the peripheral retinal vasculature and others progressing to total retinal detachment with secondary neovascular glaucoma. More severely affected patients may present in infancy or childhood with decreased visual acuity, nystagmus, or strabismus. The latter may be true strabismus or a pseudoexotropia with a large positive angle kappa due to heterotopia of the macula.

The fundus appearance can be very similar to that seen in retinopathy of prematurity; however, patients with FEVR characteristically have no history of prematurity or supplemental oxygen therapy in the neonatal period and often have a positive family history, usually in an autosomal dominant pattern. Although the disease was initially believed to be invariably progressive [1, 2], more recent studies have demonstrated that the majority of FEVR patients remain in a relatively stable, asymptomatic state (73% in the series reported by Tasman and co-workers [4] and 58% in the series of Ober and colleagues [5]). Based on the funduscopic appearance, Gow and Oliver [2] divided the clinical course of FEVR into three stages of increasing severity; Laqua [6] modified this staging system to include the characteristic fluorescein angiographic findings at each level. The stages describe mild, moderate, and severe forms of FEVR, each of which may be seen in patients of any age [7]. The disorder characteristically is bilateral but may be asymmetrical, especially in the active proliferative form [4].

Stage 1 FEVR

In stage 1 FEVR, the mildest form, affected patients are usually asymptomatic with good visual acuity. The pathological findings generally are confined to the peripheral retina on fundus examination, where peripheral avascular zones are seen. These areas resemble "white with pressure" and "white without pressure" on scleral depression. The peripheral avascular zone may be present for a complete 360 degrees, but it is always more extensive temporally. In cases with wider zones of avascularity, a wedge-shaped avascular zone in the temporal meridian with the apex directed toward the macula has been described [8]. A V-shaped area of chorioretinal atrophy or retinal opacification may be seen corresponding to this zone of avascularity. In most cases, the peripheral avascular zone persists into adulthood without regression or progression to marked neovascular proliferation [4]. This is in contrast to retinopathy of prematurity, in which the peripheral retina vascularizes with regression of the disease.

On fluorescein angiography, there may be leakage of dye, rare small hemorrhages and microaneurysms, and vitreous abnormalities. Although vitreous changes were not found in a significant portion of patients in the pedigree described by Laqua [6], stage 1 FEVR as described by Gow and Oliver [2] emphasized changes of the vitreoretinal interface, including vitreous traction on the retina, vitreous bands and membranes, and peripheral retinal cystoid degeneration. Angiographically, areas of capillary nonperfusion characteristically are seen anterior to the equator, with abrupt termination of the capillary network forming a scalloped edge. Leakage of fluorescein dye from the scalloped edge is observed often.

Angiography of the temporal periphery is extremely helpful in diagnosing milder forms of FEVR. The earliest angiographic manifestations

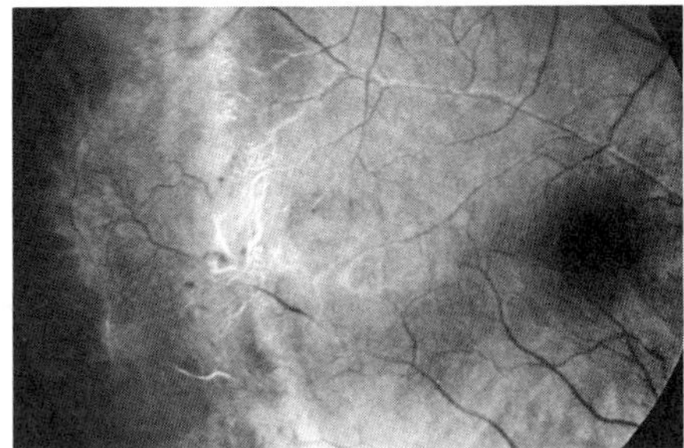

Figure 1 *Arteriovenous shunts in the temporal periphery at the border of vascularized and nonvascularized retina in a patient with stage 1 FEVR.*

include mildly dilated and leaking capillaries in the posterior pole, associated with capillary closure in the temporal retinal periphery [9]. Abnormal straightening of vessels in the temporal periphery and arteriovenous shunts at the margin of the vascularized and nonvascularized retina that anastomose in a brushlike fashion may be seen (Fig 1). Such shunts are best delineated by fluorescein angiography, although red-free light may be helpful in many cases. Feldman and co-workers [10] have described affected family members with the sole clinical finding of intraretinal deposits in the periphery or posterior pole.

Stage 2 FEVR

In stage 2 FEVR, the moderate form, proliferative and exudative changes develop. In addition to the findings of stage 1, affected patients exhibit neovascularization (Fig 2A) and both subretinal and intraretinal exudation. Fibrovascular proliferation may be seen in the retinal periphery; an elevated, exudative mass lesion may form anterior to the equator at the border of the zone of avascular retina, most commonly temporally. These fibrovascular mass lesions are fed by large-caliber arteriovenous shunt vessels. On fluorescein angiography, dye leakage into the retina is seen originating from the fibrovascular masses, dilated retinal vessels, and areas of retinal neovascularization (in a sea-fan configuration) located at the border of the vascular and avascular retina (Fig 2B, C) [9]. Reactive pigmentary changes in the vicinity of the mass lesion and overlying thick vitreous membranes have been described in a number of cases. The fibrovascular lesion may contract and exert traction on the retina, producing dragging of the major retinal vessels, heterotopia of the macula (Fig 3), reduced visual acuity, and strabismus. Localized tractional retinal detachment in the area between the equator and ora serrata may develop in some cases.

Stage 3 FEVR

In stage 3 FEVR, the advanced form, potentially blinding complications may develop due to traction from a cicatricial lesion in the temporal

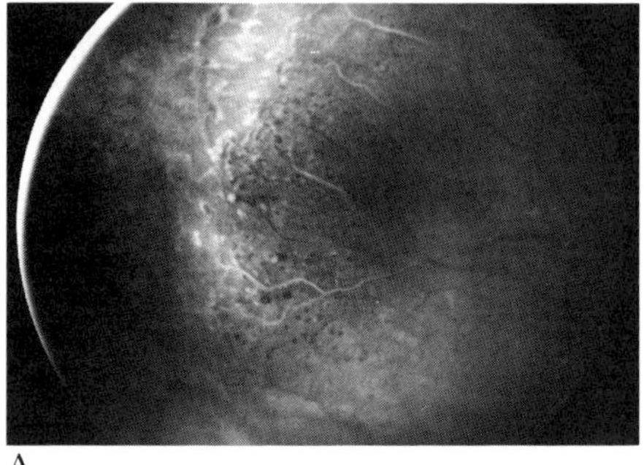

A

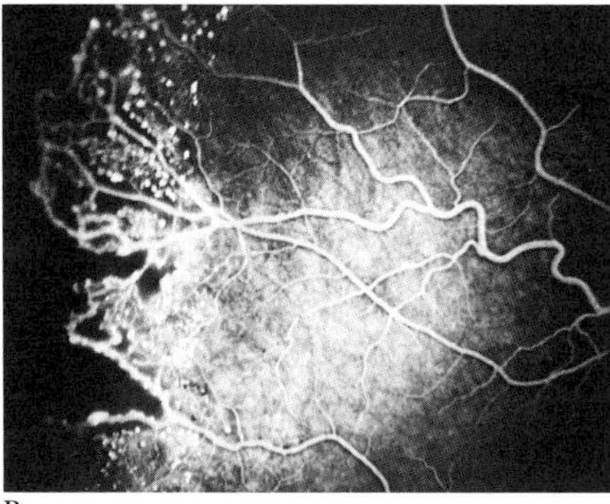

B

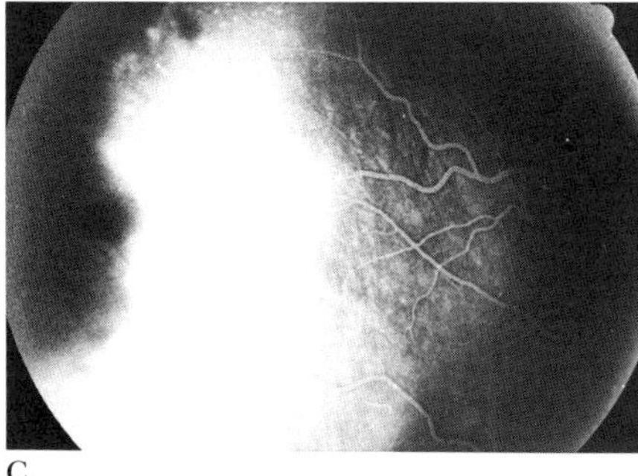

C

Figure 2 *(A) Arteriovenous shunt formation and retinal neovascularization along the margin of vascular and avascular retina in the temporal periphery in a 6-year-old boy with stage 2 FEVR. (B) Angiographic appearance of the temporal periphery in the same patient during early arteriovenous transit. (C) Late fluorescein angiographic view showing diffuse leakage of dye along the margin of vascularized and avascularized retina from dilated retinal vessels and areas of retinal neovascularization.*

periphery. Patients may present with retinal holes, tractional or rhegmatogenous retinal detachments, falciform retinal folds, or massive intraretinal and subretinal exudation (Fig 4). In the latter case, the fundus appearance may resemble Coats' disease, although the degree of exudation is usually less and exudative retinal detachments are uncommon in FEVR. Secondary anterior segment changes such as rubeosis iridis, neovascular glaucoma, cataract, and band keratopathy are also seen in patients with the advanced form of the disorder.

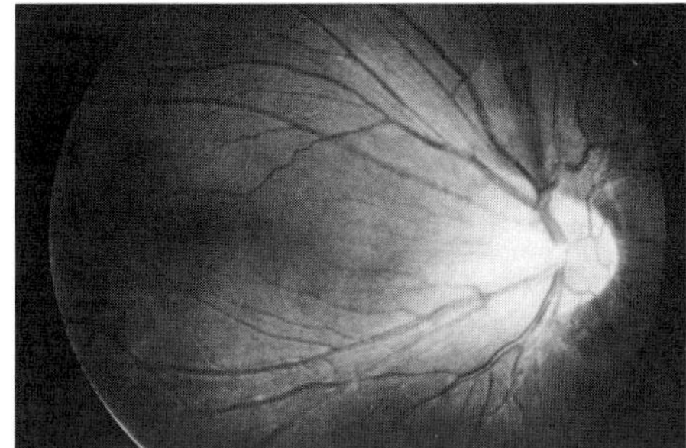

Figure 3 *Macular heterotopia in a patient with stage 2 FEVR.*

The prevalence of vitreoretinal abnormalities in affected patients was reported by Miyakubo and associates [11] in a study of 77 cases of FEVR. Vitreoretinal adhesions with fibrous bands or membranes in front of the retina, most commonly in the region of the temporal equator, were seen in 41% of the eyes studied. Areas of "white without pressure" were noted in 26% of eyes. In 62% of eyes, an avascular zone greater than 2 disc diameters was present in the peripheral retina. Another extremely common finding, seen in 81% of eyes, was a wedge-shaped avascular region in the temporal periphery with the apex pointed toward the macula. In 20%

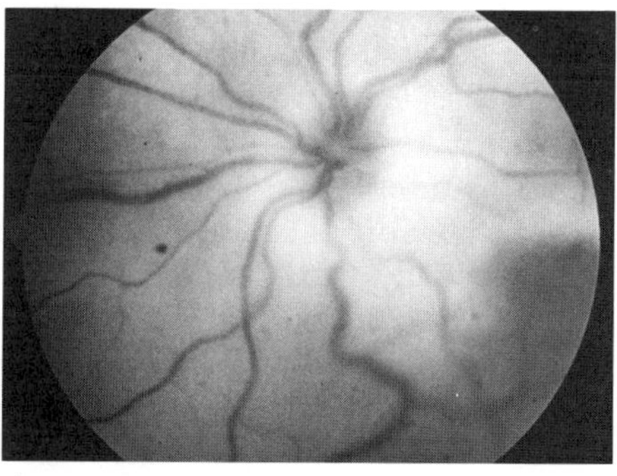

A

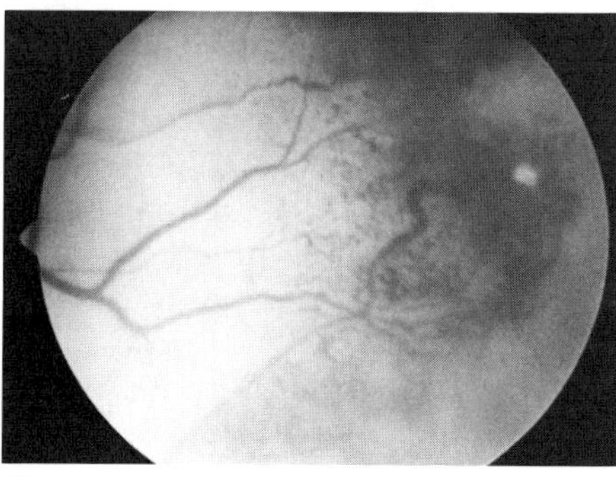

Figure 4 *(A) Massive subretinal exudation and exudative retinal detachment in a 3-year-old boy with stage 3 FEVR. (B) Exudative changes in the temporal periphery in the same patient.*

B

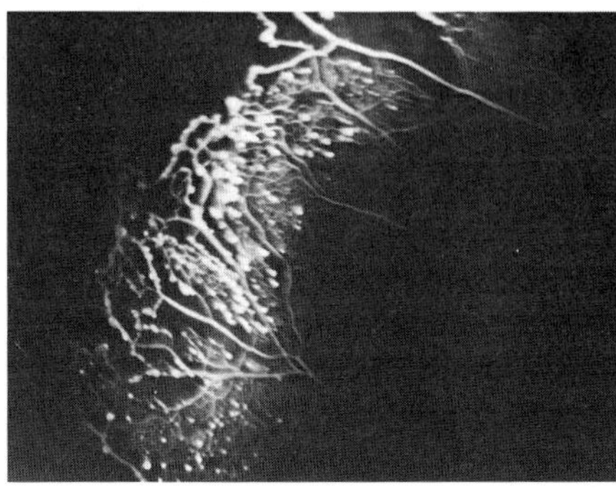

Figure 5 *Fluorescein angiographic view of the temporal periphery in a patient with FEVR, showing retinal vascular changes and neovascularization at the margin of the vascular and avascular retina.*

of eyes, neovascularization was present at the margin of the vascularized retina (Fig 5). Macular ectopia was observed in 18% of eyes secondary to traction from fibrovascular proliferations in the temporal periphery. These authors believe that the three prominent retinal vascular features of FEVR are: (1) the presence of a retinal avascular zone in the periphery and along the temporal meridian in a wedge-shaped pattern, (2) arteriovenous shunt formation along the margin of the vascular and avascular retina, and (3) retinal neovascularization [11].

Retinal detachments are seen frequently in patients with FEVR. The prevalence of this finding in published series ranges from 20% to 32% [11–13]. The detachment may be the result of traction from vitreous membranes or atrophy of the peripheral retina or, in rare cases, it may be secondary to subretinal exudation. In general, tractional retinal detachments with temporal dragging of the retina and subretinal exudation tend to occur during the first decade of life, whereas rhegmatogenous detachments usually occur in the second or third decade. Van Nouhuys [12] evaluated 90 individuals with FEVR from 17 families and noted retinal detachment in 20% of eyes. In all but one of these patients, the detachment occurred before the age of 30 years.

Tractional retinal detachments are reported to occur in 6% to 10% of eyes with FEVR. These are usually located in the temporal periphery and may be very stable; however, in patients with the active proliferative form of the disease, a total tractional detachment may develop. Tasman and co-workers [4] reported the rapid development of exudation and temporal dragging of the macula with associated significant visual loss over the course of a month in a child with FEVR.

Rhegmatogenous retinal detachments appear to be more common than tractional detachments, accounting for 25% to 63% of all retinal detachments in these patients. The break is usually located in the temporal retina. Atrophic holes, horseshoe tears, and giant tears all have been described in association with FEVR. Vitreous hemorrhage may occur in association with a retinal detachment. van Nouhuys [12] reported 2 cases with this presentation. In both instances, the hemorrhage was followed by rapid development of proliferative vitreoretinopathy and a total, closed-funnel detachment.

In the Japanese population, rhegmatogenous retinal detachments secondary to FEVR constitute a significant proportion of all rhegmatogenous detachments. Hashimoto and associates [13] reported that in 576 consecutive cases of rhegmatogenous retinal detachment, 5% were in patients with FEVR. Among patients younger than 30 years, 12% of rhegmatogenous detachments occurred in association with FEVR.

Another relatively common manifestation of FEVR is the presence of falciform retinal folds, reported in 15% to 39% of affected eyes. These folds usually extend from the region of the optic nerve and posterior pole to the temporal or inferotemporal periphery where they have cicatricial connections to the fibrovascular masses in the peripheral retina. The folds usually develop during the first decade of life and generally do not progress with age. Although Dudgeon [14] had previously postulated a link between congenital retinal folds and FEVR, van Nouhuys [15] was the first to emphasize this association in 1981. Subsequently, Nishimura and colleagues [16] studied family members of 9 patients with congenital retinal folds and found a number of them had features consistent with FEVR on fundus examination. Family members of patients with congenital retinal folds should be examined for signs of FEVR, particularly if the folds are located temporally or occur bilaterally.

■ Differential Diagnosis

The characteristic features of FEVR include nonvascularization of the retinal periphery, familial occurrence, heterotopia of the disc and macula, retinal exudation, retinal detachment, and falciform retinal folds. Clinically, the manifestations of the disorder are most analogous to retinopathy of prematurity, in which peripheral nonvascularization, fibrovascular proliferation, and cicatricial changes with resultant traction on the retina are also seen. In retinopathy of prematurity, however, there is characteristically a history of premature birth or neonatal oxygen supplementation and no family history of the disorder. In contrast to FEVR, the peripheral avascular retina in retinopathy of prematurity usually vascularizes with regression of the disease. In addition, retinal exudation is rare in retinopathy of prematurity but is seen commonly in FEVR.

The differential diagnosis of peripheral retinal nonvascularization with neovascular proliferation also includes sickle cell retinopathy, periphlebitis retinae, Eales's disease, incontinentia pigmenti, and autosomal dominant neovascularization [17].

Disorders leading to dragging of the optic disc and major vessels and heterotopia of the macula also should be included in the differential diagnosis of FEVR. Among these are persistent hyperplastic primary vitreous, Norrie's disease, incontinentia pigmenti, retinal dysplasia, congenital hereditary falciform retinal folds, and congenital toxoplasmosis. In contrast to FEVR, persistent hyperplastic primary vitreous is unilateral in more than 90% of cases and is usually present at birth; the affected eye is microphthalmic.

Causes of peripheral retinal exudation or fibrovascular mass lesions that should be considered in the differential diagnosis include Coats' disease (retinal telangiectasia), ocular toxocariasis, pars planitis (peripheral uveitis), retinal angiomatosis, and combined hamartoma. Of note, Coats' disease is usually unilateral, occurring more commonly in male children. Characteristically, no vitreous changes or extensive vitreoretinal adhesions are seen in patients with Coats' disease, and the exudates are not localized to the retinal periphery.

■ Genetic Considerations

In most cases, FEVR is inherited as an autosomal dominant trait with variable expressivity. Penetrance has been reported to be close to 100% [5]. Because of the significant phenotypical variability, some patients have only minimal manifestations of the disorder, detected only when relatives of more severely affected patients are screened carefully.

A recent report by Trese and associates [18] described an X-chromosome-linked form of the disease in 4 generations of 2 families. The pattern of inheritance in one of the families described by Criswick and Schepens [1] also was consistent with an X-linked recessive trait, with 3 brothers and a maternal uncle affected and blindness reported in a distant male relative related through females. Sporadic cases of FEVR have also been reported [16]; these may represent somatic or new germinal mutations. Careful examination of family members of any apparently sporadic case is necessary to rule out the existence of affected relatives who may be asymptomatic.

A number of investigators [5, 7, 11, 15] have suggested that FEVR is a primary disorder affecting retinal vascular development rather than a true vitreoretinopathy. Failure of the retinal periphery to vascularize, the most common finding in the mildest forms of the disorder, is believed by some researchers to be secondary to a genetic defect that induces abnormal development of the hyaloid vascular system, resulting in anomalous formation of retinal vessels, particularly small peripheral vessels. This theory is in contrast to the original hypothesis of Criswick and Schepens [1], who believed that abnormalities of vitreoretinal attachments were of primary importance in the pathogenesis.

The potential role of a vasoocclusive process in the pathogenesis of the peripheral nonvascularization has led investigators to search for hematological abnormalities in affected patients. Laqua [6] performed extensive hematological studies on one of his FEVR patients and found no abnormalities. Chaudhuri and co-workers [19] reported platelet aggregation defects in all members studied in 2 families with FEVR. The major defect was absent platelet aggregation with arachidonic acid. These authors hypothesized a possible role of this abnormality in the pathogenesis of FEVR. Defective arachidonic acid metabolism results in inadequate vasotonia and failure to protect the immature retinal blood vessels. Subsequent studies of other patients with FEVR [20] and patients with incontinentia pigmenti who have similar retinal findings [21] failed to disclose similar platelet abnormalities, although Friedrich and associates [20] did note an abnormal bleeding time and lack of adenosine triphosphate (ATP) secretion in 1 severely affected patient with FEVR.

The precise nature of the genetic defect in FEVR has not yet been identified. In recent years, a number of large kindreds of affected patients have been reported, especially in Japan, the Netherlands, Colombia, and Germany. Using a large German kindred and linkage analysis, Li and colleagues recently mapped the locus for dominant FEVR to the long arm of chromosome 11 (Li Y, personal communication, 1992). With further work in this area and the use of current molecular genetic techniques, it is hoped that researchers will be able to identify the mutations responsible for FEVR and to clarify the origin of this disorder.

■ Pathological Features

Although a few histopathological descriptions of eyes with advanced stages of FEVR have been published, no study of an eye with mild or moderate disease has been reported. The available descriptions are of eyes that were enucleated for neovascular glaucoma, acute angle closure, or phthisis or, in one 6-week-old infant, to rule out retinoblastoma. Most of the pathological findings in these end-stage eyes are typical of those seen with chronic retinal detachment, neovascular glaucoma, and phthisis bulbi.

In all published cases, retinal detachment and prominent vitreous and preretinal fibrovascular membranes were observed. Brockhurst and co-workers [22] reported the histopathological examination of 2 enucleated eyes from twins with presumed FEVR. In both eyes, a total retinal detachment was present. Prominent preretinal and vitreous membranes appeared posterior to the ora serrata, with multiple adhesions to the retina, resulting in large retinal folds.

A long-standing retinal detachment was also present in the eye of a patient with FEVR that had been enucleated secondary to neovascular glaucoma [23]. This specimen revealed a zone of focal, nodular fibrovascular proliferation, with associated necrosis and acute inflammation within the temporal portion of the retina anterior to the equator. Dense preretinal fibrovascular connective tissue was seen organized on the retinal surface. Boldrey and associates [24] noted the presence of inflammatory cells in the retina, as well as intraretinal and subretinal exudates and prominent preretinal membranes in an eye enucleated for narrow-angle glaucoma associated with FEVR.

■ Management

The identification of FEVR in patients without a known family history of the disorder often requires careful examination of the patient's blood relatives. In asymptomatic patients, observation with frequent follow-up is indicated to monitor for the development of active proliferation, retinal holes, or retinal detachment. The role of electrophysiological testing in these patients is not yet clear [10, 25].

The prophylactic treatment of areas of avascularized retina is somewhat controversial since, in many cases, these regions will remain stable and asymptomatic over extended periods of time. Treatment of the avascular areas with cryotherapy or photocoagulation may be performed in cases where there is evidence of progression of the disorder to the stage of active fibrovascular or neovascular proliferation. Active progression of the disease with associated visual loss is rare after age 20 years [5].

Loss of central vision in patients with FEVR may be secondary to heterotopia of the macula, retinal striae, cystoid retinal edema, epiretinal membrane formation, or retinal detachment. Retinal detachments are the major cause of severe visual loss in these patients. When associated with FEVR, the detachments tend to be complicated, often requiring multiple surgical procedures for repair. Rhegmatogenous retinal detachments associated with the disorder tend to have the poorest prognosis in younger children; even in adolescents, the detachments tend to recur postoperatively [12]. Release of peripheral vitreoretinal traction using painstaking membrane dissection and scleral buckling techniques is essential in the repair of retinal detachments associated with this disorder [26].

■ References

1. Criswick VG, Schepens CL. Familial exudative vitreoretinopathy. Am J Ophthalmol 1969;68:578–594
2. Gow J, Oliver GL. Familial exudative vitreoretinopathy: an expanded view. Arch Ophthalmol 1971;86:150–155
3. Canny CLB, Oliver GL. Fluorescein angiographic findings in familial exudative vitreoretinopathy. Arch Ophthalmol 1976;94:1114–1120
4. Tasman W, Augsburger JJ, Shields JA, et al. Familial exudative vitreoretinopathy. Trans Am Ophthalmol Soc 1981;79:211–226

5. Ober RR, Bird AC, Hamilton AM, Sehmi K. Autosomal dominant exudative vitreoretinopathy. Br J Ophthalmol 1980;64:112–120
6. Laqua H. Familial exudative vitreoretinopathy. Albrecht von Graefes Arch Klin Exp Ophthalmol 1980;213:121–133
7. Slusher MM, Hutton WE. Familial exudative vitreoretinopathy. Am J Ophthalmol 1979;87:152–156
8. Miyakubo H, Inohara N, Hashimoto K. Retinal involvement in familial exudative vitreoretinopathy. Ophthalmologica 1982;185:125–135
9. Nijhuis FA, Deutman AF, Aan de Kerk AL. Fluorescein angiography in mild stages of dominant exudative vitreoretinopathy. Mod Probl Ophthalmol 1979;20:107–114
10. Feldman EL, Norris JL, Cleasby GW. Autosomal dominant exudative vitreoretinopathy. Arch Ophthalmol 1983;101:1532–1535
11. Miyakubo H, Hashimoto K, Miyakubo S. Retinal vascular pattern in familial exudative vitreoretinopathy. Ophthalmology 1984;91:1524–1530
12. van Nouhuys CE. Juvenile retinal detachment as a complication of familial exudative vitreoretinopathy. Fortschr Ophthalmol 1989;86:221–223
13. Hashimoto K, Miyakubo H, Inohara N, Tada H. Juvenile retinal detachment and familial exudative vitreoretinopathy. Jpn J Clin Ophthalmol 1983;37:797–803
14. Dudgeon J. Familial exudative vitreo-retinopathy. Trans Ophthalmol Soc UK 1979;99:45–49
15. van Nouhuys CE. Congenital retinal fold as a sign of dominant exudative vitreoretinopathy. Graefes Arch Clin Exp Ophthalmol 1981;217:55–67
16. Nishimura M, Yamana T, Sugino M, et al. Falciform retinal fold as sign of familial exudative vitreoretinopathy. Jpn J Ophthalmol 1983;27:40–53
17. Gitter KA, Rothschild H, Waltman DD, et al. Dominantly inherited peripheral retinal neovascularization. Arch Ophthalmol 1978;96:1601–1605
18. Trese MT, Hartzer MR, Shastry SR. X-chromosome linked familial exudative vitreoretinopathy. Presented at the 8th International Congress of Human Genetics, Washington, DC, October 6–11, 1991
19. Chaudhuri PR, Rosenthal AR, Goulstine DB, et al. Familial exudative vitreoretinopathy associated with familial thrombocytopathy. Br J Ophthalmol 1983;67:755–758
20. Friedrich CA, Francis KA, Kim HC. Familial exudative vitreoretinopathy (FEVR) and platelet dysfunction. Br J Ophthalmol 1989;73:477–478
21. Gole GA, Goodall K, James MJ. Familial exudative vitreoretinopathy. Br J Ophthalmol 1985;69:76
22. Brockhurst RJ, Albert DM, Zakov N. Pathologic findings in familial exudative vitreoretinopathy. Arch Ophthalmol 1981;99:2143–2146
23. Nicholson DH, Galvis V. Criswick-Schepens syndrome (familial exudative vitreoretinopathy): study of a Colombian kindred. Arch Ophthalmol 1984;102:1519–1522
24. Boldrey EE, Egbert P, Gass JDM, Friberg T. The histopathology of familial exudative vitreoretinopathy. Arch Ophthalmol 1985;103:238–241
25. Ohkubo H, Tanino T. Electrophysiological findings in familial exudative vitreoretinopathy. Doc Ophthalmol 1987;65:461–469
26. Tano Y, Ikeda T. Treatment of familial exudative vitreoretinopathy with pars plana vitrectomy. Ophthalmology 1990;97(suppl):152

Is Keratoconus Genetic?

Deborah S. Jacobs, M.D.
Claes H. Dohlman, M.D.

■ Clinical Perspective on Keratoconus

Definition

Keratoconus, once called *conical cornea,* is a noninflammatory, thinning disorder of the cornea. The word *keratoconus* is derived from the Greek *keratos,* meaning "horn" and denoting relationship to horny tissue or to the cornea, and the Greek *konos,* meaning "cone." The disorder is characterized by a progressive thinning of the corneal stroma that is associated with corneal steepening and scarring. Keratoconus is most correctly classified as an ectasia (dilatation, expansion, or distension) rather than a dystrophy or degeneration. It is generally bilateral, although asymmetrical involvement of the 2 eyes is not uncommon.

Demographics

Most cases of keratoconus are diagnosed in adolescents, who present with progressive myopic astigmatism. Keratoconus occurs in all races. The demographic literature on keratoconus is reviewed in detail by Krachmer and colleagues [1] who found that the reported prevalence of keratoconus varies from 4 to 600 cases per 100,000 population. The wide range of prevalence figures probably reflects the use of different criteria for the diagnosis of keratoconus in addition to any true population differences in prevalence that might exist. The most valid prevalence figures are probably from a study from the Mayo Clinic [2], which cited a prevalence of 54.5 cases per 100,000 population in Olmsted County, Minnesota, in 1982. In many series of keratoconus patients, there is a preponderance of females to males, in a ratio of at almost 2:1 [1].

Diagnosis

The diagnosis of keratoconus is based on the presence of progressive, irregular myopic astigmatism. There are no strict diagnostic criteria. The condition in its classic form may be associated with any or all of the many signs listed in Table 1, some of which are depicted in the Figure.

Treatment and Prognosis

The treatment options for keratoconus are reviewed elsewhere [1] and are listed in Table 2. The rigid contact lens, which provides correction of irregular astigmatism, is the mainstay of therapy for keratoconus. Contact lens intolerance, contact lens instability, and axial scarring are the factors that necessitate specialized contact lenses or surgical intervention for visual rehabilitation.

Keratoconus is typically characterized by the progression of irregular astigmatism with increased steepening of the corneal curvature. Progression occurs over a period of years in the first decade or two after the time of diagnosis. With progression, there is often apical scarring at the level of Bowman's membrane. This scarring can be visually significant and can interfere mechanically with the fitting and tolerance of contact lenses. Apical touch of an ill-fitting contact lens can, in turn, lead to progressive scarring. Episodes of hydrops from rupture of Descemet's membrane occasionally lead to axial scarring and chronic edema.

The rate of progression of keratoconus is variable and very often asym-

Table 1 *Clinical Signs of Keratoconus*

Progressive, irregular, myopic astigmatism

Scissoring reflex on retinoscopy

Dark center or annulus on retroillumination of corneal cone with slit-lamp or direct ophthalmoscope

Inferotemporal steepening on keratoscopy or corneal topography

Munson's sign: angular protrusion of lower eyelid on downgaze

Rissutti's sign: triangular focusing of light in the iris plane with lateral penlight illumination of anterior segment

Vogt's striae: refractile lines in posterior stroma, often vertical but usually aligned in steepest axis

Fleischer's ring: partial or complete annular ring at base of cone formed by hemosiderin pigment deep in the epithelium

Scarring or fibrillary pattern at the level of Bowman's membrane

Prominent corneal nerves

Rupture of Descemet's membrane (acute corneal hydrops)

Scarring of Descemet's membrane

Particular patterns on computer-assisted topographical analysis

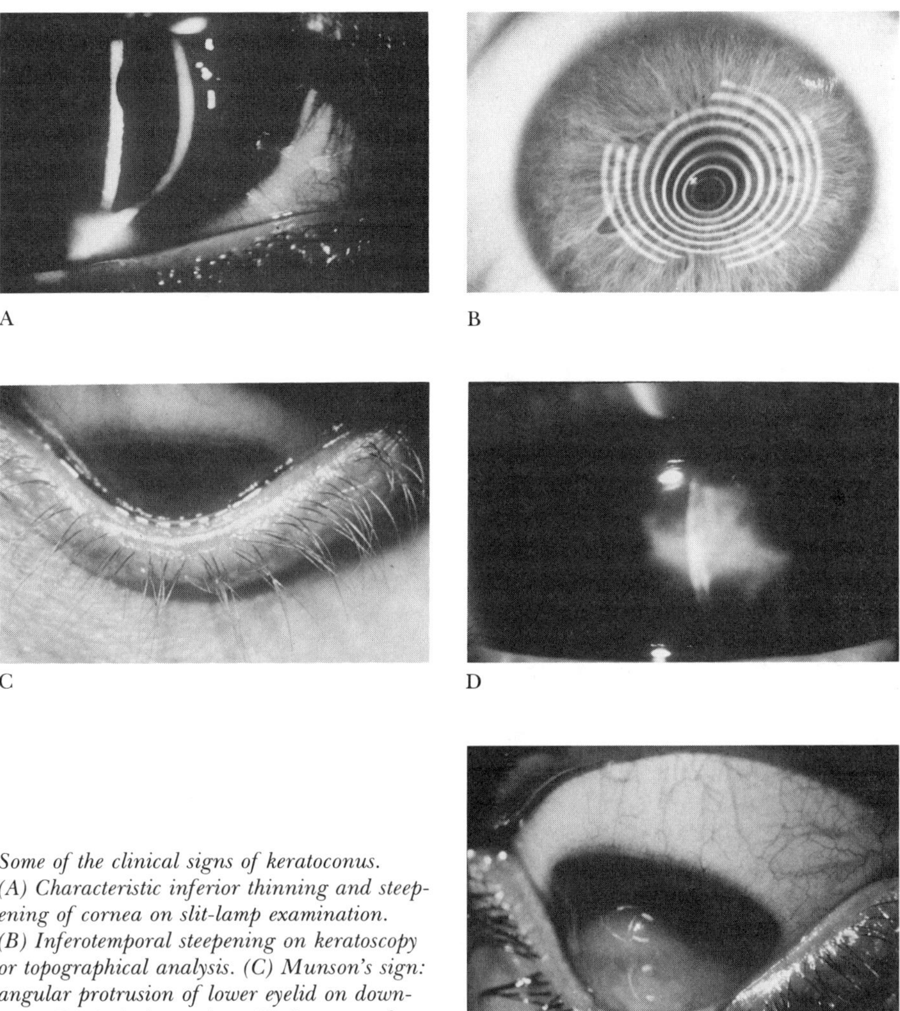

Some of the clinical signs of keratoconus. (A) Characteristic inferior thinning and steepening of cornea on slit-lamp examination. (B) Inferotemporal steepening on keratoscopy or topographical analysis. (C) Munson's sign: angular protrusion of lower eyelid on downgaze. (D) Apical scarring. (E) Rupture of Descemet's membrane (acute corneal hydrops).

metrical. Progression can stop at any level of disease severity, and it is relatively unlikely after age 30 years and rarely occurs after age 40. Corneal rupture generally does not occur but is not uncommon in keratoglobus and in keratoconus associated with the blue sclerae syndrome.

The indication for penetrating keratoplasty in keratoconus is contact lens intolerance or inadequate visual acuity with a contact lens. In the Mayo Clinic series [2], a patient with the diagnosis of keratoconus had an 80% probability of surviving 20 years after diagnosis without requiring a graft.

The prognosis for penetrating keratoplasty in keratoconus is excellent.

Table 2 *Therapeutic Options for Keratoconus*

Spectacles
Contact lenses
 Rigid lenses: polymethyl methacrylate and rigid gas-permeable
 Soper style lens: rigid lens with two posterior curves, the central one steeper to
  vault the cone
 Piggyback lenses: rigid lens on top of soft lens
Surgery
 Optical iridectomy or iridesis: most successful procedure prior to penetrating
  keratoplasty
 Penetrating keratoplasty
 Thermal keratoplasty
 Lamellar keratoplasty
 Epikeratophakia

A clear graft is obtained in more than 90% of cases, and 75% to 100% of cases result in visual acuity of 20/40 or better [1, 3].

■ Etiological Features of Keratoconus

The origin, pathogenesis, and biochemistry of keratoconus are unknown. Familial occurrence of the disease as well as associations with atopy, trisomy 21 (Down's syndrome), connective tissue disease, eye rubbing, contact lens wear, retinal degenerations, personality disturbances, and other clinical conditions have been reported. None of these associations has given rise to a unifying theory of the basis of this disease, genetic or otherwise.

A number of theorists have proposed a biochemical basis for the disease, but many of the investigations to test these theories are of questionable design and validity owing to limited numbers of pathological specimens available and the heterogeneity of the patient population. It may be that keratoconus is simply the final common pathway for a variety of clinical conditions.

In 1965, Duke-Elder and Leigh [4] wrote, regarding keratoconus:

> A multitude of theories has been put forward to account for its development, most of them relating to relatively few cases, none of them of general applicability, and all of them representing inadequate attempts to solve a problem which in our present state of ignorance is insoluble.

The determination as to whether there is a genetic basis for keratoconus can be made by observing hereditary patterns of the disease and by investigating associations with other clinical conditions that might be genetically determined. Consideration of environmental factors that might play a role in the development of keratoconus is also warranted.

Hereditary Patterns

The rate of familial involvement in keratoconus is difficult to determine. Various series use different diagnostic criteria, possibly excluding subclinical forms of the disease and including patients with ordinary astigmatism. Familial occurrence, which may involve both genetic and environmental factors, does not prove a genetic basis for the disease. Estimates of the incidence of a familial pattern of keratoconus are as high as 20% of cases [5].

Evidence from case reports on twins and from pedigree analysis suggests that there *are* heritable forms of keratoconus. The literature on keratoconus in identical twins (a total of 6 case reports) is summarized in a report of discordant keratoconus in a set of monozygotic twins [6], in which the authors suggest a role for environmental factors. In that particular case, the environmental factors postulated were reading, eye rubbing, and hormonal influences. The remaining 5 reported cases in identical twins are concordant, suggesting a heritable form of the disease [1, 6].

Duke-Elder [4] and Waardenburg and colleagues [7] review several cases in the literature in which parental consanguinity was noted, implying autosomal recessive inheritance.

Pedigrees with keratoconus in both sexes in two or three successive generations, which suggests autosomal dominant inheritance, have been reported [1, 4, 7]. In general, the dominant pattern is irregular, affecting approximately 1 in 10 blood relatives instead of the expected 1 in 2, implying variable expression or incomplete penetrance [5]. *Variable expression* means that not all aspects of a condition appear in each affected individual. *Incomplete penetrance* means that some individuals with the gene show no manifestations of the disease.

A series by Rabinowitz and co-workers [8], studying corneal topographical data in family members of patients with keratoconus, showed autosomal dominant transmission with complete penetrance but variable expression in all 5 families studied. The use of computer-assisted corneal topography in diagnosing keratoconus suggests that underdiagnosis of milder, early, or aborted forms of the disease occurs when only refractive, biomicroscopical, and keratoscopical data are used. The more accurate diagnosis of keratoconus in family members using topographical analysis may generate pedigrees suitable for biochemical and molecular biological study.

Systemic Associations

Review of the associations of keratoconus with systemic diseases of genetic origin may lend insight into the genetic basis or origin of keratoconus. Associations with connective tissue disease, atopy, human leukocyte antigen (HLA) type, and hormonal and psychiatric disturbances have been noted.

Connective Tissue Disease The association of keratoconus with connective tissue disease is reviewed in detail elsewhere [1, 3]. In summary, keratoconus associated with Marfan's syndrome and with osteogenesis imperfecta is rare and certainly not a ubiquitous feature of either syndrome. Keratoconus *is* associated with Ehlers-Danlos syndrome, particularly type VI, an autosomal recessive form in which there is lysyl hydroxylase deficiency and in which ocular manifestations predominate. Keratoconus as well as keratoglobus, microcornea, and megalocornea have been associated with Ehlers-Danlos syndrome of different types. In Ehlers-Danlos syndrome, as opposed to other forms of keratoconus, and in keratoglobus in general, spontaneous perforation and perforation from mild trauma is not uncommon, suggesting that this form of keratoconus, perhaps genetic in nature, may have a pathogenesis different from other forms. A heritable disorder may be the basis of keratoconus in association with blue sclerae [9], but the occurrence of vernal conjunctivitis in some of these cases confounds the association.

Only a small minority of cases of keratoconus are associated with these profound and obvious connective tissue disorders. Observing the association, investigators have sought to establish whether there is an association also between keratoconus and other more subtle connective tissue disorders, on the basis of a common disorder of collagen metabolism. Associations between keratoconus and abnormal connective tissue syndromes such as mitral valve prolapse have been reported [10], but a more recent study [11] does not support the hypothesis that keratoconus is part of a systemic disease syndrome consisting of mitral valve prolapse and joint hyperextensibility. Conflicting reports are probably due to the lack of standard criteria for the diagnoses involved as well as to the potential for bias in case and control selection.

Atopy A positive association between keratoconus and atopic disease (asthma, eczema, vernal conjunctivitis, hay fever, allergy) has been demonstrated and confirmed. For example, Rahi and colleagues [12] found a history of atopy in 35% of keratoconus patients and only 12% of controls. Harrison and co-workers [13] noted a history of atopic disease in more than 50% of keratoconus patients. Bietti and colleagues [14] found a statistically significant association with vernal catarrh. Studies showing a negative or no correlation between the two conditions also exist and are reviewed by Krachmer's group [1]. Comparison of these different studies is confounded by a lack of standard criteria for the diagnosis of both keratoconus and atopy. Most practitioners believe that there is an increased prevalence of atopy among keratoconus patients.

The basis for the association between atopy and keratoconus is unclear. It may be that eye rubbing from itching and ocular irritation is the link between the two conditions. It is also possible that there is some linkage between the genetic determinants of atopy and keratoconus. Clarifying such a linkage is a complex proposition because there are probably multiple genetic factors causing atopy, including HLA type, determinants of serum IgE levels, and other factors yet to be identified.

Other Systemic Associations An association between keratoconus and HLA type has been postulated, but no clear linkage has yet been demonstrated [15]. HLA type could be the link between keratoconus and atopy. In the older literature [4], endocrine disturbance was proposed as a cause of keratoconus because of the disorder's occurrence in a disproportionate number of female subjects, onset in adolescence, and association of progression with hormonal disturbances such as hypothyroidism and pregnancy. None of these associations has been found in any large series, and each is probably circumstantial rather than causal.

Some practitioners believe that there is a "keratoconic personality." A controlled study by Mannis and co-workers [16] comparing personality patterns in keratoconus patients, patients with other chronic eye disease, and normal controls could identify no specific complex of personality characteristics attributable to keratoconus. Patients with keratoconus differed from normal controls in much the same way as did patients with other chronic eye diseases, being less conforming and more passive-aggressive, paranoid, and hypomanic. The keratoconus patients tended toward more disorganized patterns of thinking and scored higher on substance abuse indicators. An earlier British study by Karseras and Ruben [17] also found no evidence for a particular psychiatric disturbance associated with keratoconus.

Ophthalmic Associations

The association of keratoconus with other types of eye disease has been observed. A statistically significant correlation between retinitis pigmentosa and keratoconus, both of which are heterogeneous entities, was demonstrated by Bietti and colleagues [14]. In infantile tapetoretinal degeneration (Leber's congenital amaurosis), an autosomal recessive condition, the incidence of keratoconus is 30% to 50% in patients older than 15 years [18]. The very high correlation between these two entities suggests a single or linked genetic determinant, perhaps expressing itself in various tissues of neuroectodermal and neural crest origin.

Mitigating against any genetic basis for association with these retinal diseases that cause early blindness are 5 reported cases of keratoconus associated with retinopathy of prematurity. All cases were unilateral but, in the absence of topographical data, subclinical forms in the fellow eye cannot be ruled out [19, 20]. Eye rubbing has been observed to be a common feature in tapetoretinal degeneration and other causes of early blindness and may be the basis for the association between these conditions and keratoconus.

Associations with Congenital Syndromes of Genetic Origin

The incidence of keratoconus in trisomy 21 (Down's syndrome) is in the region of 5% to 10% [21, 22], considerably higher than the incidence in the general population. Increased incidence of keratoconus has not been found in patients with other mental retardation syndromes in the same institutions. Increased incidence of acute corneal hydrops in the Down's syndrome subgroup of keratoconus patients is probably related to eye-rubbing behavior. Eye rubbing has been postulated as the basis for the association of keratoconus with Down's syndrome, as has the possibility of a genetic determinant of the disease existing on chromosome 21; there are no theories as to the biochemical product of such a determinant.

Environmental Associations

Contact lens wear and eye rubbing are two environmental, as opposed to genetic, factors that have been associated with keratoconus.

Rigid Contact Lenses A causal relationship has been postulated between the use of rigid contact lenses and keratoconus, based on the observation that there is an incidence as high as 26% of rigid contact lens wear in patients prior to the diagnosis of keratoconus [23]. Soft contact lens wearers have not been observed to develop keratoconus. Much of the literature on the association between keratoconus and a history of rigid contact lens wear is of questionable validity because the studies are retrospective in nature and because population groups who end up wearing rigid as opposed to soft or no contact lenses are probably more likely to include patients with subclinical keratoconus. No prospective randomized trials have been conducted. Hence, the relationship between rigid contact lens wear and keratoconus remains controversial. The analysis of serial topographical data is likely to be fruitful in attempting to understand this relationship.

Eye Rubbing Eye rubbing is common to many of the entities associated with keratoconus, including Down's syndrome, atopy, and tapetoretinal degeneration. The prevalence of eye rubbing is reported to be as high as 70% in keratoconus patients [17]. A correlation between eye rubbing and keratoconus does not, however, prove a causal relationship. There is evidence from a study by Harrison and associates [13] that unilateral keratoconus occurs more frequently on the side of the dominant hand, suggesting a correlation with eye rubbing.

■ The Genetic Defect in Keratoconus

The pathogenesis of keratoconus remains unknown. The primary pathology may lie in the basal corneal epithelium, in the stromal keratocytes, or in an extracellular matrix component elaborated by either of these cell types.

The mechanism proposed by Teng [24] and others for a basal epithelial origin involves the primary degeneration of basal epithelial cells, leading to enzymal degradation of basement membrane and stromal extracellular matrix. Stromal thinning and changes in the mechanical characteristics of the stroma are postulated to occur secondarily. An alteration in epithelial lysosomal enzyme levels has been demonstrated in keratoconus [25] and could be a primary factor in, or simply an epiphenomenon of, the abnormal basal epithelial function postulated in this mechanism.

An alternative theory is that the stromal keratocyte is the site of the primary defect in keratoconus and that the molecular basis is a defect in fibrogenesis or elaboration of ground substance. In the keratoconus cone, the thickness of the corneal lamellae is normal but the number of lamellae is reduced, suggesting that the defect is in the attachment of lamellae rather than in the lamellae themselves [26]. Conflicting reports as to the existence of abnormalities in cross-linkage of collagen as well as in the synthesis and breakdown of collagen and extracellular matrix components are reviewed elsewhere [1, 3, 27].

It is possible that keratoconus is part of an ectodermal syndrome, which would explain the disorder's association with atopy and retinitis pigmentosa. The existence of such a syndrome is not incompatible with the hypothesis that either the basal epithelium or the stromal keratocyte is the pathological locus of the disease, because the epithelium differentiates from surface ectoderm and the keratocytes differentiate from neural crest, also of ectodermal origin. The association of keratoconus with connective tissue diseases such as the Ehlers-Danlos type VI and blue sclerae syndromes, which are presumably mesodermal in origin, is not explained by an ectodermal syndrome. These forms of keratoconus often differ in clinical course, and probably in their underlying pathological basis, from the more typical forms of keratoconus.

■ Advising Patients

What should the ophthalmologist tell a patient with keratoconus who asks, "Is my condition hereditary? What's the chance that my children will have the disease?" Krachmer and co-workers [1] tell their patients that the chances are less than 1 in 10 that a blood relative will have the disease. This formulation is based on a German series [5] in which autosomal dominant inheritance was postulated and 20% penetrance observed (1 in 2 chance of inheriting the dominant gene × 1 in 5 chance of penetrant expression = 1 in 10 chance of having the disease). This formulation is not inconsistent with the findings by Rabinowitz and colleagues [8]. Furthermore, the finding that only 20% of patients with keratoconus come to keratoplasty when followed for 20 years after the diagnosis [2], coupled with the finding that 90% of keratoplasties for keratoconus result in a clear graft [1, 3], suggests that there is only a 1 in 500 chance (1/10 × 1/5 × 1/10) that a blood relative will have the disease, come to keratoplasty, and end up with a cloudy graft. Given that the disease is often asymmetrical, the possibility of good vision in the fellow eye further reduces the chance of profound bilateral visual impairment in a relative.

■ Conclusion

Is keratoconus genetic? The answer is probably not yes or no but rather sometimes. Answering this question on the basis of a review of the existing literature is fraught with pitfalls. Most clinical studies suffer from a lack of standard criteria for the diagnosis or exclusion of keratoconus and probably include many false-negative and false-positive findings. Computer-assisted corneal topographical analysis has demonstrated that there is a subclinical form of keratoconus and that keratoconus can be distinguished from ordinary astigmatism. The existence of a subclinical form means that pedigree analysis done without the use of corneal topographical analysis is likely to be erroneous, with many affected individuals not being recognized. This technology already suggests that apparently isolated cases of keratoconus may, in fact, be part of autosomal dominant pedigrees of a disease with complete penetrance but highly variable expression. Autosomal dominant keratoconus may be more prevalent than we realize.

It is also clear that keratoconus is not one disease but rather the final common pathway of several potentially pathological processes. Most pathological and biochemical studies of keratoconus use corneas from patients with various forms of the disease and, not surprisingly, have yielded ambiguous data.

Some of the clinical conditions associated with keratoconus, such as atopy, probably have at least one genetic component, and this genetic component may also be involved in the development of keratoconus. The high incidence of keratoconus in trisomy 21 and in Leber's congenital amaurosis suggests a genetic basis for the disease in these conditions.

It makes sense to confine studies of the biochemical and genetic basis of keratoconus to tissue obtained from patients with a particular form of the disease. Even if the abnormality in that form is not ubiquitous, an understanding of that form of keratoconus may lend insight into some aspects of both normal and pathological states. With the use of computer-assisted topographical analysis, autosomal dominant pedigrees might be characterized that involve a sufficient number of affected individuals to facilitate gene linkage analysis using DNA probes and restriction endonucleases. A fascinating possibility is that a gene for atopy may be in linkage disequilibrium with the keratoconus gene and hence constitute the association. A gene linkage approach could be used to study the association of keratoconus with retinitis pigmentosa, tapetoretinal degeneration, and the connective tissue syndromes. The metabolic defect in keratoconus associated with Down's syndrome is likely to be more difficult to determine. Certainly, studies assessing the role of basal epithelial cells, keratocytes, and extracellular matrix should also be confined to particular forms of keratoconus.

In 1965, Duke-Elder and Leigh [4] believed that understanding the development of keratoconus was an insoluble problem. Although our present state is not as "ignorant" as was theirs, the keratoconus problem remains unsolved. It seems likely that genetic factors are at least part of the solution. Topographical analysis for diagnosis and gene linkage studies are likely to shed some light on the origin of keratoconus, as is progress in our understanding of atopy and of the biochemistry and physiology of epithelial cells and keratocytes. A better understanding of the etiological basis of keratoconus will, in turn, help us prevent and treat this disease.

DSJ is supported by a fellowship from the Heed Ophthalmic Foundation.

■ References

1. Krachmer JH, Feder RS, Belin MW. Keratoconus and related noninflammatory corneal thinning disorders. Surv Ophthalmol 1984;28:293–322
2. Kennedy RH, Bourne WM, Dyer DA. A 48-year clinical and epidemiologic study of keratoconus. Am J Ophthalmol 1986;101:267–273
3. Maguire LJ, Meyer RF. Ectatic corneal degenerations. In: Kaufman HE, Barron BA, McDonald MB, Waltman SR, eds. The cornea. New York: Churchill Livingstone, 1988:485–510
4. Duke-Elder S, Leigh AG. Keratoconus (conical cornea). In: Duke-Elder S, ed. Diseases of the outer eye: vol 8, part 2, system of ophthalmology. St Louis: Mosby, 1965:964–976
5. Hammerstein W. Zur Genetik des Keratoconus. Albrecht von Graefes Arch Klin Exp Ophthalmol 1974;190:293–308
6. Bourne WM, Michels VV. Keratoconus in one identical twin. Cornea 1982;1: 35–37
7. Waardenburg PJ, Franceschetti A, Klein D. Genetics and ophthalmology. Springfield, IL: Thomas, 1961:452–456
8. Rabinowitz YS, Garbus J, McDonnell PJ. Computer-assisted corneal topography in family members of patients with keratoconus. Arch Ophthalmol 1990;108:365–371

9. Greenfield G, Stein R, Romano A, Goodman RM. Blue sclerae and keratoconus: key features of a distinct heritable disorder of connective tissue. Clin Genet 1973;4:8–16

10. Beardsley TL, Foulks GN. An association of keratoconus and mitral valve prolapse. Ophthalmology 1982;89:35–37

11. Street DA, Vinokur ET, Waring GO III, et al. Lack of association between keratoconus, mitral valve prolapse, and joint hypermobility. Ophthalmology 1990;98: 170–176

12. Rahi A, Davies P, Ruben M, et al. Keratoconus and coexisting atopic disease. Br J Ophthalmol 1977;61:761–764

13. Harrison RJ, Klouda PT, Easty DL, et al. Association between keratoconus and atopy. Br J Ophthalmol 1989;73:816–822

14. Bietti GB, Cambiaggi A, Del Castillo A. Sull'analisi statistica dell'associazione di malattie oculari. Bull Ocul 1962;41:3–12

15. Wachtmeister L, Ingemansson SO, Moller E. Atopy and HLA antigens in patients with keratoconus. Acta Ophthalmol (Copenh) 1982;60:113–122

16. Mannis MJ, Morrison TL, Zadnik K, et al. Personality trends in keratoconus: an analysis. Arch Ophthalmol 1987;105:798–800

17. Karseras AG, Ruben M. Aetiology of keratoconus. Br J Ophthalmol 1976;60: 522–525

18. Karel I. Keratoconus in congenital diffuse tapetoretinal degeneration. Ophthalmologica 1968;155:8–15

19. Karel I. Akutni keratokonus jako komplikace retrolentarni fibroplasie. Cesk Oftalmol 1969;25:347–351

20. Lorfel RS, Sugar HS. Keratoconus associated with retrolental fibroplasia. Ann Ophthalmol 1976;8:449–450

21. Cullen JF, Butler HG. Mongolism (Down's syndrome) and keratoconus. Br J Ophthalmol 1963;47:321–330

22. Walsh SZ. Keratoconus and blindness in 469 institutionalised subjects with Down syndrome and other causes of mental retardation. J Ment Defic Res 1981;25: 243–251

23. Gasset AR, Houde WL, Garcia-Bengochea M. Hard contact lens wear as an environmental risk in keratoconus. Am J Ophthalmol 1978;85:339–341

24. Teng CC. Electron microscope study of the pathology of keratoconus: part I. Am J Ophthalmol 1963;55:18–47

25. Sawaguchi S, Yue BYJ, Sugar J, Gilboy JE. Lysosomal enzyme abnormalities in keratoconus. Arch Ophthalmol 1989;107:1507–1510

26. Pouliquen Y, Graf B, DeKozak Y, et al. Etude morphologique du kératocone. Arch Ophtalmol (Paris) 1970;306:497–532

27. Zimmermann DR, Fischer RW, Winterhalter KH, et al. Comparative studies of collagens in normal and keratoconus corneas. Exp Eye Res 1988;46:431–442

Topographical Analysis
of Keratoconus

Harry R. Koster, M.D.
Michael D. Wagoner, M.D.

Keratoconus is a noninflammatory corneal thinning disorder. In its advanced form, conical protrusion associated with localized stromal thinning occurs at the apex of the cornea. Mild to marked impairment of vision secondary to advanced and irregular astigmatism or corneal scarring is usually present. The disease is most often bilateral but asymmetrical in severity.

■ Epidemiological Features

Estimates of the prevalence of keratoconus vary from 4 [1] to 600 [2] per 100,000 population. A prevalence rate of 54.5 per 100,000 population was identified by Kennedy and colleagues [3] in a well-controlled 48-year clinical and epidemiological study. Diagnosis was based on the examiner's description of characteristic irregular light reflexes seen on ophthalmoscopy or retinoscopy, or on irregular mires detected by keratometry with or without slit-lamp findings.

Associated clinical features included asthma, eczema, or hay fever in 36% of patients and mitral valve prolapse in 5% [3]. A history of excessive eye rubbing was reported in 26% of patients, and a prior history of hard contact lens use was present in 13% of patients with bilateral disease. Other reported associated abnormalities such as Ehlers-Danlos syndrome, osteogenesis imperfecta, Down's syndrome, and Marfan's syndrome were not present in this group, and there was no association of identical twins or consanguineous marriage.

In 6% of cases, there was a family history of keratoconus. At the time of diagnosis, 41% of patients had unilateral disease [3].

■ Methods of Examining Corneal Topography

Keratometry

Keratometers provide illuminated split-object mires reflected from the surface of the cornea (first Placido image), which acts as a convex mirror. The radius of curvature is determined by two pairs of reflected points, based on the assumption that the corneal surface is spherocylindrical. The distance between each pair of points varies with the radius of curvature from 2.6 to 3.7 mm. Power and location of the steepest meridian and that of the meridian 90 degrees away are measured with an accuracy of better than 0.25 D on a regular surface.

The major limitations of keratometers are as follows: (1) They measure only one central mire, providing no information about corneal topography central or peripheral to the points measured, and (2) they assume corneal symmetry and average corneal curvature on either side of the visual axis, thus measuring irregular astigmatism inaccurately.

Keratoscopy or Photokeratoscopy

Keratoscopy involves projecting a series of concentric circular mires that form an apparent virtual image located in the anterior chamber. Visual inspection of the size, shape, and separation of the mires gives information about the steepness and astigmatic state of a larger portion of the corneal surface than does traditional keratometry. The major limitations of this method are its insensitivity to small differences in corneal topography, making changes difficult to quantify.

Computer-Assisted Topographical Measuring Devices

Recently designed systems for computer-assisted topographical measurement digitize a typical photokeratoscopic image (16 or 32 edges) [4, 5]. Points are generated along each degree and are computer-processed to depict continuous mathematical functions describing the anterior corneal surface (Fig 1). The most common type of representation takes the form of a color-coded topographical map. Dioptric power, or radius of curvature, may be coded in absolute or relative scales. An interactive cursor allows immediate measurement of all points with precise localization. Data may be used in a variety of formulas for specific topographical assessment. The advantage of these devices is their ability to provide a complete topographical map of the cornea, which can be evaluated in many ways and compared to other computer-generated maps [4, 5].

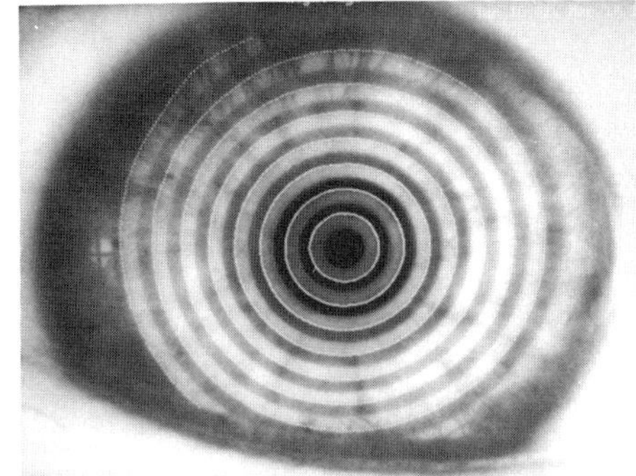

Figure 1 *Photokeratoscopic image with computer-digitized analysis used to depict corneal topography. (Courtesy of EyeSys Labs.)*

Rasterstereography

Rasterstereography uses a grid of horizontal and vertical bars projected onto the cornea. This pattern is captured by a video camera and is computer-processed. To its advantage, rasterstereography is independent of corneal reflectivity, but the technique remains in its early phases of clinical development.

Holography

Still in its developmental phase for examining corneal topography, holographic interferometry measures differences in topography related to corneal stresses. This is accomplished by interpreting interference fringes of combined wavefronts of sequential or real-time corneal images. This method may eventually aid in describing biomechanical properties of the cornea.

■ Normal Corneal Topography

The normal cornea has an aspherical surface, with progressive flattening toward the periphery. Flattening tends to occur closer to fixation on the nasal side. Overall, the nasal cornea is flatter than its temporal counterpart. The area of greatest corneal power tends to be located predominantly temporal to the visual axis, with no consistent trend in the vertical meridian. The topography of one cornea often mirrors the topography in the fellow eye.

Terms such as *apical* or *corneal cap* are anatomically arbitrary and are not based on topography.

Bogan and co-workers [6] classified normal corneal topography based on computer-assisted videokeratography. Of 399 normal corneas imaged,

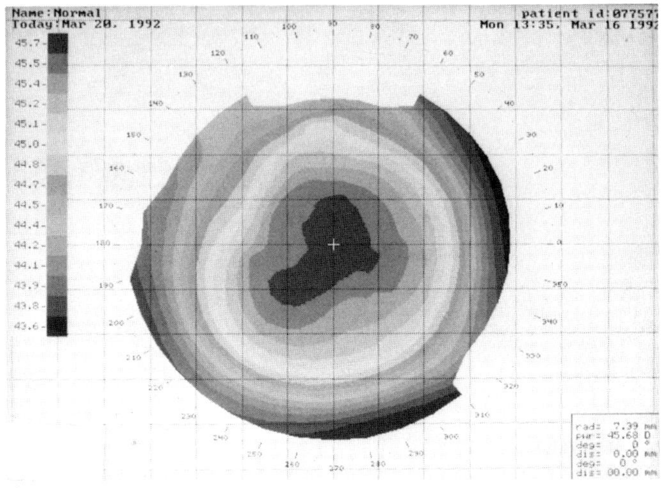

A

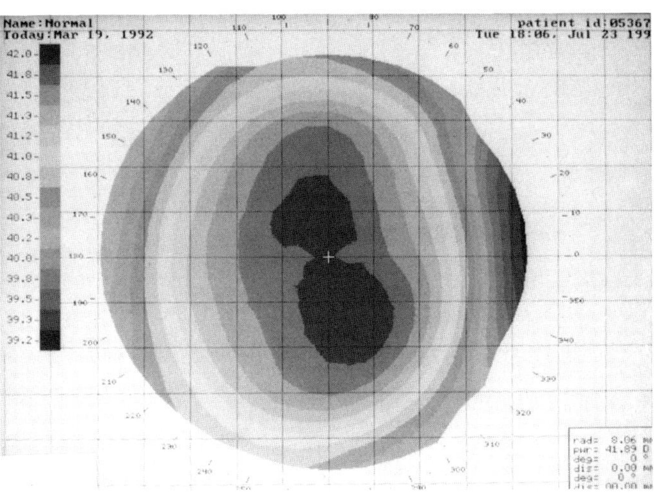

B

five patterns were discernible by objective criteria: round (22.6%), oval (20.8%), symmetrical bowtie (17.5%), asymmetrical bowtie (32.1%), and irregular (7.1%) (Fig 2). Correlation to parameters of keratometry and refraction revealed no significant astigmatic differences in the round and oval patterns, in contrast to clinically and keratometrically significant astigmatism in both bowtie patterns, which was more pronounced in the asymmetrical form. The frequency of irregular forms was believed to be overestimated as a result of eccentric fixation, tear abnormalities, or alignment system problems.

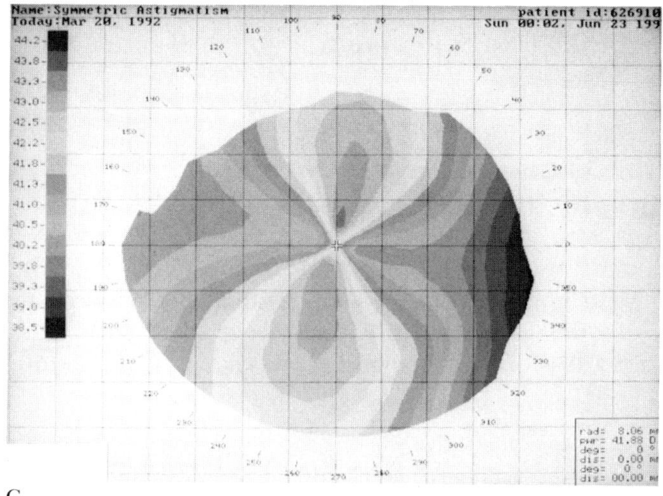

C

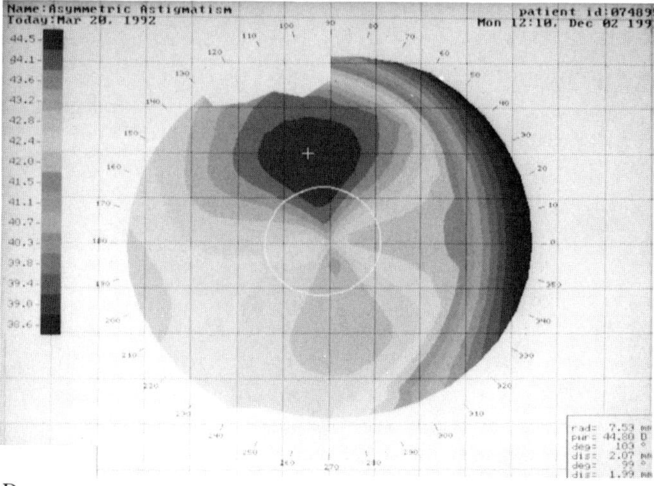

D

Figure 2 *Computer-generated examples of normal corneal topographical patterns: (A) round, (B) oval, (C) symmetrical astigmatism, and (D) asymmetrical astigmatism (note computer-generated location of pupil). Relative dioptric scales appear on left of each map; cursor reading (+) appears in lower right corner. (Courtesy of EyeSys Labs.)*

Though distinctive patterns were discernible on videokeratography, variation in corneal topography probably forms a continuum, from spherical to toroidal.

■ Traditional Classification of Corneal Topography in Keratoconus

Rowsey and colleagues [7] noted inferotemporal steepening as the earliest sign of keratoconus using the Placido disk. With progression, the steepening extends to the periphery, and eventually other quadrants are involved—first inferonasal, then superonasal and superotemporal.

■ Computer-Assisted Corneal Topographical Evaluation of Keratoconus

Rabinowitz and McDonnell [8] determined the computer-assisted topographical findings in 14 eyes of 10 patients with clinically apparent keratoconus. Three quantifiable differences from normal eyes were noted. These were (1) steepening of central corneal power; (2) marked asymmetry of corneal power between the 2 eyes of the same patient; and (3) significant steepening of the inferior compared with the superior cornea (I/S value).

The asymmetry in central power between the 2 eyes reflects the early asymmetrical progression of this disorder, as first noted by Amsler [9]. I/S values are not obtainable by conventional keratometry but involve averaging dioptric powers of five points 30 degrees apart along the superior and inferior cornea at a radius of 3 mm. The average of the superior values is subtracted from the average of the inferior values; a resulting positive value indicates a relatively steeper inferior cornea, whereas a negative value indicates a relatively steeper superior cornea.

In another study, Wilson and associates [10] imaged 63 eyes of 49 patients in whom keratoconus was diagnosed. Topographical patterns were divided into two groups, peripheral cones (72%), with steepening to the limbus in one or more quadrants, and central cones (28%). Central cones were characterized by one of two basic patterns, an asymmetrical bowtie configuration or a more symmetrical area of steepening. These patterns may represent different stages of topographical progression in keratoconus.

Steepening was most frequent in the inferior or inferotemporal quadrants, but the cone apex (point of maximal power) often did not correspond to the geometrical center of the steepened area. Seven cone apices were located superior to the visual axis.

A high degree of nonsuperimposable mirror-image symmetry of apex location and topographical alterations was noted between eyes of several patients. Despite this, there was a frequent overall asymmetry in apex power and total cylinder (mean difference of 8.2 D and 4.3 D, respectively) between the eyes of patients examined.

Several cases of bilateral disease could not be confirmed without computer-assisted topographical analysis.

Computer-Based Early Keratoconus Detection

Computerized topographical analysis may assist the clinician in diagnosing keratoconus in patients with no slit-lamp abnormalities. Maguire and Bourne [11] used this tool to screen 9 eyes of 7 patients in whom keratoconus was suspected. Five patients had keratoconus in the fellow eyes. Of the 9 eyes studied, 7 showed definite evidence of keratoconus as noted by inferior cone patterns. The topographical progression pattern of 1 patient to typical keratoconus over a 2-year span was subsequently reported in another article by Maguire and Lowry [12].

Computer-Assisted Detection of a Subclinical Familial Form of Keratoconus

In an attempt to discern subclinical topographical changes in family members of patients with keratoconus, Rabinowitz and colleagues [13] examined three groups of patients by computer-assisted topography: obvious keratoconus subjects, clinically and keratoscopically normal family members of patients with keratoconus, and normal nonfamily individuals. Quantitative measures used to separate normal, mildly abnormal, and keratoconic topographical patterns were identical to those used in these authors' previous keratoconus study [8]: central (at the visual axis) corneal power measurement, difference in central corneal power between the 2 eyes of the same patient, and relative amount of steepening of the inferior and superior cornea (expressed as the I/S value). Of the 28 clinically and photokeratoscopically normal family members of patients, 14 were considered to have abnormal topographical patterns based on these three parameters. The changes noted in normal family members of patients with keratoconus may represent incomplete or early expression of the keratoconus gene and, thus, subclinical keratoconus.

■ Current and Future Trends

The advent of computer-assisted corneal topographical instruments has vastly improved both the clinician's ability to document corneal topography and the sophistication with which corneal topography is assessed. Bogan and colleagues' [6] exhaustive effort to characterize normal corneal topography is essential to future efforts of early disease detection. Studies of the dynamics of the normal cornea over time will also help set parameters by which to detect corneal dynamics in pathological states.

Topographical characterization of a large number of clinically evident keratoconus patients has helped define the advanced parameters of this entity. Use of other measurements, such as rate of dioptric change from the visual axis along a meridian, more sensitive inferior-superior comparison, overall degree of asphericity, and surface regularity indices, may also help detect mild forms of disease. Eventually, these factors may be related to clinical variables such as optical function and biomechanical properties of the cornea.

Possible keratoconic changes due to rigid contact lenses, known to cause corneal warpage [14], may also be followed by corneal topographical assessment. It is hypothesized that rigid lenses may act as a chronic, low-grade source of trauma or pressure, especially if decentered, or as a promoter of local metabolic changes. An alternative explanation is that subclinical disease was present at the time of lens fitting and clinically evident manifestations subsequently evolved. The routine use of computer-assisted corneal topographical methods before rigid lens fitting may screen for early keratoconus, delineate groups at risk for changes, facilitate fitting, and assist clinicians in the follow-up of subtle corneal changes.

Elucidation of genetic patterns of keratoconus will involve proper epidemiological surveys and transmission pattern recognition. With keratoconus, epidemiological patterns are difficult to establish for two reasons. First, some patients may not seek medical attention, and second, there exists a spectrum of disease that, if subtle or asymptomatic, may be overlooked by the clinician. Currently, the earliest changes in keratoconus are detectable through topographical analysis. The issue as to whether and in whom subtle topographical changes lead to keratoconus remains to be fully answered. In the study of families of keratoconus patients by Rabinowitz's group [13], objective parameters helped define corneas as abnormal or at risk for progressive changes, even if slit-lamp and keratometric findings were normal. The authors pointed out that the range of age groups in which changes were seen concurs with observations first made by Amsler [9] and suggest that keratoconus may, in some instances, be abortive. Further studies of atypical topographical patterns eventually may elucidate the relation of keratoconus to regular and irregular astigmatism and may delineate progressive versus nonprogressive patterns to aid in prognosis determination and counseling.

The pedigree of families studied by Rabinowitz and colleagues [13] shows characteristics of autosomal dominant inheritance with complete penetrance, variable expression, and subclinical disease. Had members of the families who had keratoconus diagnosable by slit-lamp or photokeratoscopic examination been considered, the inheritance pattern would appear autosomal recessive. The authors contend that should dominant transmittance be the case, linkage analysis would be possible for pedigrees with vertical transmission through 3 generations and at least 10 affected members. Such a pedigree has not been described but, with the possibility of subclinical disease detection and modern molecular tools, identification of a gene or genes related to keratoconus may be possible.

Information from recognition and progression of topographical patterns as well as from molecular genetics may eventually allow keratoconus to be classified into significant subdivisions. These may include associations with systemic diseases, environmental factors, contact lens usage, and different population predilections, each with varying prognoses.

■ References

1. Duke-Elder S, Leigh AG. Diseases of the outer eye: vol 8, system of ophthalmology. London: Henry Kimpton, 1965:964–976
2. Hofstetter H. A keratoscopic survey of 13,395 eyes. Am J Optom 1959;36:3–11
3. Kennedy RH, Bourne WM, Dyer JA. A 48-year clinical and epidemiologic study of keratoconus. Am J Ophthalmol 1986;101:267–273
4. Koch DD, Foulks GN, Moran CT, Wakil JS. The corneal EyeSys system: accuracy analysis and reproducibility of first-generation prototype. Refract Corneal Surg 1989;5:423–429
5. Maguire LJ, Singer DE, Klyce SD. Graphic presentation of computer analyzed keratoscope photographs. Arch Ophthalmol 1987;94:223–230
6. Bogan SJ, Waring GO III, Ibrahim O, et al. Classification of normal corneal topography based on computer-assisted videokeratography. Arch Ophthalmol 1990; 108:945–949
7. Rowsey JJ, Reynolds AE, Brown R. Corneal topography: corneascope. Arch Ophthalmol 1981;99:1093–1100
8. Rabinowitz YS, McDonnell PJ. Computer-assisted corneal topography in keratoconus. Refract Corneal Surg 1989;5:400–408
9. Amsler M. Le keratocone fruste au javal. Ophthalmologica 1938;96:77–83
10. Wilson SE, Lin DTC, Klyce SD. Corneal topography of keratoconus. Cornea 1991;10:2–8
11. Maguire LJ, Bourne WM. Corneal topography of early keratoconus. Am J Ophthalmol 1989;108:107–112
12. Maguire LJ, Lowry JC. Identifying progression of subclinical keratoconus by serial topography analysis. Am J Ophthalmol 1991;112:41–45
13. Rabinowitz YS, Garbus J, McDonnell PJ. Computer-assisted corneal topography in family members of patients with keratoconus. Arch Ophthalmol 1990;108:365–371
14. Wilson SE, Lin DTC, Klyce SD, et al. Topographic changes in contact lens–induced corneal warpage. Ophthalmology 1990;97:734–744

Stickler's Syndrome

John H. Niffenegger, M.D.

Trexler M. Topping, M.D.

Shizuo Mukai, M.D.

Stickler's syndrome (McKusick #108300) is an autosomal dominant connective tissue disorder characterized by vitreoretinal degeneration, myopia, retinal detachment, cataract formation, hearing loss, and skeletal disorders, including premature osteoarthritis, maxillofacial hypoplasia, and spondyloepiphyseal dysplasia [1, 2, 3]. The estimated incidence is 1 per 10,000 population in the United States. Stickler's syndrome is an important cause of heritable retinal detachment.

Families with Stickler's syndrome differ from families described by Wagner [4] and Jansen [5] in that, although they share similar ocular findings, the pedigrees reported by Wagner and Jansen had no skeletal disorders.

The vitreous cavity of Wagner-Jansen-Stickler eyes is typically described as being optically empty with the exception of varying amounts of sparse intravitreal membranes and strands, especially in the periphery (Fig 1). Associated with these changes in the vitreous are latticelike changes of the peripheral retina (Fig 2). Retinal detachment is not a part of Wagner's syndrome, but its frequency is 50% in patients with Jansen's or Stickler's syndrome (Table 1) [3].

■ Related Ocular Diseases

Wagner's Syndrome

Wagner's syndrome was originally described in a Swiss family in 1938 [4]. None of the affected members had retinal detachment. The eyes did have optically empty vitreous cavities with sparse intravitreal strands and latticelike retinal changes. Most affected patients were 3 to 4 D myopic.

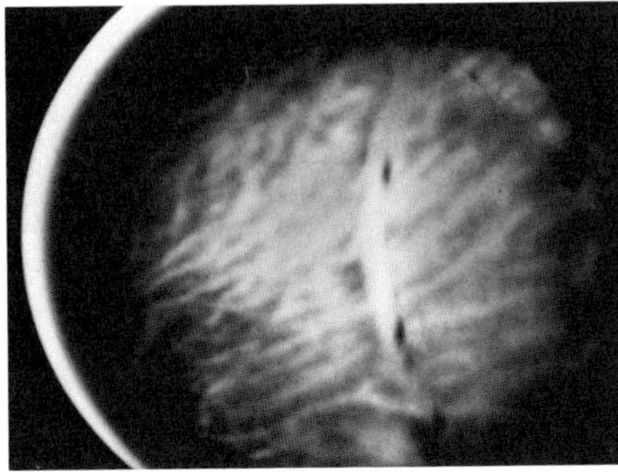

Figure 1 *Intravitreal membrane present in a patient with Stickler's syndrome.*

Pigmentary changes of the peripheral retina reminiscent of retinitis pigmentosa were also present. Retinal arteries were attenuated, and small clumps of retinal pigment were seen in the periphery in a perivascular distribution. Progressive chorioretinal degeneration with atrophy and sclerosis of the choroidal vessels was stressed by Wagner. Advanced cataract was common by age 40. A follow-up study in 1960 confirmed the absence of retinal detachment in this pedigree, despite the presence of vitreoretinal abnormalities [3].

The natural history of Wagner's syndrome has been studied by a number of investigators [3, 4]. Vision is stable until age 30 to 40 years, when there is onset of cataract formation. Cataracts typically occur as dotlike opacities in the posterior and anterior cortex [6]. Glaucoma is not uncommon after cataract extraction. With advancing age, progressive loss of vision occurs secondary to cataract, and there is chorioretinal atrophy [7]. Night blindness is inconsistently present. Electroretinography and dark adaptation are usually normal in an affected individual's youth but become progressively abnormal during adulthood [6].

Differentiation of Wagner's syndrome from Stickler's syndrome is im-

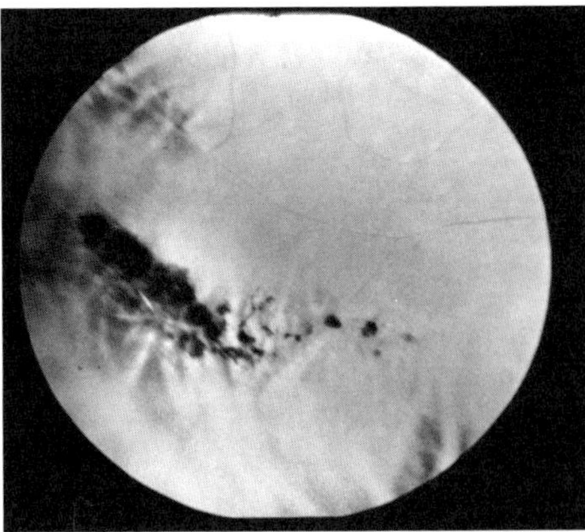

Figure 2 *Pigmented perivascular lattice in the posterior fundus is typical of Stickler's syndrome.*

Table 1 *Ophthalmic Manifestations in Wagner's, Jansen's, and Stickler's Syndromes*

Syndrome	Refractive Error	Vitreous Veils, Perivascular Lattice	Retinal Detachments	Cataract
Wagner's	Myopia 3–4 D	Yes	None in 4 generations	Onset in midchildhood, mature by age 30–40 yr
Jansen's	Normal to myopic	Yes	Approx. 50%	Cortical in teens, mature by age 30–40 yr
Stickler's	Moderately high myopia	Yes	Approx. 50%	Cortical distinctive, 50% in early adulthood

Source: Adapted from IH Maumenee, Vitreoretinal degeneration as a sign of generalized connective tissue diseases. Am J Ophthalmol 1979;88:432–449.

portant clinically because the rate of retinal detachment in Wagner's syndrome does not appear to differ from that of the normal population [3, 4]. Treatment of asymptomatic breaks is not recommended. The timing of cataract extraction is the same as that recommended for normal individuals.

Jansen's Syndrome

The condition characterized by ocular abnormalities similar to Wagner's syndrome but associated with retinal detachment can be classified as Jansen's syndrome (see Table 1) [5]. As in Wagner's syndrome, Jansen's syndrome is not associated with systemic abnormalities (Table 2). Jansen described 2 families with 30 members affected by ocular abnormalities identical to those seen in Wagner's syndrome [5]. Retinal detachment, however, was common in young patients and was sometimes bilateral. Surgical reattachment results were poor. Systemic abnormalities were absent in all the members examined [3]. All affected individuals had mild to moderate myopia. Onset of lens opacities occurred at approximately age 10, and open-angle glaucoma was common beginning in the third decade. A number of similar pedigrees of inherited retinal detachment without skeletal abnormalities have been described, often mistakenly designated as Wagner's syndrome [8–10].

■ Characteristic Findings in Stickler's Syndrome

Ophthalmological Characteristics

Stickler's syndrome is a dominantly inherited progressive arthroophthalmopathy [2]. Like Jansen's syndrome, there is a high incidence of reti-

Table 2 *Systemic Manifestations in Wagner's, Jansen's, and Stickler's Syndromes*

Syndrome	Face	Palate	Ligaments	Epiphyses
Wagner's	Normal	No clefting	Normal	No dysplasia
Jansen's	Normal	No clefting	Normal	No dysplasia
Stickler's	Midfacial hypoplasia, micrognathia	20% with cleft, high palate common	Joint laxity	Epiphyseal flattening, early arthritis

Source: Adapted from IH Maumenee, Vitreoretinal degeneration as a sign of generalized connective tissue diseases. Am J Ophthalmol 1979;88:432–449.

nal detachment. Its phenotypical expression is highly variable, and penetrance is nearly complete. Ocular findings are similar to those found in Wagner's syndrome and Jansen's syndrome (see Table 1).

Vitreous membrane structures visible with slit-lamp biomicroscopy and indirect ophthalmoscopy in an optically empty vitreous cavity are classic findings in Stickler's syndrome (see Fig 1). Vitreous liquefaction usually occurs before age 20, followed by condensation-forming bands. Sheets of vitreous condensation behind the lens may be the earliest finding [4, 6]; these later become veillike. Posterior membranes may lie on the retina. Anterior membranes may float in the vitreous, often with equatorial attachments [6, 8]. Vitreous attachments to radial perivascular lattice or typical lattice are common [11]. Histopathological evaluation reveals condensed cortical vitreous composed of acellular membranes [12].

At birth, the fundus of a Stickler's patient may appear tessellated, with diffuse circumferential areas of hypopigmentation in the periphery and in radial perivascular distribution in the posterior fundus (see Fig 2) [6, 8]. Later, pigmentation occurs in more than two-thirds of affected individuals. Retinal breaks occur in 75% [6]. Three-fourths of these patients have multiple breaks. The superotemporal quadrant is most commonly affected. One-fourth of the patients with breaks have giant tears [13], which frequently are located posteriorly. Retinal detachment occurs in nearly 50% of Stickler's syndrome patients and is bilateral in approximately 40% [6]. Detachment usually occurs by the second decade.

Myopia in Stickler's original report [1] ranged from 8 to 18 D. An increase in axial length has also been demonstrated [14]. Myopia is usually congenital and progressive [15]. Staphyloma, lacquer cracks, and choroidal neovascular membranes are rare.

Cataract occurs early in adulthood and was present in 50% to 60% of patients in two large series [4, 16]. Distinctive cortical wedge or fleck opacities are present in more than 40% of Stickler's syndrome cataracts.

Open-angle glaucoma may be associated with Stickler's syndrome. Descriptions of gonioscopy are infrequent in the literature, but those reports that appear cite normal findings [17] or patchy atrophy of the iris root

[18]. Glaucoma secondary to uveitis associated with chronic retinal detachment is well described [19].

Nonocular Characteristics

Nonocular findings initially described by Stickler included flat facies, cleft palate, and generalized arthropathy (see Table 2) [2]. Stickler's syndrome is considered the most common autosomal dominant connective tissue dysplasia in North America, and the prevalence is estimated to be 1 in 10,000 [20].

Hearing loss has subsequently been described as the most common nonocular defect [21, 22]. Most Stickler's patients with neurosensory hearing loss who are younger than 30 years are asymptomatic, whereas the majority of patients older than 50 are aware of some loss. Skull abnormalities are also believed to contribute to an increased incidence of otitis media, particularly in children with Stickler's syndrome [23].

Palate malformations are probably the most common skeletal abnormality. These range from cleft palate to submucous cleft or high arched palate. Bifid uvula or abnormal palate mobility may be the only defect in some cases [22]. Twenty percent of patients with Stickler's syndrome will have a cleft palate, and 10% of the patients screened at a cleft palate clinic had findings consistent with Stickler's syndrome [24].

Midfacial hypoplasia and skull abnormalities are common in Stickler's syndrome. Facial morphological features are shortening of the cranial base length, midfacial depth and height, maxillary depth, and mandibular depth. Supranormal total facial length and supranormal lower facial height dimensions have also been found to be characteristic for Stickler's syndrome [25]. Dental abnormalities include abnormal eruption of teeth and enamel hypoplasia.

Joint hyperextensibility of the fingers, wrists, elbows, and other joints is common [22]. Stickler [2] noted enlargement of these joints in most affected newborns. Slender or marfanoid body habitus is typical but may be subtle [17]. The most common specific radiographic findings include cox valga and widening of the femoral neck [26]. Metacarpal and phalangeal epiphyses are generally flattened. Thoracic vertebrae often manifest epiphyseal changes. Premature arthritic changes are also common.

■ Genetics

The association of retinal detachment and arthropathy has intrigued ophthalmologists and geneticists and suggested a common heritable, pathophysiological mechanism. Of the three related ocular syndromes—Wagner's, Jansen's, and Stickler's—only Stickler's is an arthroophthalmopathy.

In contrast to classification of the Wagner-Stickler syndrome as a clinical spectrum [27], Maumenee [17] subdivided these vitreoretinal degenerations according to their differentiating clinical features: ocular only (Wagner's [3] and Jansen's syndromes [6]) versus ocular plus skeletal (Stickler's syndrome [13] and others). Maumenee and others suggested the "ocular plus skeletal" group could result from abnormal type II collagen, which is present in both secondary vitreous and cartilage. Genes important in type II collagen metabolism were studied as candidate genes for Stickler's syndrome.

Initial support for this hypothesis came from pedigree studies. Collaboration of a number of investigators demonstrated genetic linkage of the disease locus to that of the structural gene for type II procollagen (COL2A1) in 2 Stickler's families [28]. The structural gene for type II procollagen is located on chromosome 12 (12q1.23-3.21). The logarithm-of-odds (LOD) score was 3.28 at a recombination fraction of 0.00 [28]. Genetic heterogeneity within the clinical phenotype became apparent when linkage was demonstrated in 2 additional families but excluded in a third by Knowlton and co-workers [29]. The LOD score was 3.52 and 1.20 in the 2 families demonstrating linkage.

Fortunately, the COL2A1 gene is rich in useful dimorphic restriction sites, allowing for a higher success rate in linkage studies. Linkage, however, could not be definitively identified or ruled out in some pedigrees that were not informative for the restriction length dimorphisms. Additional evidence linking the COL2A1 locus with that for Stickler's syndrome was obtained when the polymerase chain reaction was applied to amplify a variable region discovered just beyond the 3' end of the gene. This allowed the demonstration of probable linkage between the disease locus and the COL2A1 gene locus (LOD score of 2.86 at 0.00 recombination fraction) in a previously uninformative three-generation Stickler's family [30]. Similar techniques were used to exclude linkage of the COL2A1 locus to the disease locus in the original Swiss family studied by Wagner [31] and also in a Jansen-like pedigree [32].

One of the present authors (SM) has identified a large, four-generation family with Stickler's syndrome [33]. The affected family members have some combination of vitreoretinal degeneration, high myopia, retinal detachment, cataract, highly arched palate, and hearing loss. The maximum LOD score for this pedigree using the dinucleotide repeat polymorphism located in the 3' flanking region of type II procollagen was 0.61 at a recombination fraction of 0.10. The LOD score is only slightly positive and provides no conclusive evidence for or against linkage of the disease locus to the type II procollagen locus in this family. If one assumes linkage of the two loci, then one recombination event must have occurred. Given the large size of the type II procollagen gene, such a recombinant process could have taken place between the marker and the mutation.

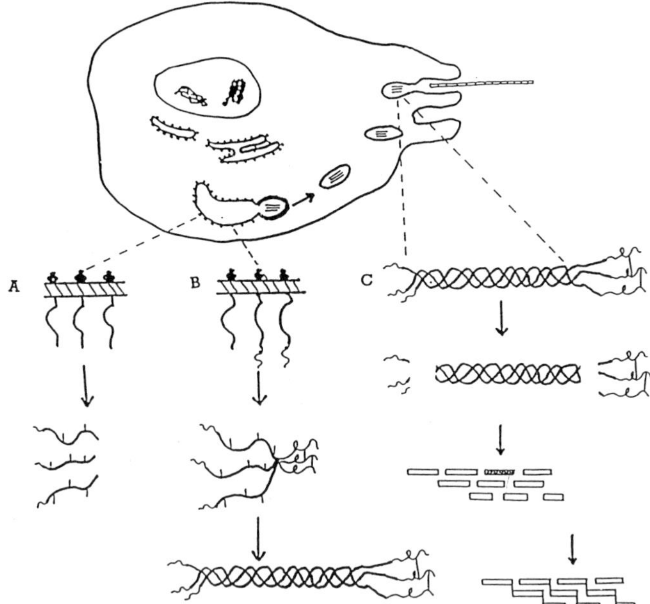

Figure 3 *(A) In the Stickler's syndrome family described by Ahmad and co-workers [33], the stop codon at the amino acid position 732 results in the synthesis of an abbreviated polypeptide that lacks a COOH-terminal propeptide. Disulfide linkage of three pro-alpha chains, nucleated growth, and zipperlike helical self-assembly are not possible due to the absence of the COOH terminus. (B) Folding of procollagen is dependent on the formation of a triple helix nucleus near the COOH terminus [34]. Normally, the propagation of the helical structure proceeds in a zipperlike fashion from the COOH terminus to the NH2 terminus after posttranslational hydroxylations, glycosylations, and disulfide bonding in the cisternae of the rough endoplasmic reticulum. (C) Proteolytic processing of the procollagen occurs through nucleated growth, self-assembly, and covalent cross-linking of the fibrils. (Adapted from DJ Prockop, Mutations that alter the primary structure of type I collagen: perils of a system for generating large structures by the principle of nucleated growth. J Biol Chem 1990;265:15349–15352.)*

Recently, the human procollagen II gene COL2A1 has been cloned, and a premature stop codon in this gene has been identified in a Stickler's family [34]. A new procedure of developing cosmid clones was employed to isolate the allele of type II procollagen linked to the disease in this family. Analysis of more than 7,000 nucleotides revealed a single base mutation converting the CGA codon for arginine at the amino acid position 732 to TGA, a "stop codon."

Ahmad and colleagues [34] propose that decreased synthesis of type II collagen results from this mutation because the truncated gene product cannot participate in the assembly of type II collagen. The stop codon at amino acid 732 results in the synthesis of an abbreviated polypeptide that lacks a COOH-terminal propeptide. Prockop [35] has demonstrated that the folding of procollagen is dependent on the formation of a triple helix nucleus near the COOH terminus. Normally, the propagation of the helical structure proceeds in a zipperlike fashion from the carboxyl to the amino terminus after posttranslational hydroxylation, glycosylation, and disulfide bonding in the rough endoplasmic reticulum (Fig 3B). Proteolytic processing of the procollagen later occurs through nucleated growth, self-assembly, and covalent cross-linking of the fibrils (Fig 3C). In patients with the premature stop codon at amino acid position 732, disulfide linkage of three pro-alpha chains is not possible due to the absence of the COOH terminus (Fig 3A).

■ Conclusion

The success of identifying a defect in the type II procollagen gene in a family with Stickler's syndrome illustrates the power of the candidate gene approach, which is based on a foundation of clinical observation and categorization. Additional studies are needed to discover whether the premature stop codon is a common genetic defect in other families with Stickler's syndrome. Although a defect in type II collagen is consistent with both arthropathy and vitreoretinal degeneration, the exact pathophysiological mechanism remains obscure. Intriguing questions concerning the role of type II collagen in the development of retinal detachment, craniofacial defects, and arthropathy remain to be answered.

■ References

1. McKusick VA. Mendelian inheritance in man: catalog of autosomal dominant, autosomal recessive, and x-linked phenotypes, ed 9. Baltimore, MD: The Johns Hopkins University Press, 1990:108–110
2. Stickler GB, Belau PG, Farrell FJ, et al. Hereditary progressive arthroophthalmopathy. Mayo Clin Proc 1965;40:433–455
3. Maumenee IH, Stoll HU, Mets MB. The Wagner syndrome versus hereditary arthroophthalmopathy. Trans Am Ophthalmol Soc 1982;80:349–365
4. Wagner H. Ein bisher unbekanntes Erbleiden des Auges (Degeneratio hyaloideoretinalis hereditaria, beobachet im Kanton Zurich). Klin Monatsbl Augenheilkd 1938;100:840–857
5. Jansen LMAA. Degeneratio hyaloideo-retinalis hereditaria. Ophthalmologica 1962;144:458–464
6. Hirose T, Lee KY, Schepens CL. Wagner's hereditary vitreoretinal degeneration and retinal detachment. Arch Ophthalmol 1973;89:176–185

7. van Nouhuys CE. Chorioretinal dysplasia in young subjects with Wagner's hereditary vitreoretinal degeneration. Int Ophthalmol 1981;3:67–77
8. Alexander RL, Shea M. Wagner's disease. Arch Ophthalmol 1965;74:310–318
9. Brown GC, Tasman WS. Vitrectomy and Wagner's vitreoretinal degeneration. Am J Ophthalmol 1978;86:485–488
10. Gillespie F, Covelli B. Hereditary high myopia with retinal detachment: a family study. Arch Ophthalmol 1963;69:733–736
11. Lisch W. Developments in ophthalmology: vol 8, hereditary vitreoretinal degenerations. Basel: Karger, 1983:46
12. Manschot WA. Pathology of hereditary conditions related to retinal detachment. Ophthalmologica 1971;162:223–234
13. Billington BM, Leaver PK, McLeod D. Management of retinal detachment in the Wagner-Stickler syndrome. Trans Ophthalmol Soc UK 1985;104:875–879
14. Weingeist TA, Hermsen V, Hanson JW, et al. Ocular and systemic manifestations of Stickler's syndrome: a preliminary report. Birth Defects 1982;18:539–560
15. Wang FM, Afran SI, Goldberg RB. Congenital myopia in Stickler's hereditary arthro-ophthalmopathy. Am J Ophthalmol 1990;110:435–436
16. Seery CM, Pruett RC, Liberfarb RM, Cohen BZ. Distinctive cataract in the Stickler syndrome. Am J Ophthalmol 1990;110:143–148
17. Maumenee IH. Vitreoretinal degeneration as a sign of generalized connective tissue diseases. Am J Ophthalmol 1979;88:432–449
18. Nielsen CE. Stickler's syndrome. Acta Ophthalmol (Copenh) 1981;59:286–295
19. Blair NP, Albert DM, Lieberfarb RM, Hirose T. Hereditary progressive arthro-ophthalmopathy of Stickler. Am J Ophthalmol 1979;88:876–888
20. Pyeritz RE. Heritable and developmental disorders of connective tissue and bone. In: McCarty DJ, ed. Arthritis and allied conditions: a textbook of rheumatology. Philadelphia: Lea & Febiger, 1989:1332–1359
21. Stickler GB, Pugh DG. Hereditary progressive arthro-ophthalmopathy: II. Additional observations on vertebral abnormalities, a hearing defect, and a report of a similar case. Mayo Clin Proc 1967;42:495–500
22. Herrmann J, France TD, Spranger JW, et al. The Stickler syndrome (hereditary arthroophthalmopathy). Birth Defects 1975;11:76–103
23. Popkin JS, Polomeno RC. Stickler's syndrome (hereditary progressive arthroophthalmopathy). Can Med Assoc J 1974;111:1071–1076
24. Kronwith SD, Quinn G, McDonald DM, et al. Stickler's syndrome in the Cleft Palate Clinic. J Pediatr Ophthalmol Strabismus 1990;27:265–267
25. Saksena SS, Bixler D, Yu PI. Stickler syndrome: a cephalometric study of the face. J Craniofac Genet Dev Biol 1983;3:19–28
26. Bennett JT, McMurray SW. Stickler syndrome. J Pediatr Orthop 1990;10:760–763
27. Liberfarb RM, Hirose T, Holmes LB. The Wagner-Stickler syndrome: a study of 22 families. J Pediatr 1981;99:394–399
28. Francomano CA, Liberfarb RM, Hirose T, et al. The Stickler syndrome: evidence for close linkage to the structural gene for type II collagen. Genomics 1987; 1:293–296
29. Knowlton RG, Weaver EJ, Struyk AF, et al. Genetic linkage analysis of hereditary arthro-ophthalmopathy (Stickler syndrome) and the type II procollagen gene. Am J Hum Genet 1989;45:681–688
30. Priestley L, Kumar D, Sykes B. Amplification of the COL2A1 3′ variable region used for segregation analysis in a family with the Stickler syndrome. Hum Genet 1990;85:525–526
31. Francomano CA, Rowan BG, Liberfarb RM, et al. The Stickler and Wagner syndromes: evidence for genetic heterogeneity. Am J Hum Genet 1988;43(suppl 3):A83

32. Fryer AE, Upadhyaya M, Littler M, et al. Exclusion of COL2A1 as a candidate gene in a family with Wagner-Stickler syndrome. J Med Genet 1990;27:91–93
33. Fine AM, Wiggs JL, De La Paz MA, et al. Linkage analysis of Stickler's syndrome and the type II procollagen gene (ARVO abstract 506-12). Invest Ophthalmol Vis Sci 1992;33(suppl):793
34. Ahmad NN, Ala-Kokko L, Knowlton RG, et al. Stop codon in the procollagen II gene (COL2A1) in a family with the Stickler syndrome (arthro-ophthalmopathy). Proc Natl Acad Sci USA 1991;88:6624–6627
35. Prockop DJ. Mutations that alter the primary structure of type I collagen: perils of a system for generating large structures by the principle of nucleated growth. J Biol Chem 1990;265:15349–15352

Index